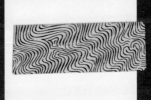

Self-Assessment in
Otolaryngology

James Paul O'Neill, MD, MB, FRCSI, MMSc, MBA, ORL-HNS
Professor of Otolaryngology, Head and Neck Surgery
Royal College of Surgeons in Ireland
RCSI Education and Research Centre
Beaumont Hospital, Beaumont
Dublin, Ireland

Jatin P. Shah, MD, PhD(Hon), DSc(Hon), FACS, FRCS(Hon), FDSRCS(Hon), FRCSDS(Hon), FRACS (Hon)
Professor of Surgery
E. W. Strong Chair in Head and Neck Oncology
Department of Surgery
Memorial Sloan-Kettering Cancer Center
New York, New York

ELSEVIER

ELSEVIER

1600 John F. Kennedy Blvd.
Ste 1800
Philadelphia, PA 19103-2899

Notices

Knowledge and best practice in this field are constantly changing. As new research and experience broaden our understanding, changes in research methods, professional practices, or medical treatment may become necessary.

Practitioners and researchers must always rely on their own experience and knowledge in evaluating and using any information, methods, compounds, or experiments described herein. In using such information or methods they should be mindful of their own safety and the safety of others, including parties for whom they have a professional responsibility.

With respect to any drug or pharmaceutical products identified, readers are advised to check the most current information provided (i) on procedures featured or (ii) by the manufacturer of each product to be administered, to verify the recommended dose or formula, the method and duration of administration, and contraindications. It is the responsibility of practitioners, relying on their own experience and knowledge of their patients, to make diagnoses, to determine dosages and the best treatment for each individual patient, and to take all appropriate safety precautions.

To the fullest extent of the law, neither the Publisher nor the authors, contributors, or editors, assume any liability for any injury and/or damage to persons or property as a matter of products liability, negligence or otherwise, or from any use or operation of any methods, products, instructions, or ideas contained in the material herein.

Library of Congress Cataloging-in-Publication Data
Names: O'Neill, James Paul, editor. | Shah, Jatin P., editor.
Title: Self-assessment in otolaryngology / [edited by] James Paul O'Neill, Jatin P. Shah.
Description: Philadelphia, PA : Elsevier, [2017] | "Each chapter contains a topic that follows the
   sequence of the chapters in Cumming's Otolaryngology, Fifth Edition."—Preface. | Includes
   bibliographical references.
Identifiers: LCCN 2015047554 | ISBN 9780323392907 (pbk. : alk. paper)
Subjects: | MESH: Otorhinolaryngologic Diseases—diagnosis | Otorhinolaryngologic Diseases—
   surgery | Examination Questions
Classification: LCC RF57 | NLM WV 18.2 | DDC 617.5/10076—dc23 LC record available at
   http://lccn.loc.gov/2015047554

Senior Content Strategist: Belinda Kuhn
Senior Content Development Specialist: Jennifer Ehlers
Publishing Services Manager: Catherine Jackson
Project Manager: Kate Mannix
Design Direction: Ashley Miner

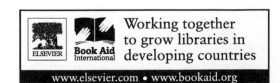

Preface

The specialty of otolaryngology has made significant strides over the past three decades, largely due to technological advances in imaging, the use of fiber-optic instrumentation for diagnosis and treatment, and the development of endoscopic and minimally invasive techniques for surgical procedures. Concurrent with this are advances in understanding of the biological processes of diseases in the ear, nose, and throat and the head and neck region. To keep pace with this advancing knowledge, major textbooks continue to bring about new editions with contributions from contemporary leaders in the specialty. One vivid example of this is the recently published fifth edition of the three-volume *Cummings Otolaryngology*. This work is considered by many as the standard textbook in contemporary otolaryngology and has remained a very popular source of learning and knowledge in the field of otolaryngology for more than 25 years.

Although textbooks such as the one mentioned previously and others are readily available for knowledge acquisition and ready reference, they do not test an individual's retention of the acquired knowledge and its reflection in improved judgment in day-to-day practice. When taking board certification or college examinations, candidates do prepare for multiple choice examinations, and there are a number of practice tests available. However, these tests are geared for an examination, and often may not have practical relevance in day-to-day practice. Therefore, one needs to have a tool for self-assessment of retained knowledge, good clinical judgment, and upkeep with advances in the specialty. We have made an attempt to fill that void through this compilation of *Self-Assessment in Otolaryngology*.

This book is by no means sufficient to measure competency in the specialty, nor is it intended to be sufficient to gain certification in the specialty. On the other hand, it introduces the reader to the process of self-assessment of knowledge and judgment, an algorithmic thinking process, and the decision-making process in dealing with day-to-day problems in the specialty of otolaryngology. Each chapter contains a topic that follows the sequence of the chapters in *Cumming's Otolaryngology,*

Fifth Edition. This standard textbook is recommended by the editors to acquire basic knowledge of the current practice of otolaryngology. The questions in this compendium are presented in three categories: (1) True or False, (2) Single Best Answer, and (3) Multiple Choice combinations. Each chapter includes a summary of the basic Core Knowledge required and has a Suggested Reading list. The answers to the questions are provided at the end of each chapter. It is our hope that the reader will benefit from taking the examination, pursuing the topic further by reviewing the Core Knowledge, and then reading the recommended references to gain further knowledge. Therefore, this compilation of self-assessment questions would be of value not only to trainees in otolaryngology but also practitioners in this specialty to remain current with state-of-the-art otolaryngology practice. We also hope that this attempt at self-assessment will stimulate the reader to remain engaged in continuing medical education to remain up-to-date with this rapidly advancing specialty.

ACKNOWLEDGMENTS

The editors wish to express their appreciation to all the contributors, who are current academic leaders in otolaryngology and represent a driving force in the specialty. They have very diligently presented thoughtful questions, keeping in mind their clinical relevance in day-to-day practice. We would also like to express our gratitude to the authors of *Cumming's Otolaryngology, Fifth Edition,* and the publisher (Elsevier), for allowing us the generous use of illustrations, figures, and diagrams in the current work. Finally, we want to acknowledge the meticulous and timely assistance from the editing and publishing staff at Elsevier, without whose help this compendium would not have been possible.

James Paul O'Neill, *MD, MB, FRCSI, MMSc, MBA, ORL-HNS*
Jatin P. Shah, *MD, PhD(Hon), DSc(Hon), FACS, FRCS(Hon), FDSRCS(Hon), FRCSDS(Hon), FRACS (Hon)*

Contributors

Sameer Ahmed, MD
Neurotology Fellow
Division of Otology-Neurotology
Department of Otolaryngology/Head and Neck
    Surgery
University of Michigan Health System
Ann Arbor, Michigan

Nafi Aygun, MD
Associate Professor of Radiology
Russel H. Morgan Department of Radiology and
    Radiological Science, Neuroradiology Division
Johns Hopkins Medical Institutes
Baltimore, Maryland

Douglas Backous, MD
Medical Director
Center for Hearing and Skull Base Surgery
Swedish Medical Center
Seattle, Washington

Fuad M. Baroody, MD
Professor
Department of Surgery,
Section of Otolaryngology-Head and Neck Surgery
Department of Pediatrics
The University of Chicago Medicine and Biological
    Sciences
Chicago, Illinois

David J. Brown, MD
Associate Professor
Pediatric Otolaryngology
University of Michigan Health System
Ann Arbor, Michigan

Jonathan Cabin, MD
Icahn School of Medicine at Mount Sinai
New York, New York

William W. Carroll, MD
Resident
Department of Otolaryngology
Medical University of South Carolina
Charleston, South Carolina

Paula Casserly, MCh, FRCS (ORL)
Department of Otolaryngology, Head and Neck
    Surgery
Royal Victoria Eye and Ear Hospital
St. James's Hospital
Dublin, Ireland

François Cloutier, MD
Departments of Otology, Neurotology
Center for Hearing and Skull Base Surgery
Swedish Medical Center
Seattle, WA;
Department of Otolaryngology, Head and Neck
    Surgery
CSSS Pierre-Boucher
Longueuil, Quebec, Canada

Chelsea Conrad, AuD
Clinical Audiologist
Hearing Rehabilitation Center
University of Michigan Health System
Ann Arbor, Michigan

Gerard Curley, MB, MSc, PhD
Assistant Professor
Departments of Anesthesia and Critical Care
St Michael's Hospital
University of Toronto
Toronto, Ontario, Canada

Adam S. DeConde, MD
Assistant Professor
Surgery, Division of Otolaryngology—Head and Neck
    Surgery
University of California at San Diego
San Diego, California

Colleen Heffernan, MB
Department of Otolaryngology/Head and Neck
    Surgery
Mater Misericordiae University Hospital
Dublin, Ireland

David M. Hogan, MD
Otolaryngology Head and Neck Surgery Fellow and
    Lecturer
Department of Otolaryngology, Head and Neck
    Surgery
Beaumont Hospital
The Royal College of Surgeons in Ireland
Dublin, Ireland

Matthew D. Johnson, MD
Assistant Professor, Facial Plastic & Reconstructive
    Surgery
Division of Otolaryngology—Head and Neck Surgery
Southern Illinois University School of Medicine
Springfield, Illinois

Karan Kapoor, FRCS, MEd
Consultant Head and Neck Surgeon
Queen Victoria Hospital
East Grinstead, United Kingdom;
Surrey and Sussex Hospital Trust
Redhill, United Kingdom;
Royal Hospital for Neuro-disability
London, United Kingdom

Robert M. Kellman, MD
Professor and Chair
Department of Otolaryngology and Communication
    Sciences
SUNY—Upstate Medical University
Syracuse, New York

S. Guan Khoo, MD
Consultant Otolaryngologist/Head and Neck Surgeon
Otolaryngology/Head and Neck Surgery
St. Vincent's University Hospital
Dublin, Ireland

Paul R. Kileny, PhD
Professor of Otolaryngology and Head and Neck
    Surgery
Academic Program Director, Audiology and
    Electrophysiology
University of Michigan Health System
Ann Arbor, Michigan

Ericka King, MD
Assistant Professor
Otolaryngology—Head and Neck Surgery
Oregon Health and Science University
Portland, Oregon

Philip D. Knollman, MD
Resident
Department of Surgery, Section of Otolaryngology—
    Head and Neck Surgery
The University of Chicago Medicine and Biological
    Sciences
Chicago, Illinois

Salvatore V. Labruzzo, DO
Clinical Fellow
Russel H. Morgan Department of Radiology and
    Radiological Science, Neuroradiology Division
Johns Hopkins Medical Institutes
Baltimore, Maryland

Derek J. Lam, MD, MPH
Assistant Professor
Otolaryngology—Head and Neck Surgery
Oregon Health and Science University
Portland, Oregon

Paul Lennon, FRCS (ORL-HNS)
Specialist Registrar in Otolaryngology, Head and Neck
    Surgery
St. James's Hospital
Dublin, Ireland

Douglas Mattox, MD
William Chester Warren, Jr., MD Professor and Chair
Otolaryngology—Head and Neck Surgery
Emory University School of Medicine
Atlanta, Georgia

J. Scott McMurray, MD
Associate Professor Pediatric Otolaryngology
University of Wisconsin School of Medicine and Public
    Health
Madison, Wisconsin

Howard Meng, MD
Anesthesia Resident
University of Toronto
Toronto, Ontario, Canada

Anna H. Messner, MD
Professor and Vice Chair
Otolaryngology/Head and Neck Surgery
Stanford University
Stanford, California

James Paul O'Neill, MD, MB, FRCSI, MMSc, MBA, ORL-HNS
Professor of Otolaryngology, Head and Neck Surgery
Royal College of Surgeons in Ireland
RCSI Education and Research Centre
Beaumont Hospital, Beaumont
Dublin, Ireland

Tara Ramachandra, MD
Otolaryngology Head and Neck Surgery Fellow and
    Lecturer
Department of Otolaryngology, Head and Neck
    Surgery
Beaumont Hospital
The Royal College of Surgeons in Ireland
Dublin, Ireland

Virginia Ramachandran, AuD, PhD
Senior Staff Audiologist and Research Coordinator,
    Division of Audiology
Department of Otolaryngology—Head and Neck
    Surgery
Henry Ford Hospital
Detroit, Michigan

Gregory W. Randolph, MD
Director
Divisions of General Otolaryngology and Thyroid and
    Parathyroid Surgery
Massachusetts Eye and Ear
Boston, Massachusetts

Guri Sandhu, MD
Consultant Otolaryngologist/Airway Surgeon
Charing Cross Hospital
Imperial College
London, United Kingdom

Anthony P. Sclafani, MD
Department of Otolaryngology—Head and Neck
    Surgery
Weill Cornell Medical College
New York, New York

Neville Patrick Shine, FRCS(ORL-HNS)
Consultant, Head and Neck
Thyroid and Parathyroid Surgeon
Otolaryngology Head and Neck Surgery
University Hospital Limerick
Limerick, Ireland

Catherine F. Sinclair, MD
Assistant Professor
Department of Otolaryngology
Mount Sinai—Roosevelt
New York, New York

Timothy L. Smith, MD
Professor and Director
Department of Otolaryngology—Head and Neck
    Surgery
Oregon Sinus Center
Oregon Health and Science University
Portland, Oregon

Brad A. Stach, PhD
Director, Division of Audiology
Department of Otolaryngology—Head and Neck
    Surgery
Henry Ford Hospital
Detroit, Michigan

Shawn M. Stevens, MD
Fellow, Neurotology Otology and Skull Base Surgery
Department of Otolaryngology, Head and Neck
    Surgery
University of Cincinnati
Cincinnati, Ohio

Mai Thy Truong, MD
Clinical Assistant Professor
Lucile Packard Children's Hospital, Stanford
Stanford, California

Esther Vivas, MD
Assistant Professor
Otolaryngology—Head and Neck Surgery
Emory University School of Medicine
Atlanta, Georgia

Contents

Contents

Embryology and Anatomy

1

Paul Lennon | James Paul O'Neill

TRUE OR FALSE QUESTIONS

EMBRYOLOGY

T/F   1. Neural crest cells arise from the midbrain.

T/F   2. The buccopharyngeal membrane consists of bilateral opposed ectoderm and endoderm, which initially separates the stomodeum from the foregut.

T/F   3. The primitive stomodeum is initially bound rostrally by the frontal process, caudally by the developing heart, and laterally by the second pair of branchial arches.

T/F   4. The inner aspect of the first branchial arch is covered by endoderm because it forms in front of the buccopharyngeal membrane.

T/F   5. The central core of the branchial arches is invaded by mesoderm from the neural crest known as ectomesenchyme, which condenses to form a bar of cartilage (arch cartilage).

T/F   6. The cartilage of the second arch is called Meckel cartilage and gives rise to the muscles of facial expression.

T/F   7. The floor of the mouth is formed by the epithelium covering the mesenchyme of the first, second, and third branchial arches.

T/F   8. The frontonasal process and bilateral medial nasal processes give rise to the middle portion of the nose, the middle portion of the upper lip, the anterior portion of the maxilla, and the secondary palate (Figure 1-1).

T/F   9. The formation of the secondary palate commences between 7 and 8 weeks and is completed the 6th month of gestation.

T/F 10. In the development of the tongue, the tuberculum impar arises prior to lingual swellings (Figure 1-2).

T/F 11. The posterior one third of the tongue develops from mesenchyme of the 2nd (copula), 3rd, and 4th (hypobranchial eminence) branchial arches.

T/F 12. The anterior aspect of the 6th brachial arch gives rise to the epiglottis.

T/F 13. Motor innervation of the tongue by the hypoglossal nerve is due to the muscles of the tongue arising from occipital somites.

T/F 14. The mandible develops in cartilage from Meckel cartilage, which also gives rise to the incus, malleus, and the sphenomandibular ligament.

T/F 15. The maxillary sinus develops at 24 weeks' gestation and is still a rudimentary structure at birth, approximately the size of a pea.

ANATOMY

The Orbit

T/F 16. The bony orbit is made up of the frontal, lacrimal, zygomatic, ethmoid, temporal, and zygomatic bones, along with the greater and lesser wings of the sphenoid.

T/F 17. The orbital septum, also known as the palpebral fascia, is continuous with the periosteum of the bony orbit, and inserts into the eyelids, thus preventing infection spreading from skin to the orbit.

T/F 18. The tarsal plates lie deep to the orbital septum and provide support to the eyelids by attaching to the medial and lateral canthal ligaments.

T/F 19. Hasner valve (plica lacrimalis) is the nasal opening of the nasolacrimal duct located one-fourth the way back from the front border of the inferior meatus.

T/F 20. The optic canal is bounded laterally by the greater wing of the sphenoid bone.

The Temporal Bone/Ear

T/F 21. The tympanomastoid fissure contains the canal of Huguier for the anterior tympanic artery and the chorda tympani nerve.

T/F 22. When present, the fissure of Santorini is located in the tragal cartilage.

T/F 23. The foramen of Huschke is located in the anterosuperior bony external auditory meatus in children and may allow spread of infection to and from the parotid gland.

T/F 24. Ceruminous glands are found mainly on the superior and inferior walls of the external auditory canal and lie in the dermis superficial to the sebaceous glands.

T/F 25. Acute mastoiditis will cause a subperiosteal abscess, whereas infection of postauricular lymph nodes will cause an abscess superficial to the periosteum.

T/F 26. The roof of the middle ear separates the tympanic cavity from the posterior cranial fossa.

T/F 27. The ponticulus (little bridge) is a ridge located between the pyramidal eminence and the promontory, while the subiculum is a ridge between the styloid eminence and the posterior aspect of the round window niche.

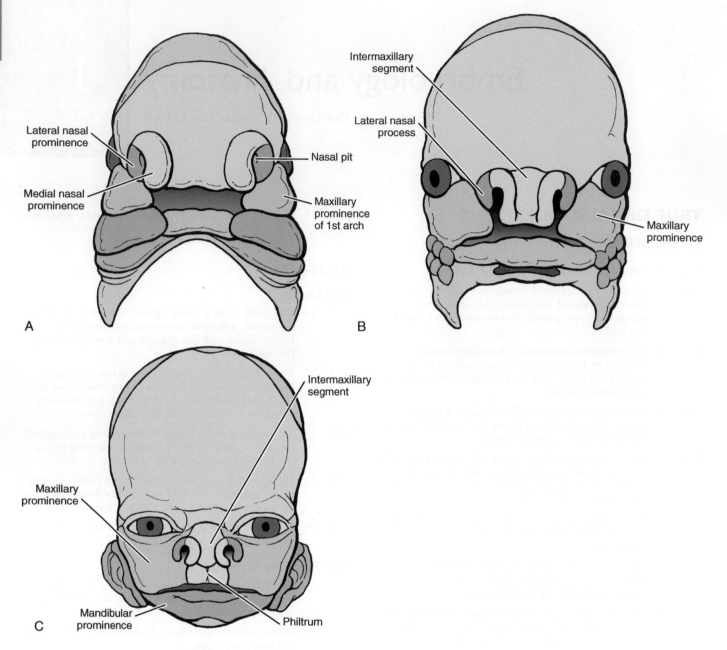

FIGURE 1-1 Developmental anatomy of the face. **A,** Week 5. **B,** Week 6. **C,** Week 8.

T / F 28. Obesity can cause eustachian tube dysfunction due to enlargement of the fat pad of Ostmann.

T / F 29. The endolymphatic duct is formed as an extension of the utricular and the saccular ducts in a groove on the posterolateral wall of the vestibule, and passes through the vestibular aqueduct to the endolymphatic sac.

T / F 30. At the fundus of the internal auditory meatus the facial nerve lies in the superior-posterior quadrant (Figure 1-3).

The Facial Nerve

T / F 31. Removal of bone along the lateral surface of the digastric ridge is a useful technique for identification of the facial canal at the stylomastoid foramen.

T / F 32. The cochleariform process is the insertion point for the stapedius tendon.

T / F 33. The pyramidal ridge divides the facial recess and sinus tympani.

T / F 34. Key landmarks to the posterior tympanic segment are the stapes and round window.

T / F 35. Geniculate ganglion branches include the greater superficial petrosal nerve, the lesser petrosal nerve, and the external petrosal nerve (Figure 1-4).

The Parotid

T / F 36. Stensen duct passes deep to masseter and superficial to buccinator.

T / F 37. The parasympathetic supply of the parotid proceeds as follows: preganglionic fibers: superior salivary nucleus—glossopharyngeal

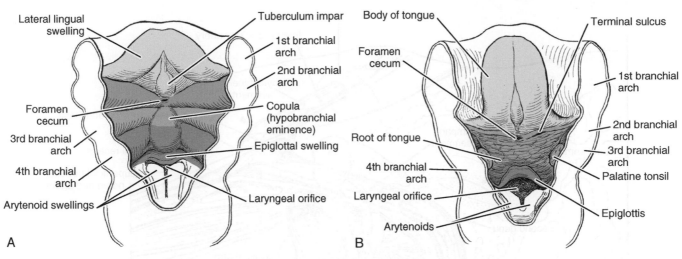

FIGURE 1-2 Development of the tongue. **A,** At weeks 4-5, the 1st arch forms the medial tuberculum impar and the lateral lingual swellings. The 2nd, 3rd, and 4th arches form the copula, or hypobranchial eminence. **B,** The 1st arch forms the anterior tongue, whereas the 3rd arch primarily contributes to the posterior tongue. The 4th arch forms the root of the tongue and epiglottis.

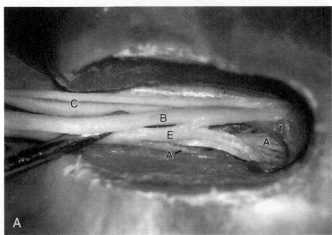

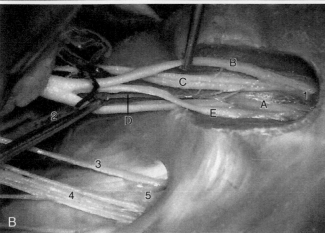

FIGURE 1-3 **A,** Close-up posterior view of the nerves in the internal auditory canal (right side). **B,** Close-up posterior view of the midface showing the petrous bone and internal auditory canal with nerve dissection. *1,* Transverse crest; *2,* anterior inferior cerebellar artery; *3,* cranial nerve IX (glossopharyngeal nerve); *4,* cranial nerve X (vagus nerve); *5,* dural septum; *A,* cochlear nerve; *B,* superior vestibular nerve; *C,* facial nerve and nervus intermedius (of Wrisberg); *D,* internal auditory artery; *E,* inferior vestibular nerve. (Courtesy Oswaldo Laércio M. Cruz, Helder Tedeschi, and Albert Rhoton.)

nerve—tympanic plexus—greater petrosal nerve—postganglionic fibers: otic ganglion—auriculotemporal nerve—parotid.

T / F 38. The sympathetic supply proceeds as follows: preganglionic fibers: interomediolateral horn nucleus between T1 and T3—enter sympathetic chain—postganglionic fibers: superior cervical ganglion following external carotid to the parotid.

T / F 39. The lesser petrosal nerve carries postganglionic parasympathetic secretory fibers to the parotid gland via the otic ganglion.

T / F 40. The nerve of the pterygoid canal synapse in the pterygopalatine ganglion and postsynaptic fibers via V2 maxillary nerve supply the lacrimal gland and mucous glands of the nasal and oral cavities.

Thyroid/Parathyroid

T / F 41. The Cernea classification describes the course of the external branch of the superior laryngeal nerve in relation to the cricothyroid muscle.

T / F 42. Each parathyroid gland weighs approximately 2 g.

T / F 43. Parathyroid hormone has a half-life of 15 minutes approximately.

T / F 44. Osteoclastic action is indirectly stimulated in bone by parathyroid hormone (PTH), thereby increasing calcium levels in the bloodstream. In the kidney PTH enhances resorption of calcium and magnesium within the distal tubules and thick descending limb.

T / F 45. The thyroid gland begins embryological development within the fetal oropharynx at 3 weeks.

Vocal Cords

T / F 46. Reinke space is a "potential" anatomical space.

T / F 47. The squamous epithelium and superficial lamina propria serve as the vocal mucosal vibratory component in phonation.

T / F 48. The posterior cricoarytenoid muscle abducts the vocal cords by adducting the rima glottidis.

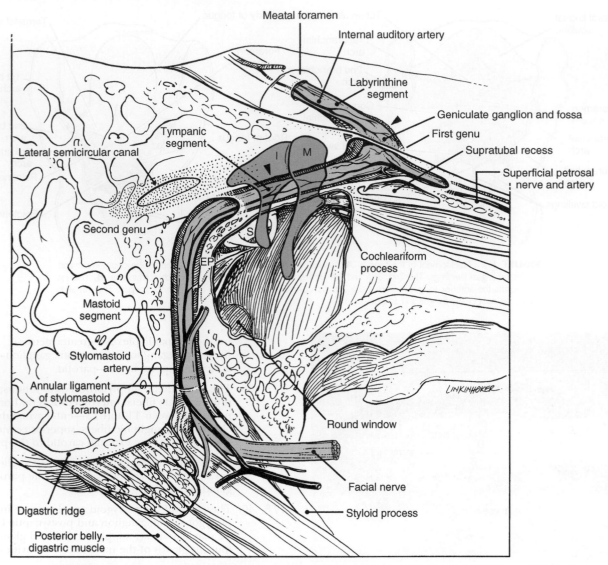

FIGURE 1-4 Anatomy of the infratemporal portion of the facial nerve and associated middle ear structures. Shown are sites of vulnerability to injury *(arrowheads)*. *Perigeniculate region:* Susceptibility of the genicular fossa to fracture also increases the risk of nerve injury due to nerve compression and ischemia in the narrow meatal foramen and labyrinthine segment. The first genu of the facial nerve is tethered by the greater superficial petrosal nerve, which increases susceptibility to shearing injuries. The geniculate ganglion is susceptible to injury during surgical dissection in the supratubal recess of the anterior epitympanum. *Tympanic segment:* The nerve is most frequently dehiscent above the oval window and distal tympanic segment; the second genu is susceptible to injury in cholesteatoma surgery because of pathologic dehiscence or distorted anatomy and failure to identify important surgical landmarks. *Mastoid segment:* In the lower portion of its vertical course and just distal to the stylomastoid foramen, the nerve is positioned lateral to the tympanic annulus and is therefore susceptible to injury during surgery of the external auditory canal. *EP,* Eminence pyramidale; *I,* incus; *M,* malleus; *S,* stapes. (From Francis HW. Facial nerve emergencies. In: Eisele D, McQuone S, eds. Emergencies of the Head and Neck. St Louis: Mosby; 2000.)

T/F 49. The vocal ligament is the superficial and intermediate layers of lamina propria.

T/F 50. The "body" of the vocal cord is the thyroarytenoid and vocalis muscles.

SINGLE BEST ANSWER QUESTIONS

EMBRYOLOGY

51. Implantation of human embryos typically occurs:
    a. Approximately 1 day after fertilization
    b. Approximately 1 week after fertilization
    c. Approximately 2 weeks after fertilization

d. Around the same time as neural tube closure
e. None of the above

52. The most correct sequence of early development following fertilization is:
    a. Zygote, morula, blastocyst, embryo
    b. Blastocyst, fetus, morula, zygote
    c. Morula, embryo, fetus, blastocyst
    d. Blastocyst, zygote, morula, fetus

53. The endoderm gives rise to all of the following *EXCEPT*:
    a. Thyroid follicles
    b. Endothelial lining of blood vessels
    c. Epithelial lining of the respiratory tract

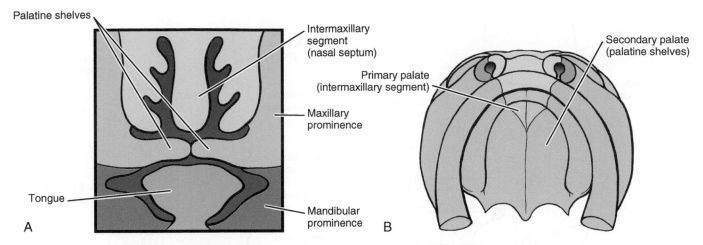

FIGURE 1-5 Development of the palate. **A,** Coronal section. **B,** Transverse section.

   d. Mucosa of the oral cavity
   e. Epithelium of the eustachian tube and tympanic cavity

54. Neural crest cells give rise to all of the following *EXCEPT:*
   a. Spinal cord
   b. Melanocytes
   c. Ultimobranchial bodies
   d. Dentine of the teeth
   e. Choroid, sclera, and iris of the eye

55. The embryonic cartilage that develops in the first pharyngeal arch is derived from:
   a. Somite mesoderm
   b. Unsegmented paraxial mesoderm
   c. Lateral plate mesoderm
   d. Neural crest
   e. Sclerotome

56. Derivatives of which embryonic structure give rise to medullary thyroid cancer?
   a. Second branchial pouch
   b. Foramen cecum
   c. Third branchial pouch
   d. Fourth branchial pouch
   e. Fifth/sixth branchial pouch

57. The hypobranchial eminence contributes to formation of tissue innervated by the nerve of which branchial arch?
   a. First
   b. Second
   c. Third
   d. Fourth
   e. Fifth/sixth

58. A unilateral cleft lip and a unilateral cleft of the primary palate (Figure 1-5) are most likely the result of:
   a. Failure of fusion of the mandibular prominences
   b. Failure of fusion of the medial nasal processes
   c. Failure of fusion of the maxillary prominence with the medial nasal prominence
   d. Failure of fusion of the lateral palatine processes with the nasal septum
   e. None of the above

59. Sensation to the auricle is via all *EXCEPT:*
   a. Cranial nerve V (auriculotemporal nerve)
   b. Cranial nerve VII (nerve of Wrisberg [anterior auricular nerve])
   c. Cranial nerve X (Arnold nerve)
   d. Anterior branch of great auricular nerve (C2/3)

   e. Lesser occipital nerve and greater occipital nerves (C2)

60. Structures formed from cartilage of the first branchial arch include all of the following *EXCEPT:*
   a. The ramus of the mandible (Meckel cartilage)
   b. The sphenomandibular ligament
   c. Anterior malleolar ligament
   d. The malleus (except for the manubrium)
   e. The long process of the incus

61. Choose the correct anatomical site per American Joint Committee on Cancer classifications:

a. Supraglottis	i.	The free border of the soft palate
b. Glottis		
c. Subglottis	ii.	Vallecula
d. Oropharynx	iii.	Aryepiglottic folds
e. Hypopharynx	iv.	Fossa of Rosenmüller
f. Nasopharynx	v.	Postcricoid
g. Oral cavity	vi.	Glossotonsillar sulci
	vii.	Retromolar trigone
	viii.	Upper margin of cricoid
	ix.	Posterior hard palate
	x.	Lingual aspect of epiglottis

62. Match the single best anatomical structure of the tongue and floor of mouth with the list below:

a. Mylohyoid muscle	i.	Gag reflex
b. Anterior belly of digastric	ii.	Protrudes the tongue
c. Lingual nerve	iii.	Somatic information from the mucous membranes of the anterior two-thirds of the tongue
d. Genioglossus		
e. Hypoglossal nerve		
f. Submandibular gland	iv.	First pharyngeal arch
g. Mandibular canal	v.	Ducts of Rivinus
h. Intrinsic tongue musculature	vi.	Papillary thyroid cancer
i. Thyroglossal duct cyst	vii.	Separates the deep and superficial lobes of the submandibular gland
j. Afferent fibers of the glossopharyngeal nerve	viii.	Passes deep to the belly of digastric
k. Sublingual gland	ix.	The superficial component comprises the majority of the gland.
	x.	Inferior alveolar artery

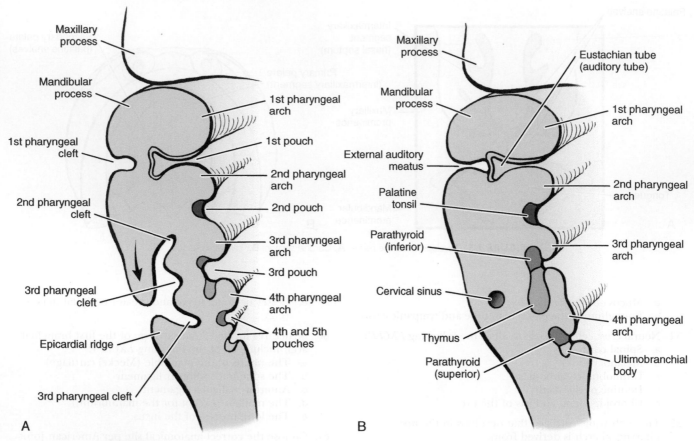

FIGURE 1-6 A, Derivatives of the pharyngeal pouches and formation of the cervical sinus. **B,** Maturation of the pharyngeal pouches.

63. Regarding the larynx and phonation, which statement is *INCORRECT*?
    a. The larynx ascends as a child grows.
    b. The laryngeal cartilaginous skeleton consists of three paired and three single cartilages.
    c. The vocal process provides attachment to the posterior end of the true vocal cords.
    d. The corniculate and cuneiform cartilages are nonfunctional in humans.

64. Regarding the paranasal sinuses, which statement is correct?
    a. The sphenoid ostium is located posterolateral to the superior turbinate in 85% of the population and should be safely opened inferolaterally.
    b. A Haller cell exists between the maxillary sinus and the floor of the orbit.
    c. The anterior and middle ethmoidal cells are innervated by the maxillary division of the trigeminal nerve.
    d. The intersphenoidal septum may insert into the external carotid artery.

65. Match the branchial arch with the anatomical structure (Figure 1-6):
    a. 1st branchial arch
    b. 2nd branchial arch
    c. 3rd branchial arch
    d. 4th branchial arch

    i. Internal carotid artery
    ii. Posterior belly of digastric muscle
    iii. Mandibular arch
    iv. Stapes
    v. Parotid, submandibular, and sublingual glands

66. Match the boundaries of the sinus tympani with the anatomical structures:
    a. Superiorly
    b. Posteriorly
    c. Inferiorly
    d. Medially
    e. Laterally

    i. Pyramidal eminence and facial nerve
    ii. Ponticulus and lateral semicircular canal
    iii. Bony labyrinth
    iv. Subiculum, styloid eminence, and jugular wall
    v. Posterior semicircular canal

67. Match the boundaries of the infratemporal fossa with the anatomical structures (Figure 1-7):
    a. Superiorly
    b. Posteriorly
    c. Inferiorly
    d. Medially
    e. Laterally
    f. Anteriorly

    i. Infratemporal surface maxilla
    ii. Greater wing of the sphenoid
    iii. Articular surface of the temporal and spine of sphenoid
    iv. Medial pterygoid muscle
    v. Ramus of the mandible
    vi. Lateral pterygoid plate

ANATOMICAL CORRELATIONS

You perform a clinical examination including panendoscopy and observe the following tumor characteristics. Provide the correct TNM staging in questions 68 to 80.

68. A 2.5-cm tumor on the soft palate involving the left tonsil. You can palpate two cervical nodes approximately 3 cm in size in the left levels 2 and 3.
    a. T4N2B
    b. T4N2C
    c. T2N2C
    d. T2N2B

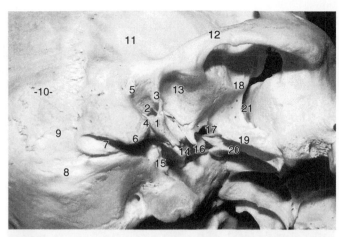

FIGURE 1-7 Cranium, lateral inferior view *(right side)*: *1*, Tympanic bone; *2*, external auditory canal; *3*, tympanosquamous suture; *4*, tympanomastoid suture; *5*, suprameatal spine; *6*, mastoid tip; *7*, digastric sulcus; *8*, occipital bone; *9*, occipitomastoid suture; *10*, parietomastoid suture; *11*, squamous portion of the temporal bone; *12*, zygoma; *13*, glenoid fossa; *14*, styloid process; *15*, jugular foramen; *16*, carotid canal; *17*, sphenopalatine foramen; *18*, greater wing of the sphenoid bone; *19*, lateral pterygoid process; *20*, medial pterygoid process; *21*, pterygomaxillary fossa. (Courtesy Oswaldo Laércio M. Cruz, Helder Tedeschi, and Albert Rhoton.)

69. A 3.0-cm tumor on the floor of mouth with evidence of mandibular erosion and cervical lymph nodes in bilateral levels 1 and 2.
    a. T4aN2B
    b. T2N2C
    c. T4aN2C
    d. T4aN3

70. A 1.5-cm tumor on superior and inferior aspect of the right vocal cord. No cervical lymph nodal disease is palpable.
    a. T1aN0
    b. T4N0
    c. T2N0
    d. T1bN0

71. A 3.5-cm tumor in the postcricoid region extending to the left pyriform fossa with one 4-cm cervical node in left level 3.
    a. T2bN2a supraglottic tumor
    b. T2N2a hypopharyngeal tumor
    c. T3N2a supraglottic tumor
    d. T2aN2b hypopharyngeal tumor

72. A right-sided 2.5-cm anterolateral tongue tumor with extension onto the lower alveolar margin and multiple cervical nodes along the right jugular chain.
    a. T4aN2B
    b. T3N2C
    c. T2N2C
    d. T2N2B

73. A 2.0-cm central nasopharyngeal mass extending to the right lateral oropharyngeal wall. Two cervical lymph nodes (3- and 2-cm) can be palpated in right level 3 and 4.
    a. T1N1
    b. T2N2B
    c. T1N2B
    d. T3N2B

74. A 1.5-cm squamous cell carcinoma on the lingual surface of the epiglottis with bilateral nodal disease <6 cm.
    a. T1N2C oropharyngeal
    b. T1N2C supraglottic
    c. T1N2B oropharyngeal
    d. T1N2B supraglottic

75. A 3.5-cm nasopharyngeal tumor with extension into the left nasal cavity and a 4.5-cm mass in the left supraclavicular region.
    a. T1N1
    b. T1N3
    c. T2N3
    d. T2N1

76. A 3.0-cm maxillary sinus tumor with extension into the posterior maxillary sinus wall and the pterygoid fossa.
    a. T3N0
    b. T4aN0
    c. T4bN0
    d. T2N0

77. A 2.5-cm ethmoidal squamous cell carcinoma with extension and erosion of the medial wall and floor of the orbit.
    a. T2N0
    b. T4aN0
    c. T3N0
    d. T2bN0

78. A 3.0-cm glottic tumor, involving both cords, with radiological evidence of paraglottic space invasion, normal vocal fold movement on fiberoptic endoscopy, and two cervical lymph nodes in the right levels 2 and 3.
    a. T3N2B
    b. T1bN2B
    c. T4aN2B
    d. T3N1

79. A 2.5-cm medullary thyroid carcinoma with extrathyroidal extension and four nodes positive in level 6 in a 55-year-old woman.
    a. T3N1A
    b. T2N2B
    c. T2N1
    d. T3N2B

80. A 3.0-cm anaplastic thyroid carcinoma with no extrathyroidal extension and multiple bilateral lateral neck disease <6 cm.
    a. T2N2C
    b. T4bN2C
    c. T4aN1B
    d. T4aN2C

81. "Preseptal" cellulitis anatomically refers to a cellulitic insult:
    a. Anterior to the orbital septum
    b. Posterior to the orbital septum
    c. Both anterior and posterior to the orbital septum
    d. Resulting in cavernous sinus thrombosis

82. The orbital septum is best described as:
    a. A perforated membranous sheet extending from the orbital rim to the eyelid incorporating the levator palpebrae superioris superiorly and the tarsal plate in the lower eyelid inferiorly
    b. A membranous sheet extending from the orbital rim to the eyelid anastomosing with the superior and inferior tarsal plates
    c. A continuous fibrous sheet extending from the orbital rim to the lower tarsal plate
    d. A perforated membranous sheet extending posterior to the levator palpebrae superioris and lower tarsal plate

83. The following structures pass through the cavernous sinus:
    a. Medially the internal carotid artery (ICA) with its sympathetic plexus and laterally the VI cranial nerve
    b. Medially the ICA and laterally the VI cranial nerve
    c. Laterally the ICA with its sympathetic plexus and medially the VI cranial nerve
    d. Medially the sympathetic plexus and laterally the VI cranial nerve

84. Thrombosis of the cavernous sinus readily occurs due to infection of:
    a. The maxillary sinus
    b. The ethmoid sinus
    c. The agger nasi cell
    d. The sphenoid sinus

85. Gradenigo syndrome is:
    a. Otorrhea, VI cranial nerve paralysis, and retroorbital pain due to involvement of V_1
    b. Otorrhea, IV cranial nerve palsy, and retroorbital pain due to involvement of V_1
    c. Otorrhea, VII cranial nerve paralysis, and retroorbital pain due to involvement of V_1
    d. Otorrhea, X cranial nerve palsy, and retroorbital pain due to V nerve involvement

86. Regarding the superficial muscular aponeurotic system (SMAS), which statement is *INCORRECT*?
    a. In the parotid region, SMAS is superficial to the branches of the facial nerve.
    b. In the mandibular area, loose fibrous connections exist between the SMAS and the platysma muscle.
    c. The main facial artery and vein are located deep to the SMAS.
    d. The SMAS is completely separate from the parotid fascia in the pretragal region.

87. The sensation of the tongue:
    a. Is largely mediated by the V_1 nerve and taste by the chorda tympani (VII)
    b. Is largely mediated by the V_3 and IX nerves and taste by the chorda tympani (VII)
    c. Is mediated by the V_2 and IX nerves and taste by the lingual nerve (VII)
    d. Is mediated by the chorda tympani and taste by the lingual nerve (VII)

88. Taste loss after a tonsillectomy is likely related to a damaged:
    a. Lingual nerve
    b. Vagus nerve
    c. Glossopharyngeal nerve
    d. Chorda tympani

89. Regarding the hypoglossal nerve, which statement is *INCORRECT*?
    a. The nerve emerges between the internal cranial artery and internal jugular vein.
    b. The nerve travels superficial to the anterior belly of the digastric muscle.
    c. The nerve travels deep to the stylohyoid and posterior belly of the digastric muscle.
    d. The nerve innervates the intrinsic and extrinsic muscles of the tongue.

90. The sublingual gland:
    a. Lies between the mucosa of the floor of the mouth and above the mylohyoid muscle
    b. Is drained by the Wharton duct
    c. Is drained by anterior sublingual ducts, which may fuse to form a single duct called the duct of Rivinus.
    d. Abuts the hyoid bone

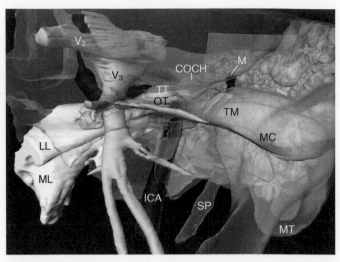

FIGURE 1-8 Lateral view of the left eustachian tube shows the relationship to adjacent structures. *COCH*, Cochlea; *ICA*, internal carotid artery; *LL*, lateral cartilaginous lamina; *M*, head of malleus; *MC*, mandibular condyle; *ML*, medial cartilaginous lamina; *MT*, mastoid tip; *OT*, osseous eustachian tube; *SP*, styloid process; *TM*, tympanic membrane; *TT*, tensor tympani muscle; *V₂*, maxillary division, trigeminal nerve; *V₃*, mandibular division, trigeminal nerve. (Courtesy Michael Teixido, MD, Mads Sorensen, and Haobing Wang.)

91. Regarding the middle ear, which statement is *INCORRECT*?
    a. The stapedius muscle is innervated by the VII cranial nerve.
    b. The tensor tympani is innervated by the V cranial nerve.
    c. The tegmen tympani separates the tympanic cavity from the middle cranial cavity.
    d. The tegmen tympani may be dehiscent in up to 15% of people.

92. Regarding the eustachian tube (Figure 1-8), which statement is correct?
    a. It is 52 mm in length in adults.
    b. The bony portion is in the posterolateral third.
    c. The fibrocartilaginous portion is in the posterolateral third.
    d. The fossa of Rosenmüller is situated anterior to the torus.

93. Eustachian tube dysfunction may cause the following *EXCEPT*:
    a. Autophony
    b. Serous otitis media
    c. Nasal polyposis
    d. Palatal myoclonus

94. The eustachian tube opens during swallowing or yawning due to the following muscles, *EXCEPT*:
    a. Palatopharyngeus
    b. Tensor veli palatine
    c. Salpingopharyngeus
    d. Levator veli palatine

95. True Ludwig angina is an infection of the:
    a. Buccal space
    b. Submandibular space
    c. Parotid space
    d. Digastric space

96. Ludwig angina is commonly caused by:
    a. Alpha-hemolytic streptococci
    b. *Streptococcus agalactiae*
    c. Rhinovirus
    d. *Haemophilus influenzae* type B

97. A 52-year-old patient with a right Bell palsy cannot close her right eye, thus the House-Brackmann score is:
    a. 2
    b. 3
    c. 4
    d. 5

98. Common causes of VII nerve palsy include the following *EXCEPT*:
    a. Herpes zoster oticus
    b. Neurosarcoidosis
    c. Acoustic neuroma
    d. Amyloidosis

99. Which of the following pairings is incorrect?
    a. CN III and Edinger-Westphal nucleus
    b. CN VII and inferior salivatory nucleus
    c. CN X and dorsal motor nucleus
    d. CN IX and inferior salivatory nucleus

100. Which of the following pairings is incorrect?
    a. CN VII and greater superficial petrosal nerve
    b. CN IX and greater superficial petrosal nerve
    c. CN IX and tympanic plexus
    d. CN VII and chorda tympani

CORE KNOWLEDGE

EMBRYOLOGY

Branchial Apparatus

* This appears in the third to fourth weeks of fetal development as neural crest cells. Analogous to gills in a fish, the branchial apparatus consists of pairs of embryologic arches separated externally by grooves (clefts) and internally by paired pharyngeal pouches. The fifth arch is noncontributory in humans, while the rest give rise to muscle/cartilage, an artery, and a nerve (Table 1-1).

Palate

* The face is formed from a single medial premaxillary bud and two lateral maxillomandibular buds. The lateral buds give rise to the mandibular (fusing inferiorly to form the mandible) and maxillary processes, which fuse with the premaxilla to form the maxilla. The maxillary processes also give rise to the upper lips and the zygomatic arches. Failure of the premaxilla and maxillary process to fuse results in a cleft deformity. This may be simple, involving only the lip, or complex, where the hard palate is also involved.

External Ear

* At 4-6 weeks' gestation, six mesenchymal condensations (hillocks of His) appear and fuse by 8-9 weeks with all adult structures evident by 28 weeks. The first three are from the first branchial arch and give rise to the tragus, helical root, and helical crus. Hillocks 4-6 are derived from the 2nd branchial arch and give rise to the antihelix, antitragus, and lobule. The first branchial pouch expands to form the tubotympanic recess, whereas the first cleft forms the external auditory canal. These structures meet to form the tympanic membrane. Failure of a meatal plug to be reabsorbed by 28 weeks leads to congenital aural atresia.

ANATOMY

Oral Cavity Subsites

* These are hard palate/floor of mouth/alveolar margin/anterolateral tongue/buccal mucosa.

Pharynx

* *Nasopharynx:* Anteriorly at the posterior choana to free border of the soft palate. It includes the vault, the lateral wall (including fossa of Rosenmüller and mucosa covering the torus tubarius) and the posterior wall.
* *Oropharynx:* Superior border of soft palate to vallecula (hyoid). Base of tongue/the inferior (anterior) surface of the soft palate/uvula/anterior and posterior tonsillar pillars/pharyngeal tonsils/posterior wall/lateral wall.
* *Hypopharynx:* Vallecula (superior border of the hyoid) to the lower border of the cricoid. Pyriform sinus/lateral wall/posterior wall/post cricoid wall (which is the anterior wall of the hypopharynx).

Table 1-1	**Branchial Apparatus**			
Arch	**Muscular Contributions**	**Skeletal Contributions**	**Nerve**	**Artery**
1st	Muscles of mastication Anterior belly of digastric, mylohyoid Tensor tympani Tensor veli palatini	Meckel cartilage Premaxilla, maxilla, mandible, zygomatic bone, squamous part of the temporal bone, incus, malleus sphenomandibular ligament, EAC	Trigeminal nerve (V_2 and V_3)	Maxillary, external carotid
2nd	Muscles of facial expression, stapedius Stylohyoid Posterior belly of the digastric Auricular	Reichert cartilage Stapes, LPI, styloid process Hyoid (lesser horn and upper part of body), stylohyoid ligament	Facial nerve (VII)	Stapedial, hyoid
3rd	Stylopharyngeus	Hyoid (greater horn, lower part of body), thymus, inferior parathyroids	Glossopharyngeal nerve (IX)	Common carotid, internal carotid
4th	Cricothyroid muscle, soft palate muscles, except tensor veli palatini	Thyroid cartilage, superior parathyroids, epiglottic cartilage	Vagus Superior laryngeal nerve (X)	Subclavian Aortic arch
6th	All intrinsic muscles of larynx except cricothyroid muscle	Cricoid cartilage, arytenoid cartilages, corniculate cartilage, cuneiform cartilages	Vagus Recurrent laryngeal nerve (X)	Pulmonary artery, ductus arteriosus

EAC, External auditory canal; *LPI,* long process of incus.

Larynx

- *Supraglottic larynx:* Epiglottis (both lingual and laryngeal aspect)/suprahyoid epiglottis/infrahyoid epiglottis/aryepiglottic fold (laryngeal aspect)/arytenoids/false cords. The supraglottis inferior boundary is the horizontal plane through the lateral margin of the ventricle at its junction with the superior surface of the vocal cord.
- *Glottic larynx:* Includes the superior and inferior aspect of the true cords/anterior and posterior commissures. It occupies a horizontal plane of 1 cm in thickness.
- *Subglottic larynx:* Extends from the lower boundary of the glottis to the lower margin of the cricoid cartilage.

Esophagus

- *Cervical esophagus* starts at 15 to 20 cm from incisors. *Upper thoracic esophagus* starts at 20 to 25 cm. *Middle thoracic esophagus* starts at 25 to 30 cm. *Lower thoracic esophagus and esophagogastric junction* starts at 30 to 40 cm.

Cervical Fascia

- *Superficial fascia:* Is a continuous layer of fatty subcutaneous tissue. In the face, this invests the muscles of expression. In the neck, it invests the platysma muscle. The deep cervical fascia is broken up into the superficial (SLDF); middle (MLDF), which has a muscular and visceral subdivision; and deep cervical layer (DLDF), which is also subdivided into the prevertebral and alar divisions. The SLDF arises from the spinous process of the vertebral column and encases the neck. It envelops the trapezius and sternocleidomastoid muscles. A single sheet of fascia covers the posterior belly of the omohyoid, fixing it to the clavicle, and a thin sheet passes in front of the strap muscles. Above the hyoid it covers the mylohyoid and anterior belly of the digastric to split into two layers investing the mandible. It envelops the parotid and submandibular gland before extending up to cover the masseter and ultimately insert into the zygomatic arch. MLDF forms a continuous sheet deep to the SLDF and has a muscular and visceral division. The muscular division invests the sternohyoid, sternothyroid, thyrohyoid, and the omohyoid muscles. This layer extends from the hyoid and thyroid cartilages to the sternum, clavicle, and scapula. The visceral layer invests the thyroid gland, trachea, pharynx, and esophagus. Included within the MLDF is the buccopharyngeal fascia, which lies posterior to the pharynx and covers the constrictor muscles extending from the outer buccinator muscle fascia down to continue as the fibrous pericardium and covering to the thoracic esophagus and trachea. The DLDF is a complete fascial ring around the neck. This covers the posterior compartment of the neck deep to the more superficial visceral compartment. It lies deep to the great vessels of the neck but superficial to the phrenic nerve. The prevertebral division is anterior to the vertebral bodies enclosing the vertebral musculature and inserting into the transverse processes. It extends from the skull base to the coccyx. The alar division extends across the midline from transverse process to transverse process. This extends from skull base to T2 where it fuses with the MLDF. In the neck from the midline it extends in an anterolateral direction to form the medial, posterior, and lateral border of the carotid sheath (the anterolateral aspect consists of the SLDF and, to a lesser degree, MLDF).

Parapharyngeal Space

- This space was previously divided into the prestyloid and poststyloid space. This terminology is now incorrect. The prestyloid space is the true parapharyngeal space. The parapharyngeal space is an inverted cone-shaped space that extends from the skull base to the level of the hyoid bone on either side of the pharynx. The carotid space is the designation given to the previously named poststyloid space and is separated from the prestyloid space by the tensor vascular-styloid fascia overlying the tensor veli palatini muscle.

Carotid Space

- This space is contained by the carotid sheath and is formed from all three layers of the deep cervical fascia, spanning the entire neck and extending from the skull base to the aortic arch. The carotid space communicates with the carotid canal and jugular foramen superiorly at the skull base and contains the carotid artery; internal jugular vein; cranial nerves IX, X, XI, and XII; and the sympathetic chain.

Masticator Space

- This space is enclosed by the split layers of the superficial layer of the deep cervical fascia and extends from the skull base to the inferior border of the mandible. It contains the ascending mandibular ramus, the posterior body of the mandible, the muscles of mastication (masseter, medial and lateral pterygoids, and temporalis), the motor and sensory branches of mandibular branch of the trigeminal nerve (V_3), and the inferior alveolar artery and vein.

Pterygopalatine Fossa

- This is bounded by the pterygopalatine fissure laterally and the perpendicular plate of the palatine bone and orbital sphenoidal process medially. Anterior is the infratemporal face of the maxilla and posterior the root of the pterygoid process and greater wing of the sphenoid. The distal or terminal third of the internal maxillary artery (IMAX) crosses the pterygopalatine fossa terminating as the sphenopalatine artery. The pterygopalatine fossa connects with seven anatomical zones: anteriorly the inferior orbital fissure; inferiorly the palatine foramen; posteriorly the foramen rotundum, vidian canal, and palatovaginal canal; laterally the pterygomaxillary fissure; and medially through the sphenopalatine foramen.

Infratemporal Fossa

- The boundaries are the ramus of the mandible laterally, the lateral pterygoid plate medially, the infratemporal surface of the maxilla anteriorly, the superior wing of the sphenoid and undersurface of the squamous portion of the temporal bone superiorly, the spine of the sphenoid and the articular tubercle of the temporal bone posteriorly. The inferior aspect is the medial pterygoid muscle. The contents include the chorda tympani; otic ganglion and the mandibular nerve, which supplies all muscles of mastication (and the mylohyoid, digastric anterior belly, tensores veli palati, and tympani); the IMAX, which runs on the lower border of the lateral pterygoid muscle only to cross through its two heads of origin; the pterygoid venous plexus; the medial and lateral pterygoid muscles; and the lower aspect of the temporalis muscle.

PAROTID

- Parasympathetic supply: preganglionic fibers: inferior salivary nucleus (pre—glossopharyngeal nerve—tympanic plexus—lesser petrosal nerve—postganglionic fibers: otic ganglion—auriculotemporal nerve—parotid).

- Sympathetic supply: preganglionic fibers: anteromediolateral horn nucleus between T1 and T3—enter sympathetic chain—postganglionic fibers: superior cervical ganglion following external carotid to the parotid.

GENICULATE GANGLION

- This has three branches: the greater superficial petrosal nerve, the lesser petrosal nerve, and the external petrosal nerve. In the pterygoid canal, the greater petrosal nerve (preganglionic parasympathetics) joins the deep petrosal nerve (postganglionic sympathetics) to become the nerve of the pterygoid canal. The nerve of the pterygoid canal synapse in the pterygopalatine ganglion and postsynaptic fibers via V_2 maxillary nerve supply the lacrimal and mucous glands of the nasal and oral cavities. The external petrosal nerve is an inconstant neural branch. The lesser petrosal nerve carries preganglionic secretory fibers, joins the otic ganglion, and then proceeds to the parotid gland as postganglionic fibers that travel with the (mixed) auriculotemporal nerve. This is a branch of V_3, which carries sympathetic nerves to vasculature and sweat glands of the scalp, and parasympathetic fibers to the parotid. Frey syndrome is where aberrant regeneration of parasympathetic nerves to local vessels and sweat glands following superficial parotidectomy results in a "sympathetic response" of facial sweating and erythema instead of the normal gustatory response, hence "gustatory sweating."

FACIAL NERVE

- The facial nerve within the epitympanum passes medial to the necks of the malleus and incus. The posterior portion of the tympanic segment has a constant anatomical association with the inferior margin of the lateral semicircular canal. The most common sites of facial nerve injury are at the second genu and mastoid segment. Removal of bone along the lateral surface of the digastric ridge is a useful technique for identification of the facial canal at the stylomastoid foramen. The cochleariform process is the attachment point for the tensor tympani muscle (V_3), which inserts into the manubrium of the malleus, pulling it medial and thereby reducing vibration and amplitude of sound. The pyramidal ridge (a cone-shaped bony prominence in the posterior wall of the tympanic cavity) gives rise to the stapedius tendon (VII). The facial recess and sinus tympani are divided by the pyramidal ridge. The sinus tympani is of variable depth, extending posterior to the facial nerve. Key landmarks to the posterior tympanic segment are the stapes and oval window. The facial nerve exits the stylomastoid foramen and gives rise to the posterior auricular nerve entering the parotid fossa and passing between the stylohyoid and the posterior belly of the digastric. The superior aspect of the posterior belly of digastric is the key surgical landmark in the identification of the pes anserinus. The trajectory of the posterior belly indicates the anatomical level of dissection for the pes.

TRIGEMINAL NERVE

- The gasserian ganglion is a sensory ganglion within "Meckel cave," or the cavity of the dura at the apex of the petrous temporal bone. V_1 is the ophthalmic branch, which passes through the superior orbital fissure and is exclusively sensory. V_2 is the maxillary branch, which passes through foramen rotundum and is also exclusively sensory. V_3, the mandibular nerve, is a mixed nerve and passes through the foramen ovale. The motor component joins the mandibular nerve outside the cranium. Within

the infratemporal fossa, smaller branches include the meningeal nervus spinosus and the nerve to the medial pterygoid muscle. V_3 then branches into the anterior (4) and posterior (4) branches.

MUSCLES

- Anterior digastric. First pharyngeal arch. Mandibular nerve innervation. Originates from the digastric fossa on the lower border of the mandible. Posterior digastric originates from the mastoid process and digastric groove (between the styloid process and the mastoid process), second pharyngeal arch and facial nerve innervates. Contraction of the digastric elevates the hyoid. The sternocleidomastoid (SCM) muscle originates from the sternal manubrium and the clavicle to insert into the mastoid. Innervation is via the XI nerve. The blood supply to the SCM muscle can be divided into three parts: upper, middle, and lower. The upper third of the SCM muscle is supplied by branches of the occipital artery. The middle third is supplied by the superior thyroid artery; the external carotid (or branches of both) and the lower third are supplied by the suprascapular artery (thyrocervical trunk). The omohyoid muscle extends from the scapula to the hyoid. It is innervated by ansa cervicalis (cervical plexus) and is an important landmark in neck surgery.

PHARYNGEAL POUCH

- Also called Zenker diverticulum, this is a pharyngeal mucosal herniation at Killian dehiscence that occurs between the propulsive oblique fibers of the thyropharyngeus and the horizontal fibers of the cricopharyngeus, which have a sphincteric action.

THYROID GLAND

- Embryological development begins between the 1st and 2nd pouches at 18 to 24 days gestation between the tuberculum impar and the copula at the foramen cecum, which is the opening of the thyroglossal duct into the tongue. This duct obliterates by weeks 7 to 10 following the descent of the thyroid. The pyramidal lobe represents persistence of the inferior aspect of the thyroglossal duct. The ultimobranchial body originates from the ventral portion of the 4th pharyngeal pouch. Neural crest cells infiltrate the ultimobranchial body. This then fuses with the thyroid and its parafollicular C cells disperse within it and hence are of neural crest origin (Figure 1-9).

PARATHYROID GLANDS

- The superior parathyroid gland originates from the 4th pouch and the lower parathyroid from the 3rd pouch. The blood supply for both glands is from the inferior thyroid artery, a branch of the thyrocervical trunk. The parathyroids weigh between 25 and 40 mg and produce PTH, which is a polypeptide containing 84 amino acids. PTH acts in the bones, kidneys, and intestine. In bone it indirectly stimulates osteoclasts, thereby increasing calcium resorption by directly stimulating osteoblastic activity. PTH results in osteoblasts binding to a protein called RANKL (receptor activator of nuclear factor kappa-B ligand). This reduces their expression of a protein called osteoprotegerin, which inhibits osteoclasts. RANKL then binds with its receptor RANK resulting in increased osteoclastic formation. In the intestine, PTH results in 1-alpha-hydroxylase activating vitamin D to 1,25-dihydroxycholecalciferol. This acts with the protein

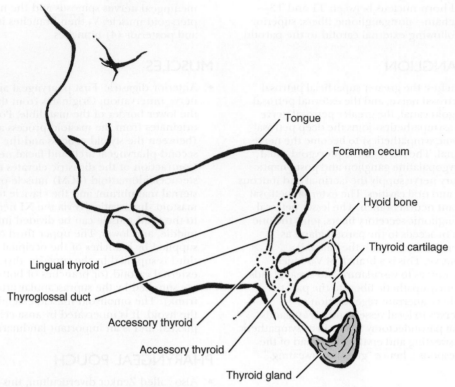

Tongue

Foramen cecum

Hyoid bone

Thyroid cartilage

Lingual thyroid

Thyroglossal duct

Accessory thyroid

Accessory thyroid

Thyroid gland

FIGURE 1-9 Migration of thyroid tissue.

calbindin to increase calcium absorption. In the kidneys, PTH increases resorption of calcium and magnesium in the proximal tubules and thick ascending limb and reduces the resorption of phosphate. The treatment of hypoparathyroidism is limited by the fact that there is no artificial replacement form of the hormone.

VOCAL CORDS

- There are five layers to the vocal cords: the epithelial, the superficial, intermediate and deep lamina propria, and the muscular layers. The Reinke space is only a potential space that becomes pathological when fluid accumulates within the superficial lamina propria. This is commonly attributed to smoking. Speech is impaired, as the vibratory components of the cords are the epithelial and superficial lamina propria layers. The vocal ligament is the intermediate and deep layers of the vocal fold, and the "body" is the thyroarytenoid and vocalis muscles. The superior laryngeal nerve (SLN) has an external branch that supplies the cricothyroid muscle and an internal branch that pierces the thyrohyoid membrane, offering sensory innervation above the glottis. The vocal cords receive dual sensory innervation between the recurrent laryngeal nerve (RLN) and the internal branch of the SLN. The RLN is recurrent because it loops around the arch of the aorta on the left and the right subclavian artery on the right. It supplies sensation at and below the cords and also has a motor function supplying all laryngeal muscles except for the cricothyroid.

LARYNGEAL SUPERSTRUCTURE

- The cartilaginous structure is made of three paired cartilages (arytenoids, cuneiform, corniculate) and three single structures (cricoid, thyroid, epiglottis). The intrinsic

membranes of the larynx include the conus elasticus (cricovocal membrane), which extends laterally deep to the cricothyroid ligament attaching inferiorly to the cricoid cartilage and extends to the inner surface of the thyroid cartilage and posteriorly to the arytenoid cartilage. The superior free edge bilaterally forms the vocal ligament. The quadrangular membrane extends from the side of the epiglottic cartilage to the corniculate and arytenoid cartilages. This forms the aryepiglottic fold of the larynx and false (vestibular) folds. There are two spaces within the larynx of importance: the preepiglottic and paraglottic spaces. The preepiglottic space is bounded by the thyrohyoid membrane anteriorly, the thyroepiglottic ligament and valleculae superiorly, and the anterior surface of the epiglottis and petiole posteriorly. The paraglottic space is bounded anterolaterally by the conus elasticus, the quadrangular membrane, and the thyroid cartilage. Posteriorly lies a reflection of the pyriform sinus mucosa. The paraglottic space extends anterosuperiorly into the preepiglottic space and is a route of glottic cancer extralaryngeal progression.

THE ARTERIAL SUPPLY TO THE NOSE

- This is from the anterior and posterior ethmoid arteries, which are branches of the ophthalmic artery. The sphenopalatine artery (terminal branch of IMAX) branches into the posterior septal artery and the posterior lateral nasal artery. The greater palatine arteries originate from IMAX, and the sublabial artery is a branch of the facial artery.

MAXILLARY SINUS

- This grows according to a biphasic pattern at 0 to 3 years and at 6 to 12 years. The roof of the maxillary sinus is the floor of the orbit, and there is a pyramidal orientation to the sinus. The posteromedial wall aspect of the sinus is the pterygopalatine fossa, and the infratemporal fossa lies behind the posterolateral wall. The maxillary sinus is supplied by branches of the IMAX, including the infraorbital, alveolar, greater palatine, and sphenopalatine arteries. Innervation is through branches of V_2 (infraorbital and greater palatine nerves).

ETHMOID SINUS

- Present at birth; it grows and pneumatizes up to the age of 12 years. The agger nasi is the first anterior ethmoidal cell to undergo pneumatization. The ethmoid sinuses are supplied by the anterior and posterior ethmoidal arteries (ophthalmic artery) and the sphenopalatine artery (terminal branches of IMAX). The Keros classification divides the ethmoid roof into three configurations: shallow type I (1-3 mm), medium type II (4-7 mm), and deep type III (8-16 mm). A Haller cell, or infraorbital cell, is an anterior ethmoidal cell that pneumatizes into the maxillary sinus ostium below the inferior orbital wall. The ethmoid bulla lies posterior to the uncinate process, superior to the infundibulum, and anterior to the basal lamella. The two-dimensional space between the bulla and the uncinate is the hiatus semilunaris. Anterior ethmoidal cells drain into the middle meatus via the ethmoid infundibulum. Posterior ethmoidal cells drain into the superior meatus. The osteomeatal complex is lamina papyracea laterally, the middle turbinate medially, the frontal recess superiorly, and the maxillary sinus ostium inferiorly.

MIDDLE TURBINATE

- This has an anterior and posterior buttress, a horizontal and a vertical lamella. The anterior buttress is a point of attachment of the turbinate to the lateral nasal wall in the agger nasi region. The posterior buttress is a point of attachment to the lateral nasal wall near the posterior end of the middle turbinate. The vertical lamella attaches to the lateral cribriform plate lamella and marks the boundary between the cribriform plate and the ethmoid roof. The horizontal lamella (also called the *ground lamella*) attaches to the lateral nasal wall and marks the division between the anterior and posterior ethmoid air cells. The uncinate process originates from ethmoid bone and has three potential attachments. It usually attaches to the medial orbital wall superiorly but may attach to the skull base or the middle turbinate.

FRONTAL SINUS

- This is formed by the upward movement of anterior ethmoid cells after the age of 2. The growth of the sinus is largely between ages 6 to teenage years. The frontal sinus is supplied by the supraorbital and supratrochlear arteries of the ophthalmic artery (the first branch of the supraclinoid internal carotid artery). It is innervated by the supraorbital and supratrochlear nerves of V_1. The frontal recess is bounded anteriorly by the posterior wall of the agger nasi cell, superiorly by the frontal sinus, medially by the lateral cribriform plate lamella, laterally by the lamina papyracea, and posteriorly by the anterior wall of the ethmoidal bulla.

SPHENOID SINUS

- This has three potential orientations: sellar (67%), presellar, and conchal. This sinus does not reach full size until teenage years. The ostium is located on the anterosuperior surface of the sphenoid face, usually medial to the superior turbinate. The sphenopalatine artery supplies the sinus, except for the planum sphenoidale, which is supplied by the posterior ethmoidal artery. Innervation of the sphenoid sinus comes from branches of V_1 and V_2.

ANSWERS

TRUE OR FALSE QUESTIONS

1. T	14. F	27. T	40. T
2. T	15. F	28. T	41. F
3. F	16. F	29. T	42. F
4. F	17. T	30. F	43. F
5. T	18. T	31. T	44. T
6. F	19. T	32. F	45. T
7. T	20. F	33. T	46. T
8. F	21. F	34. F	47. T
9. F	22. T	35. T	48. F
10. T	23. F	36. F	49. F
11. T	24. T	37. F	50. T
12. F	25. T	38. T	
13. T	26. F	39. F	

SINGLE BEST ANSWER QUESTIONS

51. c	59. e	63. a	70. a
52. a	60. e	64. b	71. b
53. b	61. i, d; ii, d; iii, a; iv, f; v, e;	65. i, c; ii, b; iii, a; iv, b; v, a	72. d
54. a	vi, d; vii, g; viii, c; ix, g;	66. i, e; ii, a; iii, d; iv, c; v, b	73. a
55. d	x, a	67. i, f; ii, a; iii, b; iv, c; v, e;	74. b
56. e	62. a, vii; b, iv; c, iii; d, ii; e,	vi, d	75. b
57. c	viii; f, ix; g, x; h, v; i, vi;	68. d	76. a
58. c	j, i	69. c	77. c

78. a	84. d	90. a	96. a
79. a	85. a	91. d	97. c
80. c	86. d	92. b	98. d
81. a	87. b	93. c	99. b
82. a	88. c	94. a	100. b
83. a	89. b	95. b	

SUGGESTED READINGS

1. Janfaza P. *Surgical Anatomy of the Head and Neck.* Lippincott Williams & Wilkins; 2001.
2. Shah J. *Head and Neck Surgery and Oncology.* 4th ed. Mosby; 2012.
3. Patel SG, Meyers P, Huvos AG, et al. Improved outcomes in patients with osteogenic sarcoma of the head and neck. *Cancer.* 2002;95(7):1495-1503.
4. Netter F. *Atlas of Human Anatomy.* 5th ed. Saunders; 2010.
5. Mohebati A, Shaha AR. Anatomy of thyroid and parathyroid glands and neurovascular relations. *Clin Anat.* 2012;25(1):19-31.
6. Pinheiro-Neto CD. Anatomical correlates of endonasal surgery for sinonasal malignancies. *Clin Anat.* 2012;25: 129-134.
7. Rhoton AL Jr. The anterior and middle cranial base. *Neurosurgery.* 2002;51:S273-S302.
8. Pravin KP, Shyamsunder NB. Head and Neck Embryology. Medscape. WebMD Health Professional Network. <emedicine.com>.
9. Stambuk H, Patel S. Imaging of the parapharyngeal space. *Otolaryngol Clin N Am.* 2008;41:77-101.
10. Logan B, Reynolds P, Hutchings R. *McMinns Color Atlas of Head and Neck Anatomy.* 4th ed. Elsevier; 2010.

Otolaryngology Radiology 2

Salvatore V. Labruzzo | Nafi Aygun

TRUE OR FALSE QUESTIONS

GENERAL RADIOLOGY

T/F 1. Iodinated contrast material is routinely used for neck computed tomography (CT) unless it is contraindicated.

T/F 2. Gadolinium-based contrast material in magnetic resonance imaging (MRI) is contraindicated in advanced chronic kidney disease.

T/F 3. Artifacts from dental amalgam are less problematic in MRI than CT.

T/F 4. Fluorodeoxyglucose (FDG)-positron emission tomography (PET) is superior to MRI and/or CT in T-staging of head and neck cancer.

T/F 5. FDG-PET is superior to MRI and/or CT in assessment of recurrent head and neck cancer.

TEMPORAL BONE/PETROUS APEX/SKULL BASE

T/F 6. Contrast-enhanced CT is the modality of choice for assessment of malignant external otitis.

T/F 7. Keratosis obturans is commonly associated with erosion of the bony cortex in the external acoustic canal.

T/F 8. CT is the modality of choice for the assessment of conductive hearing loss.

T/F 9. Bezold abscess is an intracranial complication of acute mastoiditis.

T/F 10. Coalescent mastoiditis refers to resorption of the bony septa separating mastoid air cells in the setting of acute mastoiditis.

T/F 11. In a chronically infected ear, ossicular erosion demonstrated on CT is strongly suggestive of cholesteatoma.

T/F 12. Asymmetric pneumatization of the petrous apices occurs in 3% of the population.

T/F 13. CT is the study of choice for stapes fixation in chronic otitis media.

T/F 14. Dehiscence of the tegmen tympani demonstrated on CT indicates cerebrospinal fluid (CSF) leak or meningoencephalocele.

T/F 15. Noncontrast-enhanced CT of the temporal bone is sufficient for the diagnosis of an aberrant carotid artery.

T/F 16. Dehiscence of the facial nerve canal along its tympanic segment on CT scans is a contraindication for oval window surgery.

T/F 17. Facial nerve hemangiomas most frequently occur at the mastoid segment of the nerve.

T/F 18. The prevalence of superior semicircular canal dehiscence on CT is much higher than the prevalence of superior semicircular canal dehiscence syndrome.

T/F 19. Tinnitus is caused by dehiscence of the jugular canal.

T/F 20. Otic capsule sparing fractures are the most common type of temporal bone fractures.

T/F 21. A narrow internal auditory canal (IAC) is the CT finding that best predicts absence of the cochlear nerve.

T/F 22. Small vestibular schwannomas can be detected by noncontrast-enhanced MRI.

T/F 23. MRI readily differentiates cerebellopontine angle cistern arachnoid cysts from the more common schwannomas.

T/F 24. Following resection of a vestibular schwannoma, newly appearing enhancement on MRI scan in the cochlea indicates recurrent tumor in the labyrinth.

T/F 25. In most cases, a skull base schwannoma can be differentiated from a paraganglioma on CT and MRI, obviating the need for catheter angiography.

PARANASAL SINUSES AND NASAL CAVITY

T/F 26. The nasolacrimal duct drains into the nasal cavity via the middle meatus.

T/F 27. On MRI, a mildly T2 hyperintense mass that is not separated from the sinus wall by mucosa is concerning for malignancy.

T/F 28. Eosinophilic mucin is responsible for the high density in the sinuses of patients with allergic fungal sinusitis.

T/F 29. The basal lamella of the middle turbinate separates the posterior ethmoid sinus from the sphenoid sinus.

T/F 30. A concha bullosa is pneumatization of a turbinate, most frequently the middle turbinate.

FACE (INCLUDING FACIAL TRAUMA)

T/F 31. Naso-orbital-ethmoidal fractures result in injury to the medial canthus ligament complex.

T/F 32. The ipsilateral sphenopalatine foramen is lateral to the pterygopalatine fossa.

T/F 33. MRI of the brain is indicated in a neonate with a severe cleft palate.

T/F 34. Congenital nasolabial cysts arise from epithelial remnants from the nasolacrimal duct extending between the lateral nasal process and the maxillary prominence.

T/F 35. A direct blunt force injury to the orbit results in orbital floor fractures more frequently than medial orbital wall fractures.

PEDIATRIC NECK/CONGENITAL

T/F 36. Type 1 branchial cleft cysts arise in the periparotid region.

T/F 37. A midfacial mass at the bridge of the nose in a 1-year-old requires CT and/or MRI for further evaluation of the brain.

T/F 38. The first-line imaging modality for the evaluation of cervical lymphadenopathy in a 4-year-old is CT.

T/F 39. A cystic mass along the course in the medial canthus region of a 2-month-old is most likely a dermoid.

T/F 40. An enhancing mass in the neck of a patient with neurofibromatosis type 1 is most likely to be a schwannoma.

LYMPH NODES

T/F 41. Lymphadenopathy associated with Kawasaki disease is more often unilateral than bilateral.

T/F 42. Lymphoma and leukemia are the most common cause of chronic lymphadenopathy in children.

T/F 43. Infections are the most likely cause of isolated posterior triangle lymphadenopathy in a 70-year-old male.

T/F 44. According to the American Joint Committee on Cancer, regarding oropharyngeal cancer, a lymph node greater than 6 cm is N2.

T/F 45. Human papilloma virus (HPV)-related squamous cell carcinomas tend to have homogeneously enhancing lymph nodes.

THYROID/PARATHYROID

T/F 46. Parathyroid adenomas may be found within the thyroid gland.

T/F 47. The incidence of malignancy in a cold thyroid nodule is 10% to 15%.

T/F 48. On iodine-131 scans cold thyroid nodules are less likely to be malignant than hot or warm nodules.

T/F 49. Hurthle cell tumors of the thyroid take up more iodine than papillary thyroid carcinoma.

T/F 50. The parathyroid glands wash out faster than the thyroid gland on technetium-99m sestamibi scans.

SINGLE BEST ANSWER QUESTIONS

51. In CT, the unit of measured radiograph attenuation is:
    a. Sievert
    b. Gray
    c. Hounsfield
    d. Window level
    e. Window width

52. ALARA (*as low as reasonably achievable*) principle is related to:
    a. Appropriateness of diagnostic imaging
    b. Allergic reactions to radiologic contrast material
    c. Cost of radiologic imaging
    d. Risks of radiologic imaging

53. CT's advantages compared with MRI include all *EXCEPT*:
    a. Less costly
    b. Quicker
    c. Higher contrast resolution
    d. Higher spatial resolution
    e. Can be performed in patients with cardiac pacemakers

54. FDG used in PET imaging is taken up by:
    a. Malignant tumors only
    b. Malignant and benign tumors only
    c. Malignant and inflammatory tissue only
    d. All tissues that can metabolize glucose

55. The most common mass seen in the external auditory canal (EAC) is:
    a. Keratosis obturans
    b. Cholesteatoma
    c. Cholesterol granuloma
    d. Squamous cell carcinoma
    e. Hemangioma

56. A child with congenital atresia of the external ear canal is least likely to have:
    a. Bony atresia
    b. Auricle dysplasia
    c. Ossicular anomalies
    d. Cochlear dysplasia
    e. Aberrant facial nerve canal

57. The most common location for acquired middle ear cholesteatoma is:
    a. Mesotympanum medial to the ossicles
    b. Mesotympanum lateral to the ossicles
    c. Hypotympanum
    d. Medial wall
    e. Lateral epitympanum

58. The most specific MRI sequence for the diagnosis of recurrent cholesteatoma in the middle ear is:
    a. T2-weighted
    b. T1-weighted
    c. Diffusion weighted
    d. Postcontrast T1-weighted
    e. Gradient echo

59. The most common site of otospongiosis (otosclerosis) involvement on CT is:
    a. Anterior to the stapes foot plate
    b. Posterior to the stapes foot plate
    c. Round window
    d. Cochlea
    e. Semicircular canal

60. A patient with improved hearing following stapedotomy and prosthesis placement for otosclerosis experiences worsening of hearing. Her CT is most likely to show:
    a. Vestibular perforation
    b. Progressive otosclerosis
    c. Prosthesis displacement
    d. Incus fracture
    e. Cholesteatoma

61. CT of a person with sound-induced vertigo, nystagmus, and oscillopsia is most likely to show:
    a. Perilymphatic fistula
    b. Vestibular schwannoma
    c. Superior semicircular canal dehiscence

d. Otospongiosis
e. Paget disease

62. The facial nerve segment that is least likely to enhance on contrast-enhanced MRI is:
    a. Labyrinthine
    b. Geniculate
    c. Tympanic
    d. Mastoid

63. MRI of a woman with facial nerve weakness and a whitish mass behind the tympanic membrane shows an avidly enhancing mass associated with the tympanic segment of the facial nerve. The most likely diagnosis is:
    a. Schwannoma
    b. Hemangioma
    c. Paraganglioma
    d. Cholesterol granuloma
    e. Cholesteatoma

64. A purple mass behind the tympanic membrane is least likely to be a:
    a. Glomus tumor
    b. Cholesterol granuloma
    c. Cholesteatoma
    d. Dehiscent jugular bulb
    e. Aberrant carotid artery

65. Gradenigo syndrome is caused by spread of mastoid infection to the:
    a. Middle ear tegmen
    b. Inferior mastoid
    c. Petrous apex
    d. Sigmoid sinus
    e. Orbit

66. What is the most common abnormality of the petrous apex seen in imaging studies?
    a. Cholesterol granuloma
    b. Congenital cholesteatoma
    c. Meningoencephalocele
    d. Effusion
    e. Metastasis

67. Hyperintense T1 signal in an expansile petrous apex lesion is characteristic for:
    a. Cholesterol granuloma
    b. Congenital cholesteatoma
    c. Meningoencephalocele
    d. Effusion
    e. Metastasis

68. A mass demonstrating marked heterogeneity of MRI signal due to blood by-products centered in the dorsal petrous ridge is most likely to represent a:
    a. Cholesterol granuloma
    b. Cholesteatoma
    c. Meningioma
    d. Endolymphatic sac tumor
    e. Choristoma

69. An expansile petrous apex mass that shows fluid signal and no enhancement on MRI is most likely to be a:
    a. Schwannoma
    b. Cholesteatoma
    c. Meningocele
    d. Effusion
    e. Cholesterol granuloma

70. Which of the following is a contraindication for cochlear implantation?
    a. Absence of the cochlear nerve on MRI
    b. Enlarged vestibular aqueduct

c. Michel anomaly
d. Anomalous cochlea
e. Anomalous vestibule

71. The most common imaging abnormality in a child with sensorineural hearing loss is:
    a. Semicircular canal anomaly
    b. Cochlear anomaly
    c. Vestibular anomaly
    d. Enlarged vestibular aqueduct
    e. Enlarged cochlear aqueduct

72. Which of the following structures exits the cranium outside the jugular foramen?
    a. Glossopharyngeal nerve
    b. Vagus nerve
    c. Spinal accessory nerve
    d. Hypoglossal nerve
    e. Internal jugular vein

73. The most common mass in the jugular foramen is:
    a. Paraganglioma
    b. Schwannoma
    c. Meningioma
    d. Metastasis
    e. Chondrosarcoma

74. The incidence of multicentric paraganglioma in a patient with a family history of neck masses is:
    a. 2%
    b. 7%
    c. 15%
    d. 20%
    e. 25%

75. The most common site of CSF leak at the anterior skull base is:
    a. Cribriform plate
    b. Fovea ethmoidalis
    c. Lateral lamella
    d. Frontal plate
    e. Crista galli

76. The middle meatus is part of the drainage pathway for which sinuses?
    a. Sphenoid and posterior ethmoid
    b. Anterior and posterior ethmoid
    c. Frontal, maxillary, and sphenoid
    d. Frontal, maxillary, and anterior ethmoid

77. The modality of choice for the evaluation of chronic rhinosinusitis and planning of surgery is:
    a. MRI
    b. Radiography
    c. Fluoroscopy
    d. CT

78. The imaging characteristics of silent sinus syndrome include:
    a. A clear sinus airspace
    b. Sinus wall thickening
    c. Bulging of the anterior wall of the sinus
    d. Exophthalmos
    e. Patent infundibulum

79. Identification of sphenoethmoidal (Onodi) air cells is made by the presence of:
    a. Pneumatization of the anterior clinoid processes
    b. Large sphenoid sinuses pneumatized posterior to the sella turcica
    c. A transverse bony septum within the sphenoid with separation of superior and inferior airspaces
    d. A deviated or absent intersinus septum

80. Which of the following CT findings would best characterize chronic rhinosinusitis rather than an acute sinusitis?
    a. Osteitis
    b. Fluid levels
    c. Orbital inflammation
    d. Intracranial abscess

81. Regarding mucoceles and mucus retention cysts, which statement is correct?
    a. A mucocele is caused by an obstructed seromucinous gland within the sinus lining.
    b. A mucus retention cyst is caused an obstructed sinus ostium.
    c. Mucoceles are more common than mucus retention cysts.
    d. A mucocele is associated with expansion of the sinus.
    e. Mucoceles most commonly occur in the maxillary sinus.

82. Regarding the LeFort classification of maxillofacial fractures, which statement is correct?
    a. The pterygoid processes may be intact.
    b. The mandibular condyles are fractured in type IV.
    c. Type I results in the "floating face" configuration.
    d. Type III fracture does not include a fracture of the nasal septum.
    e. Type II fracture extends through the inferior orbital rim and orbital floor.

83. Regarding the parotid gland, which statement is most correct?
    a. Neoplasms are more often malignant than those arising in the submandibular gland.
    b. T2 hypointense masses are likely to be benign.
    c. The eponymous name for the parotid duct is Wharton duct.
    d. Cystic changes can be seen in both Sjögren disease and HIV.
    e. Glandular calcifications are infrequent in chronic sialoadenitis.

84. The most specific test to identify the location of a CSF leak due to trauma is:
    a. Contrast-enhanced MRI
    b. B2 transferrin analysis
    c. CT cisternography
    d. Nuclear cisternography

85. Regarding nasal fractures, which statement is most correct?
    a. The use of plain radiographs has a critical role in the management of nasal fractures.
    b. CT is indicated in minor, uncomplicated nasal fractures because physical examination is insensitive.
    c. CT is indicated to determine the extent of bony injury in more complicated injury.
    d. Septal hematomas are more often seen in adult trauma than pediatric trauma.

86. The most common congenital neck cyst is:
    a. 1st branchial cleft cyst
    b. 3rd branchial cleft cyst
    c. Thyroglossal duct cyst
    d. Epidermal inclusion cyst
    e. Cystic hygroma/lymphatic malformation

87. Normal lymph nodes tend to have _____ signal on T1 and _____ signal on T2-weighted MRI.
    a. High, high
    b. Low, low
    c. High, low
    d. Low, high
    e. None of the above

88. The most common location for a thyroglossal duct cyst is:
    a. Infrahyoid
    b. Suprahyoid, excluding intralingual
    c. At the level of the hyoid
    d. In the hyoid
    e. In the tongue base

89. Imaging characteristics of venous malformations in the face and neck include:
    a. Hyperintensity on T2-weighted images
    b. No enhancement with contrast material
    c. Foci of low signal on T2-weighted images and high density on CT
    d. a and c
    e. a, b, and c

90. Select the most common association for the cancer location and nodal basin involved.
    a. Nasopharyngeal and supraclavicular
    b. Floor of the mouth and ipsilateral level III
    c. Oral tongue and ipsilateral level III
    d. Tonsillar and ipsilateral level II
    e. Supraglottic and ipsilateral level I

91. Necrotic and cystic lymph nodes are least often associated with:
    a. Squamous cell carcinoma
    b. Nasopharyngeal carcinoma
    c. Tuberculosis
    d. Hodgkin lymphoma

92. The least likely cause of a calcified lymph node is:
    a. Metastatic mucinous adenocarcinoma
    b. Treated lymphoma
    c. Granulomatous disease
    d. Squamous cell carcinoma of the larynx
    e. Papillary thyroid carcinoma

93. In a patient with vocal cord paralysis, an avidly enhancing mass is identified in the neck splaying the internal carotid artery and the internal jugular vein. This is most likely a:
    a. Carotid body tumor
    b. Glomus vagale
    c. Glomus jugulare
    d. Glomus tympanicum
    e. Lymph node metastasis of lung carcinoma

94. Regarding retropharyngeal lymph nodes in adults with nasopharyngeal carcinoma, the most likely characteristic to indicate benignity is a:
    a. 4 mm medial lymph node
    b. Cystic lymph node
    c. Cluster of lymph nodes
    d. 4 mm lateral lymph node

95. Concerning lymph nodes in level II, what characteristic would be most specific for pathology?
    a. Short axis greater than 5 mm
    b. Long axis greater than 10 mm
    c. Absence of fatty hilum with thin cortex
    d. Poorly defined capsule and surrounding inflammation

96. Regarding the recurrence of well-differentiated thyroid cancer assessed by elevation of thyroglobulin, the first-line imaging modality is:
    a. Iodine-131 scan
    b. PET-CT
    c. MRI
    d. Iodine-123 scan
    e. Neck ultrasound

97. The most common histology of thyroid cancer to be associated with calcifications in metastatic lymph nodes is:
    a. Papillary
    b. Medullary
    c. Anaplastic
    d. Hürthle

98. The most concerning characteristic of a thyroid nodule at imaging is:
    a. Size of 2 to 4 cm
    b. Growth greater than 20% in two dimensions in less than 18 months
    c. Multiple nodules
    d. Hyperechoic nodule
    e. Wider than tall orientation

99. Imaging evaluation for parathyroid adenoma would less likely include:
    a. Technetium-99m sestamibi scintigraphy
    b. Multiphase CT
    c. Ultrasound
    d. MRI

100. Regarding parathyroid adenomas, which statement is correct?
    a. The parathyroid adenoma should have a lower attenuation on CT than the thyroid prior to contrast.
    b. Enhancement should be evident in the arterial phase.
    c. Polar vessel sign is present in the majority.
    d. There should be delayed washout on nuclear scintigraphy.
    e. All of the above

CORE KNOWLEDGE

GENERAL RADIOLOGY

- Cross-sectional imaging such as CT and MRI has replaced the use of conventional radiography in the head and neck.
- Modern CT techniques and hardware allow for rapid imaging of the head and neck. A single scan, usually in the axial plane, utilizing spiral (or helical) techniques allows for volumetric data acquisition. Sophisticated postprocessing of this data utilizing algorithms to accentuate bone or soft tissue characteristics can be performed, and multiplanar reformations can be provided for improved visualization of anatomy and pathology.
- In CT, the unit of measured radiograph attenuation is the Hounsfield. Those tissues or materials that inhibit transmission of x-rays to the detector, such as bone or metal, have higher Hounsfield measurements than those tissues or materials that do not, such as air and fat.
- Contrast-enhanced techniques are frequently utilized on both CT and MRI. Contrast is useful when imaging the neck and orbits with either modality. CT of the temporal bones and paranasal sinuses is most commonly performed without intravenous contrast administration. Advanced MRI techniques often utilized for evaluation of tumors in these locations may include postcontrast sequences. MRI with contrast utilizing high-resolution techniques is particularly useful in the evaluation of masses and associated perineural spread.
- Allergic reactions and diminished renal function are the main contraindications for contrast use in both CT and MRI.
- MRI is often more prone to artifacts than CT. Probably the most recognized artifact in both modalities is motion. Dental amalgam-related artifacts are also common and affect CT generally more than MRI.
- CT is generally less costly, quicker, and more readily available in most communities and has higher special resolution than MRI, although MRI's contrast resolution—the ability that helps differentiate various soft tissues—is much superior. There are no contraindications for utilizing CT associated with pacemakers, which are a relative contraindication of MRI. Some institutions have protocols in place whereby some patients with pacers can be imaged.
- Chemical shift artifact arising from the differences in the tissue properties between fat and water are unique to MRI, which results in spatial misregistration.
- When determining the most appropriate imaging modality to use for evaluation of otolaryngologic pathology, the medical community should adhere to the principles of ALARA. This means making every reasonable effort to maintain exposures to ionizing radiation as low as possible.
- Common hyperintense or bright substances on T1-weighted MRI are fat, blood, purulent debris, proteinaceous fluid, melanin, and gadolinium-based contrast agents.
- Common hyperintense or bright substances on T2-weighted MRI are fat and substances with high water content.
- The signal from fat can be suppressed on both T1 and T2 MRI, resulting in dark signal from fat, which can help to increase conspicuity of other tissues. This is particularly helpful in the neck and orbits.
- Ultrasound is a valuable imaging modality in the field of otolaryngology. It allows for reliable assessment of cystic lesions, lymph nodes, and vascularity of lesions. Ultrasound is highly operator dependent. It is relatively inexpensive and usually readily available. Ultrasound is useful for imaging guidance during biopsy and fine-needle aspiration.
- Nuclear medicine techniques provide biochemical data and physiological assessment of the organ(s) examined. PET is often coupled with CT imaging (PET-CT) to provide anatomic localization of metabolic activity. Depending on the radiopharmaceutical used, the metabolism or accumulation of variable compounds or elements can be identified. In the head and neck, the most commonly used radiopharmaceutical is ^{18}F-FDG, which is a glucose analog.
- T-staging of head and neck cancer is best accomplished by CT or MRI, as assessment of small structures with PET is limited because of the low spatial resolution available. PET offers advantages in nodal staging as well as distant metastases particularly when it is performed in conjunction with CT. In the posttreatment setting, PET-CT is the most accurate imaging test available.
- Other nuclear medicine agents and techniques include technetium-99m pertechnetate scanning for evaluation of salivary gland function, iodine-123 and iodine-131 scanning for the evaluation of thyroid dysfunction and cancer, and technetium-99m sestamibi for the evaluation of parathyroid adenomas.

TEMPORAL BONE/PETROUS APEX

- The most common mass seen in the EAC is keratosis obturans, which represents circumferential accumulation of desquamated epithelium in the external auditory canal,

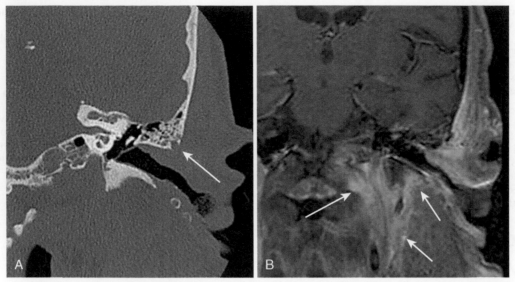

FIGURE 2-1 Malignant otitis externa. Coronal computed tomographic image **(A)** of the left temporal bone shows soft tissue thickening in the left external auditory canal with erosion of the mastoid cortex *(arrow)*, indicating an aggressive process. Coronal postcontrast T1-weighted magnetic resonance image **(B)** much better depicts the deep extension of infection into the skull base and craniocervical junction *(arrows)*.

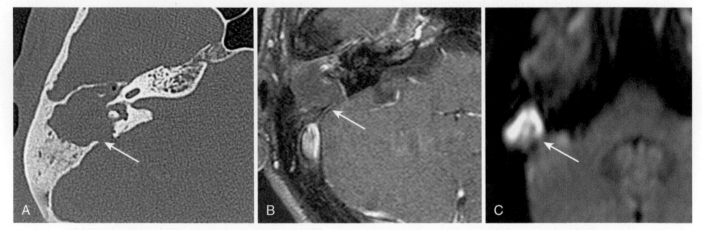

FIGURE 2-2 Cholesteatoma. Axial computed tomography **(A),** postcontrast T1-weighted magnetic resonance image (MRI) **(B),** and diffusion-weighted (DWI) MRI **(C)** images of the right temporal bone show a mass occupying the middle ear cavity with destruction of the ossicles and petrous ridge and invasion of the lateral semicircular canal *(arrows)*. Mass shows no enhancement **(B)** and markedly elevated DWI signal **(C)**, which is characteristic of cholesteatoma.

which is similar to, although distinct from, cholesteatoma. Keratosis obturans results in conductive hearing loss from obstruction of the EAC by a keratin plug. It more commonly affects young people presenting with pain and can result in secondary otitis externa.

- Malignant otitis externa (Figure 2-1) is a *Pseudomonas aeruginosa* infection of the external ear canal seen in diabetic elderly patients. It has a high propensity to spread through the skull base and is best evaluated with MRI.
- Cholesteatoma (Figure 2-2) is a nonneoplastic proliferation of squamous epithelium that most frequently occurs in the middle ear in the setting of chronic otitis media. These lesions show marked restricted diffusion, allowing a specific diagnosis on MRI. They are generally low signal intensity on T1 and bright on T2, with no enhancement on postcontrast sequences.
- The most common imaging abnormality seen in the petrous apex region is trapped fluid (effusion) in pneumatized cells, which is asymptomatic in most cases.

Effusion in the petrous apex does not expand the bone, and the bony trabeculae or septae between air cells are maintained. No enhancement is present on postcontrast images. About one-third of the population has aeration of the petrous apex, the presence and degree of which are frequently asymmetric between the two sides.

- Cholesterol granuloma (Figure 2-3) is the most common expansile lesion of the petrous apex. These are bright on both T1 and T2 MRI. There may be faint peripheral enhancement without central enhancement. There is no restricted diffusion, unlike cholesteatoma.
- An expansile lesion in the petrous apex that shows fluid signal on MRI and no enhancement with contrast is most compatible with a meningocele (Figure 2-4). High-resolution MRI may show CSF tracking from the Meckel cave region.
- Endolymphatic sac tumor is a rare aggressive tumor centered in the vestibular aqueduct region. It usually presents as a large and destructive mass in the posterior fossa with heterogeneous signal on MRI secondary to

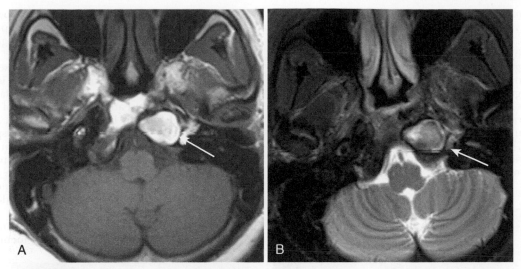

FIGURE 2-3 Cholesterol granuloma. Axial T1-weighted (T1W) magnetic resonance image (MRI) **(A)** and T2-weighted MRI **(B)** show a very bright mass on T1W image in the left petrous apex (arrows), which is expanded compatible with a cholesterol granuloma. The T2 signal of cholesterol granuloma is heterogeneously hyperintense.

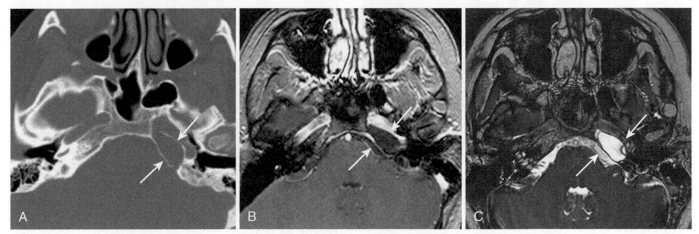

FIGURE 2-4 Petrous apex meningocele. Axial computed tomography **(A),** postcontrast T1-weighted magnetic resonance image (MRI) **(B),** and high-resolution T2-weighted MRI **(C)** show a slightly expansile lesion (arrows) in the left petrous apex that shows no enhancement and fluid signal in all MRI pulse sequences compatible with a meningocele. Coronal images (not shown) revealed a connection between the petrous apex and Meckel cave.

blood by-products. It can be seen in the setting of von Hippel-Lindau syndrome.

- EAC atresia may be sporadic or part of a syndrome such as Crouzon, Treacher Collins, Goldenhar, and Pierre Robin syndromes. In cases of EAC atresia, the auricle is always dysplastic and there are frequently anomalies of the middle ear ossicles, facial nerve canal, and mastoid, although the cochlea and vestibule, including the stapes foot plate, are usually spared because these structures have distinct embryologic origins.
- Otosclerosis/spongiosis is a metabolic bone disease resulting in abnormal bony proliferation most commonly occurring at the fissula ante fenestram, which is anterior to the oval window. Otosclerosis presents with conductive hearing loss. When it occurs around the cochlea and vestibule it is referred to as retrofenestral otosclerosis, which is associated with sensorineural hearing loss. The treatment is stapedotomy with placement of a stapes piston prosthesis. The most common cause for recurrent conductive hearing loss after treatment is displacement of the prosthesis (Figure 2-5).
- Semicircular canal dehiscence may result in Tullio syndrome characterized by vertigo, nystagmus, and

oscillopsia. The superior canal is most frequently dehiscent. Incidental detection of dehiscence of the superior canal is common on CT examinations obtained for other reasons.
- It is common to see enhancement of the 7th nerve on MRI between the labyrinthine and mastoid segments because of a perineural arteriovenous plexus. Enhancement should not be seen proximal to the labyrinthine or distal to the mastoid segments. An enhancing mass seen along the facial nerve is most commonly a schwannoma. Facial nerve hemangiomas (Figure 2-6) occur in the geniculate ganglion and have a characteristic honeycomb appearance on CT.
- Common masses occurring in the middle ear include cholesteatomas, paragangliomas, cholesterol granulomas, hemangiomas, and schwannomas. Less common masses include carcinomas and adenomas. Pars flaccida cholesteatomas occur in the Prussak space, which is in the epitympanum lateral to the ossicles and are tan masses on otoscopy. Paragangliomas of the middle ear often occur at the medial wall and appear as red masses behind the tympanic membrane. Schwannomas may occur on the facial nerve, Jacobson nerve, or the chorda tympani.

- Aberrant carotid artery is a vascular anomaly that may present as a red pulsatile mass mimicking glomus tympanicum. The aberrant course of the carotid is depicted in high-resolution CT of the temporal bone. A dehiscent jugular bulb may also cause a purple hue on otoscopy. Although an increased rate of occurrence of dehiscent jugular canal is reported in the setting of tinnitus, a causal relationship has not been established.
- Most temporal bone fractures involve multiple oblique planes and are difficult to describe as transverse or longitudinal. Whether a fracture involves the otic capsule is an important prognostic feature. The majority of temporal bone fractures spare the otic capsule.

- Gradenigo syndrome is characterized by abducens nerve palsy, trigeminal neuralgia, and petrous capacities, which is caused by extension of mastoiditis through pneumatized petrous bone.
- In the MRI/CT evaluation of a child with sensorineural hearing loss, enlarged vestibular aqueduct is the most common imaging finding. If cochlear implant is a consideration for treatment, the absence of a cochlea such as in Michel anomaly is a contraindication. Absence of the cochlear nerve on MRI portends a poor response to cochlear implantation, although it is not an absolute contraindication. Absence of the cochlear nerve canal (aperture) at the base of the cochlea is the CT finding that best predicts absence of the cochlear nerve. A narrow IAC is also associated with cochlear nerve deficiency (Figure 2-7).
- Complications of acute otomastoiditis include Gradenigo syndrome, labyrinthitis, facial neuritis, meningitis, cerebral

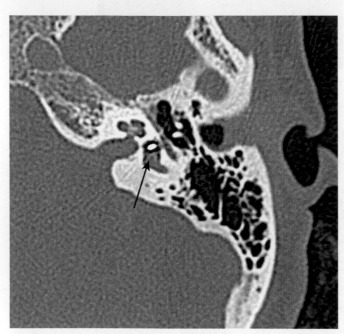

FIGURE 2-5 Stapes prosthesis migration. Axial computed tomographic scan of the left temporal bone shows the tip of the prosthesis inserting into the vestibule *(arrow)* in this patient with otosclerosis status-post stapedotomy and new symptoms. Prosthesis extension more than 2 mm from the oval window is considered abnormal.

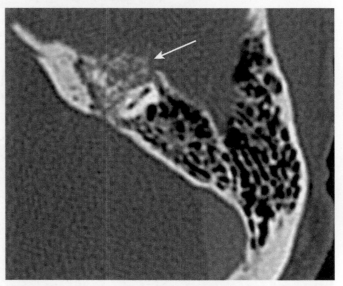

FIGURE 2-6 Facial nerve hemangioma. Axial computed tomographic image of a patient with facial nerve paralysis shows a mass in the geniculate ganglion region *(arrow)* with characteristic "honeycomb" appearance compatible with hemangioma.

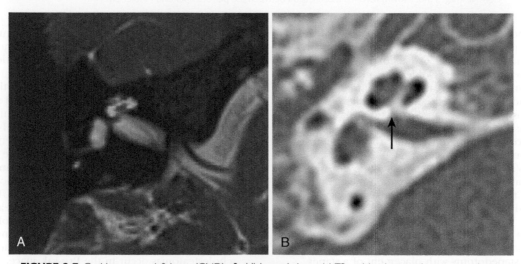

FIGURE 2-7 Cochlear nerve deficiency (CND). **A,** High-resolution axial T2-weighted magnetic resonance image shows absence of the cochlear nerve within the right internal auditory canal (IAC) despite a normal appearing cochlea and cochlear nerve canal at the base of the cochlea. **B,** Axial computed tomographic (CT) image of a different patient with congenital sensorineural hearing loss shows obliteration of the cochlear nerve canal *(arrow)* compatible with CND. Note that a normal cochlear nerve canal on CT does not necessarily mean that the cochlear nerve is intact, as illustrated in image **(A).** Note that the IAC is narrow, which is another CT sign that is predictive of CND.

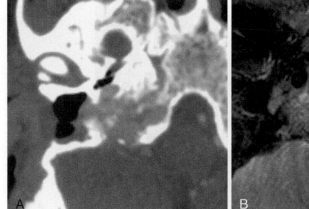
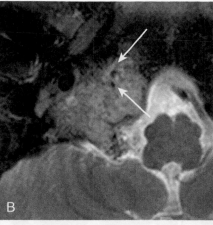
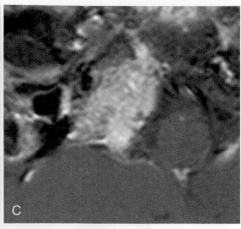

FIGURE 2-8 Glomus jugulare (paraganglioma). Axial computed tomographic image **(A)** shows a destructive mass centered in the right jugular foramen. On axial T2-weighted magnetic resonance imaging **(B)**, the mass is hyperintense but shows multiple small hypointense foci *(arrows)* compatible with intratumoral blood vessel, which is characteristic of glomus tumor. The mass shows marked enhancement on postcontrast T1-weighted image **(C).**

abscess, subdural empyema, and venous sinus thrombosis. Additionally when infection is seen in fully pneumatized mastoid cells, a Bezold abscess, which is a deep neck abscess extending along the sternocleidomastoid muscle, may occur.

- Vestibular schwannomas are common masses arising from the IAC or the labyrinth. Contrast-enhanced MRI is considered the definitive study in diagnosis, although recently developed high-resolution T2-weighted images can also effectively diagnose even small schwannomas without the need for contrast. Enhancement in the labyrinth in the postoperative MRI evaluation of IAC schwannomas is a common finding that may be attributable to ischemic damage to the membranous labyrinth rather than recurrent tumor.

ANTERIOR/CENTRAL/POSTERIOR SKULL BASE

- The jugular foramina are paired openings at the skull base between the occipital bone and the petrous temporal bone through which the cranial nerves IX, X, and XI transmit as well as the jugular bulb and the inferior petrosal sinus. The hypoglossal canal, which transmits the hypoglossal nerve, is slightly medial and inferior to the jugular canal.
- Masses encountered at the jugular foramen include most commonly paraganglioma (glomus jugulare) (Figure 2-8), schwannoma, and meningioma followed by chondrosarcoma and metastasis. Dural venous sinus thrombosis extending through the jugular bulb is not infrequently encountered at this location. Hereditary forms of paragangliomas may be multicentric in up to 30% of the cases.
- Hoarseness is a commonly encountered symptom and has multiple causes aside from diseases of the vocal folds. There are multiple locations of potential disease secondary to the course of the vagus nerves and the recurrent laryngeal nerves. Common locations of diseases causing vocal cord paralysis include the jugular foramen, high carotid space, mediastinum, and thyroid.
- The lateral lamella is the thinnest bone of the anterior skull base and most prone to CSF leak (Figure 2-9). Other common locations for CSF leak include the fovea ethmoidalis, cribriform plate, sphenoid sinus, and tegmen tympani.

PARANASAL SINUSES

- The primary imaging modality for the evaluation of chronic rhinosinusitis is CT. Noncontrast technique is most often adequate for accurate characterization of disease and anatomy. When there is concern for tumor or disease extension beyond the sinuses, MRI with high-resolution precontrast and postcontrast sequences may be indicated. For cases of occult postoperative CSF leak, CT cisternography (see Figure 2-9) is both sensitive and specific for identifying the location of CSF leak. Other adjunct techniques include nuclear cisternography, MRI, and high-resolution noncontrast CT.
- MRI can help discern a mass within the sinus from inflammatory disease. When the lesion is separated from the wall by potentially thickened, but otherwise normal mucosa, neoplasm is much less likely. The negative predictive value of this finding is increased if there is no enhancement in the lesion at question. If there is disruption of the mucosa on MRI and there are changes to the bony wall of the sinus, extension of disease beyond the wall of the sinus, or mass-like enhancement, a more aggressive process, possibly neoplastic, is likely.
- Drainage patterns of the paranasal sinuses: Each of the sinuses ultimately drains into the nasopharynx:
  - Frontal sinus: into the frontal recess→ethmoid infundibulum/middle meatus complex→posterior nasal cavity
  - Maxillary sinus: maxillary ostium→ethmoidal infundibulum→middle meatus→posterior nasal cavity
  - Anterior ethmoid sinuses: variable ostia: commonly through the middle meatus
  - Posterior ethmoid and sphenoid sinus→through their respective ostia→sphenoethmoidal recess→superior meatus
- The nasolacrimal duct drains from the medial orbit to the inferior meatus through the Hasner valve.
- Mucosal thickening, fluid levels, and foamy secretions are the imaging findings that suggest acute sinusitis, although the diagnosis of sinusitis should be made on the clinical grounds. Imaging is discouraged for noncomplicated acute sinusitis.
- Osteitis, thickening of the bony sinus walls, and circumferential thickening of the mucosa are the imaging findings of chronic sinusitis that may be seen in addition to the characteristics of acute sinusitis.

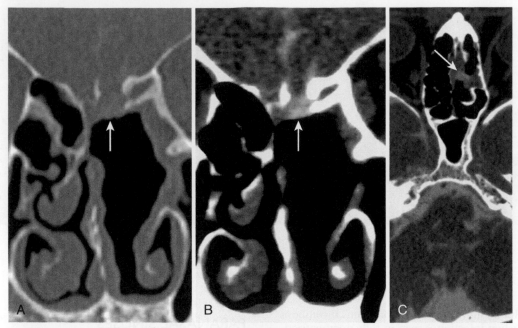

FIGURE 2-9 Computed tomographic cisternogram for cerebrospinal fluid (CSF) leak. Coronal bone **(A)**, soft tissue **(B)**, and axial soft tissue **(C)** images show the intrathecally administered contrast material accumulating in a sac inferior to the cribriform plate *(arrows)*, confirming the location of CSF leak in this patient with prior surgery.

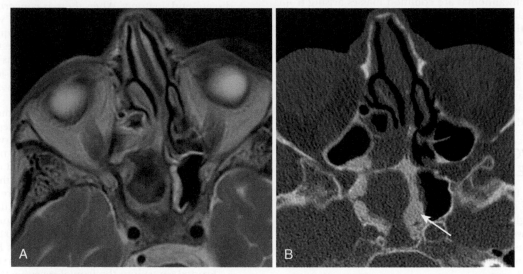

FIGURE 2-10 Chronic sinusitis. Axial T2-weighted magnetic resonance image **(A)** and computed tomography **(B)** show opacification of the right sphenoid sinus with markedly hypointense material compatible with thick mucin with or without fungal by-products. Marked thickening (osteitis) *(arrow)* of the sinus wall indicates a chronic process.

- Complicated acute sinusitis imaging findings include intracranial and intraorbital extension of disease as well as inflammatory stranding in the retroantral and premaxillary fat.
- Eosinophilic mucin of fungal sinusitis, inspissated secretions, and blood may all appear as high-density opacity on CT. Fungal products and the high protein secretions within the sinuses are characteristically low signal intensity on T2-weighted MRI (Figure 2-10).
- Sinonasal polyposis is a pattern of chronic sinusitis with extensive polyps obliterating the sinuses and the nasal cavity. Bone remodeling or erosion may occur, and fungal infection is common (Figure 2-11).
- There are three paired "tight spots" where obstruction of sinus outflow most commonly occurs. When there is anterior ethmoid and or maxillary sinusitis, the common areas affected by mucosal thickening and narrowing are the primary maxillary sinus ostia, ethmoid infundibulum, and the middle meatus. In cases of frontal sinusitis, the frontal recess and middle meatus are most commonly affected. For posterior ethmoid and sphenoid sinusitis, the obstruction to outflow is commonly at the sphenoethmoidal recess.
- A concha bullosa, pneumatization of a turbinate, and most frequently the middle turbinate may result in narrowing of the ipsilateral nasal cavity, specifically the middle meatus. When large, these are usually found with nasal septum deviation and spurring. Spurs/focal deviations of the nasal septum occur in an anterior-inferior to posterior-superior distribution at the junction of the vomer with the perpendicular plate of the ethmoid posteriorly and the cartilaginous septum anteriorly.

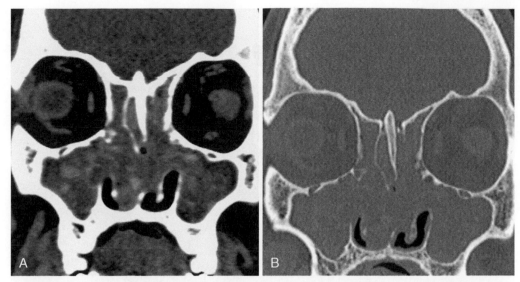

FIGURE 2-11 Sinonasal polyposis. Coronal computed tomography in soft tissue **(A)** and bone **(B)** algorithms show extensive heterogeneous opacification of the sinuses and nasal cavity. The high density components may be due to inspissated mucus and/or coexisting fungal components.

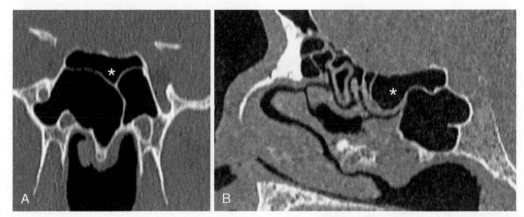

FIGURE 2-12 Sphenoethmoidal (Onodi) cell. Coronal **(A)** and sagittal **(B)** computed tomographic images show a transversely oriented septum intersecting the vertical sphenoid intersinus septum indicating an Onodi cell (asterisks) extending superior and posterior to the sphenoid sinus. The sphenoid intersinus septa are always vertically oriented.

- For surgical and radiologic terminology, the anterior ostiomeatal unit is comprised of the maxillary sinus ostium, the ethmoidal infundibulum, the uncinate process, the hiatus semilunaris, and the middle meatus. The ethmoid bulla forms the posterior/superior wall of the ethmoidal infundibulum.
- Certain anatomic features of the sphenoid sinus are important to identify prior to surgical intervention. These include:
  - Sphenoethmoidal (Onodi) cells (Figure 2-12): If unrecognized, the potential for undertreatment is increased, especially if not utilizing intraoperative CT navigation. Also, if not recognized, there is increased risk of anterior skull base penetration. To identify the presence of sphenoethmoidal (Onodi) cells, the coronal images of the CT data set should be used. If there is a transverse bony septum within the sphenoid, the airspaces above this septum represent the ethmoid air cells that have pneumatized into the sphenoid.
  - Pneumatization of the anterior clinoid processes (Figure 2-13): In the presence of allergic fungal rhinosinusitis, if adequate debridement is not performed and disease remains, recurrence is more

likely. Also, when present, the optic canal often traverses the sphenoid sinus, increasing the risk of optic nerve injury. Pneumatization of the anterior clinoid processes may or may not occur when sphenoethmoidal cells are present.
  - Extensive lateral pneumatization, potentially into the pterygoid processes: It is difficult to access laterally at the time of functional endoscopic sinus surgery (FESS), and the potential for pterygoid (vidian) canal injury increases. The pterygoid nerve can be uncovered and traverse the sinus cavity without bony protection. It can also be found on a bony septum extending from the wall of the sinus.
  - The posterior extent of pneumatization relative to the sella turcica: Especially in cases of extensive pneumatization, the posterior wall of the sinus may be thin.
  - The internal carotid artery prominence and potential dehiscence of the sinus wall at the level of the internal carotid artery: The risk of injury to the artery with disastrous results is increased.
  - The optic nerve canal and potential dehiscence of the canal wall (see Figure 2-13): Optic nerve injury,

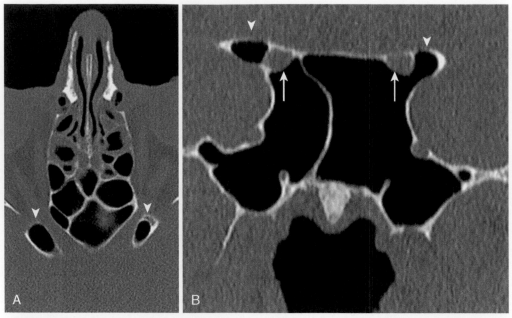

FIGURE 2-13 Pneumatized anterior clinoid processes. Axial **(A)** and coronal **(B)** computed tomographic images of the sphenoid sinus show pneumatized anterior clinoid processes *(arrowheads)* with bilateral optic nerves protruding into the sinus cavity with apparent dehiscence of the walls of the optic canals *(arrows)*.

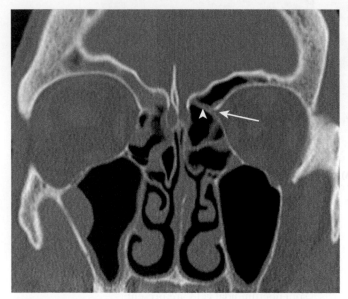

FIGURE 2-14 Coronal computed tomographic (CT) image shows the anterior ethmoid artery sulcus *(arrow)*, which is a small notch usually located in the lamina papyracea where the muscle bellies of the medial rectus and superior oblique are thickest. In this case, the artery traverses an ethmoid air cell in a mesentery *(arrowhead)* instead of being safely embedded in the skull base. This configuration increases the risk for transection of the artery during surgery and should be noted in CT reports and at surgery.

although a small risk, increases when there is pneumatization of the anterior clinoid process, sphenoethmoidal cells, bony dehiscence, and extensive disease in the sphenoid, limiting intraoperative visualization.
- The anterior ethmoidal artery sulcus should be identified on preoperative CT scan (Figure 2-14). The anterior ethmoidal artery exits the orbit through a small notch in the lamina papyracea, usually found on the coronal plane where the muscle bellies of the medial rectus and medial oblique are thickest. It then travels embedded in the skull base before proceeding intracranially, although in some cases the artery may traverse the ethmoidal airspace within a bony mesentery or may be uncovered, creating a surgical hazard. If the artery is inadvertently transected, the vessel may retract into the orbit and form a potentially blinding hematoma if not addressed.
- Silent sinus syndrome is a distinct clinical entity resulting from atelectasis of the ethmoidal infundibulum. This is the hallmark finding accompanied with decreased volume of the maxillary sinus, which is opacified; centrifugal bowing of the sinus walls; enophthalmos from downward bowing of the orbital floor; and enlargement of the ipsilateral nasal cavity.
- A mucocele forms when a sinus ostia is obstructed. These are characterized by complete opacification of the sinus involved, expansion and thinning of the sinus walls, and often inspissation of the sinus secretions.
- Mucus retention cysts form when there is obstruction of an epithelial secretory gland that progressively accumulates secretions, resulting in a round/oval focal mucosal thickening in the sinus. Depending on the protein content, chronicity, and associated sinusitis, the density on CT and signal intensity on MRI can be variable. These can be fleeting findings on CT and can regress/resolve spontaneously.
- Maxillary sinusitis can occur in the setting of dental disease. Dental etiologies of sinusitis can be identified on CT and should be addressed as the potentially causative or comorbid disease.

FACE (INCLUDING FACIAL TRAUMA)

- There are different fracture complexes that may occur in isolated patterns, although they often occur in more complex ways with combined features even on the same side of the face. The fractures are named depending on the structures involved. High-resolution noncontrast CT of the facial bones is the modality of choice to image facial

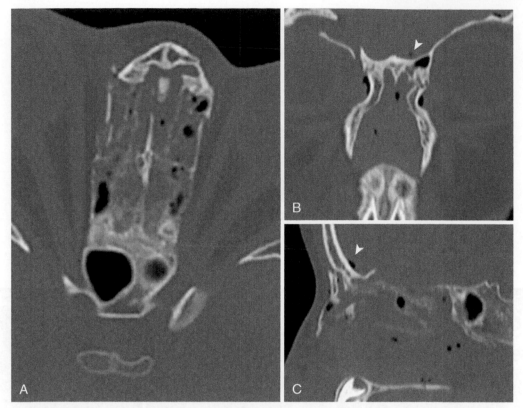

FIGURE 2-15 Nasoorbitoethmoid complex fracture. Axial **(A),** coronal **(B),** and sagittal **(C)** computed tomographic images show moderately comminuted multiple fractures involving the nasal bones, nasal septum, lamina papyracea, cribriform plate, and the right orbital roof. The status of the medial canthal ligament is critical in classification and treatment planning of nasoorbitoethmoid complex fractures. Note pneumocephalus *(arrowheads).* Intracranial injury and cerebrospinal fluid leaks are common in this setting.

fractures. Some commonly described facial fracture patterns are outlined as follows.

- Le Fort classification: These invariably involve fractures of the pterygoid processes.
  - I: Transmaxillary fracture: This separates the hard palate from the remainder of the face.
  - II: Pyramidal fracture: There are fractures through the zygomatico-maxillary suture area, inferior and medial orbits, and frontal nasal suture region isolating the maxilla, portions of the ethmoid, and the nasal bones from the remainder of the face.
  - III: Craniofacial dissociation: There are fractures through the zygomatic arch, lateral and medial orbits, nasal frontal region, and the sphenoid.
- Zygomaticomaxillary complex: There is dissociation of the zygoma from the remainder of the face and head. Fractures and/or sutural diastasis at or near the zygomaticofrontal suture, zygomaticomaxillary suture, zygomaticotemporal suture, and the zygomaticosphenoid suture are present.
- Naso-orbital-ethmoidal (Figure 2-15): This includes comminuted fractures of the nasal bones, septum, ethmoid sinuses, and medial orbital walls. Injury to the medial canthus ligament or its bony attachment is invariable. CSF leak and exophthalmos frequently occur.
- Orbital blowout: This occurs when the intraorbital pressure is increased acutely, resulting in lamina papyracea and/or orbital floor fractures with displacement centripetally away from the orbit.
- Mandible fractures: These occur anywhere along the mandible, and since it is a ring-like structure associated with the temporomandibular joints, there are often two discrete fractures and/or a dislocation. Transient dislocation of the temporomandibular joint accounts for cases where there is only one fracture identifiable at CT.
- Nasal bone fractures: Imaging is deferred from the acute setting for isolated asymptomatic nasal bone fractures and indicated when contemplating surgical repair/revision or if there are chronic symptoms attributable to the facial injury. Physical examination is highly reliable for identifying nasal bone fractures. Radiographs have little role in the identification of nasal bone fractures. Children are more prone to nasal septal hematomas than adults.
- CSF leaks in the setting of facial trauma are often at the level of the cribriform plate. The lateral lamella of the cribriform plate is the thinnest bone of the anterior skull base. CSF leaks have traditionally been evaluated with a multimodality approach utilizing CT, MRI, and nuclear medicine scanning. CT cisternography is both highly sensitive and specific for identifying the location of a CSF leak. This would be the imaging modality of choice following a positive β-2 transferrin test.
- Parotid neoplasms (Figure 2-16) are more often benign than malignant when compared with minor salivary gland tumors or those arising in the submandibular gland. Common histologies include benign mixed tumors (pleomorphic adenomas), which are usually T2 hyperintense; malignancies such as mucoepidermoid carcinoma or adenoid cystic carcinoma usually show areas of T2 hypointensity on MRI. In fact, identifying

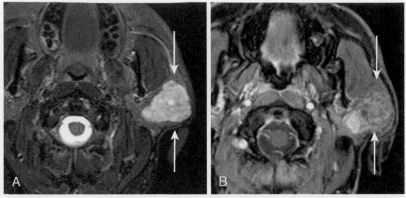

FIGURE 2-16 Pleomorphic adenoma. Axial T2-weighted **(A)** and postcontrast T1-weighted **(B)** magnetic resonance images of the left parotid gland show a hyperintense T2, heterogeneously enhancing mass in the superficial parotid gland with lobulated and well-defined margins *(arrows)*. If there were areas of low T2 signal within the mass, malignancy would have to be suspected.

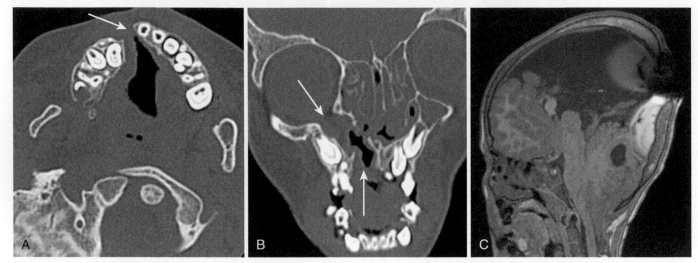

FIGURE 2-17 Complex craniofacial malformation. Axial **(A)** and coronal **(B)** computed tomographic images of the face through the maxilla show a cleft extending from the hard palate to the inferomedial right orbit *(arrows)*. A smaller palatal cleft (not shown) on the left is also present in this patient. Sagittal T1-weighted **(C)** image shows dysgenesis of the corpus callosum and Chiari 1 malformation of the posterior fossa. Additional anomalies (not shown) include rhombencephalosynapsis and Klippel-Feil anomaly of the cervical spine. Midline facial anomalies are often associated with midline intracranial anomalies; depending on the severity of the facial malformation, further imaging may be indicated.

T2 hypointensity in a salivary gland mass suggests malignancy.

- Two common diseases resulting in cystic changes in the parotid gland are HIV/AIDS and Sjögren disease.
- Calcifications within the salivary glands can be seen with or without ductal dilation and are frequently seen in chronic sialoadenitis.
- Schwannomas are usually hyperintense on T2-weighted MRI and enhance avidly with the exception of cystic areas, which are common. When small, these can be identified by a fusiform elongate morphology with tapered/pointed ends.
- HPV-related head and neck cancers are associated with cystic lymph nodes more commonly than non-HPV-related head and neck cancer.
- Intracranial malformations/anomalies occur at higher frequency with midline facial malformations. MRI and/or CT is recommended to evaluate the intracranial anatomy, especially if the child is not meeting developmental milestones. Facial clefts (Figure 2-17) are just one example of midface malformations.

PEDIATRIC NECK/CONGENITAL

- Regarding congenital neck masses, the most common is a thyroglossal duct cyst. These occur most commonly within 2 cm of midline and immediately below the hyoid, next to the thyroid cartilage.
- The second branchial cleft cyst is the most common of the branchial cleft anomalies, usually presenting when infected as a cystic mass anterior to the sternocleidomastoid muscle and posterior to the submandibular gland.
- Congenital vascular malformations include venous (Figure 2-18), lymphatic (Figure 2-19), and mixed malformations. These have variable enhancement characteristics and are often transpatial. Venous malformations often contain phleboliths identified as round calcifications within the lesion on CT and on MRI as low signal intensity foci on both T1 and T2 within the lesion, which otherwise enhances avidly and is hyperintense on T2.
- Dermoids of the orbit most often occur in the superolateral quadrant.

- A cystic lesion showing a blue/purple hue on physical examination in the medial canthal region in a young child usually represents a dacryocystocele.
- Lymphoma and leukemia are the most common causes of chronic lymphadenopathy in a child.

LYMPH NODES

- Normal lymph nodes tend to have low signal on T1-weighted and high signal on T2-weighted images.
- Absence of the normal fatty hilum, thickening of the lymph node cortex, and perinodal stranding with ill-defined cortical margins are suspicious findings when evaluating lymph nodes. A normal lymph node should have an intact, fat-containing hilum, a thin cortex, a reniform shape, and well-defined margins.
- Lymph node metastasis patterns are predictable based on the primary tumor location.
  - Nasopharynx: Ipsilateral and contralateral levels II-IV and retropharyngeal
  - Floor of mouth and oral tongue: Ipsilateral levels I and II

- Base of tongue and tonsil and supraglottic larynx: Ipsilateral levels II and III, and contralateral level II
- Soft palate: Ipsilateral and contralateral level II, ipsilateral level III
- Glottis: Ipsilateral levels II and III
- Retropharyngeal lymph nodes are not included in the levels of the neck. Normal retropharyngeal lymph nodes should be less than 6 mm in adults. Clusters of retropharyngeal lymph nodes are suspicious.
- Hodgkin lymphoma most commonly occurs as bulky, solid lymphadenopathy unilaterally or bilaterally. Cystic nodes are uncommon with Hodgkin lymphoma, although they occur in squamous cell carcinoma, nasopharyngeal carcinoma, thyroid carcinoma, and tuberculosis, as well as other granulomatous diseases.
- Lymph node calcifications occur in metastatic mucinous carcinomas, treated lymphoma, granulomatous diseases, and papillary thyroid carcinoma.
- Paragangliomas of the head and neck are named for their location of occurrence. Carotid body paragangliomas occur at the bifurcation of the common carotid artery splaying the internal carotid and external carotid artery. Glomus vagale paragangliomas occur posterior to the carotid sheath and splay the internal carotid artery from the internal jugular vein. Glomus jugulare paragangliomas occur at and usually extend inferiorly from the skull base at the pars nervosa of the jugular foramen. Glomus tympanicum paragangliomas occur in the middle ear along the tympanic segment of the facial nerve.
- Laryngeal carcinoma arising from the glottis usually presents with hoarseness rather than lymphadenopathy.
- Sinus histiocytosis (Rosai-Dorfman) (Figure 2-20) is a rare benign idiopathic proliferative disease occurring in young adults and presenting as massive painless cervical lymphadenopathy.

THYROID AND PARATHYROID

- Neck ultrasound is the first-line imaging modality for assessing recurrence of well-differentiated thyroid carcinoma suspected based on elevated thyroglobulin.
- Papillary carcinoma of the thyroid is the most frequent histology of thyroid cancer and often contains calcifications within the primary tumor as well as its lymph node metastases.
- Imaging alone has poor sensitivity and specificity for determining malignancy of thyroid nodules; thus, fine-needle aspiration is often necessary.

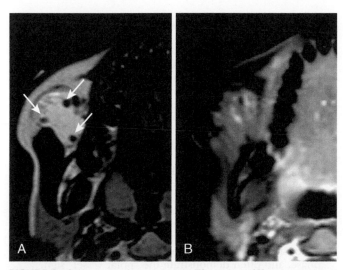

FIGURE 2-18 Venous malformation. Axial T2-weighted **(A)** and postcontrast T1-weighted **(B)** magnetic resonance images show a T2 hyperintense and heterogeneously enhancing mass in the right buccal space with multiple hypointense round structures within the mass (arrows) compatible with phleboliths, which are hallmarks of venous malformations.

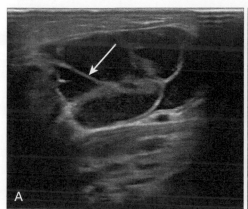
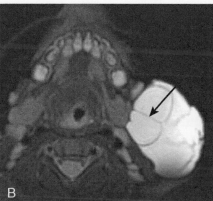
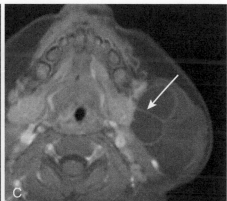

FIGURE 2-19 Lymphatic malformation. Transverse ultrasound **(A)**, T2-weighted magnetic resonance imaging (MRI) **(B)**, and postcontrast T1-weighted MRI **(C)** show a multiloculated cystic mass with thin septa (arrows) and no significant enhancement in the left neck, compatible with lymphatic malformation in this young child.

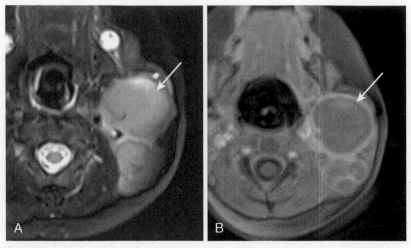

FIGURE 2-20 Rosai-Dorfman disease. Axial T2-weighted **(A)** and postcontrast T1-weighted **(B)** magnetic resonance images show an enlarged lymph node in the left neck *(arrows)* with a cluster of nodes posteriorly that show increased T2 signal and mild peripheral enhancement. Biopsy revealed "sinus histiocytosis with massive lymphadenopathy," also known as Rosai-Dorfman disease.

- Sonographic features associated with benign thyroid nodules include:
  - Purely cystic or a cystic component containing colloid (hyperechoic foci with a "ring-down" sign)
  - Spongiform or honeycomb appearance (microcystic spaces with thin walls, comprising >50% of the nodule)
  - Eggshell-type calcification around the periphery
  - Isoechoic or (mildly) hyperechoic in relation to the surrounding normal thyroid tissue and typically with a surrounding hypoechoic halo
  - Comet tail artifact
  - Peripheral vascularity on color flow or power Doppler
- Sonographic features associated with malignant thyroid nodules (papillary and medullary) include:
  - Solid hypoechoic in relation to the surrounding normal thyroid tissue, which may contain hyperechoic foci (i.e., microcalcifications)
  - Irregular or spiculated margins

- Intranodular vascularity and absence of an associated halo
  - A "taller than wide" shape referring to anterior/posterior dimension greater than those dimensions parallel to the transducer
  - Eggshell-type calcification around the periphery with a broken calcified rim where there is extension beyond the calcified rim of a hypoechoic mass/nodule
- Growth of a thyroid nodule greater than 20% in two dimensions in less than 18 months is concerning for malignancy.
- Imaging evaluation of parathyroid adenomas most often includes ultrasound followed by technetium-99m sestamibi scintigraphy. Multiphase CT is gaining popularity as a guide to minimally invasive surgery. Parathyroid adenomas demonstrate delayed washout of the radiopharmaceutical, are of lower CT density than the thyroid gland prior to contrast administration, enhance avidly in the arterial phase, and often demonstrate the "polar vessel" sign.

ANSWERS

TRUE OR FALSE QUESTIONS

1. T	14. F	27. T	40. F
2. T	15. T	28. T	41. T
3. T	16. F	29. F	42. T
4. F	17. F	30. T	43. F
5. T	18. T	31. T	44. F
6. F	19. F	32. F	45. F
7. F	20. T	33. T	46. T
8. T	21. F	34. T	47. T
9. F	22. T	35. F	48. F
10. T	23. T	36. T	49. F
11. T	24. F	37. T	50. T
12. F	25. T	38. F	
13. F	26. F	39. F	

SINGLE BEST ANSWER QUESTIONS

51. c	64. c	77. d	90. d
52. d	65. c	78. b	91. d
53. c	66. d	79. c	92. d
54. d	67. a	80. a	93. b
55. a	68. d	81. d	94. d
56. d	69. c	82. e	95. d
57. e	70. c	83. d	96. e
58. c	71. d	84. c	97. a
59. a	72. d	85. c	98. b
60. c	73. a	86. c	99. d
61. c	74. e	87. d	100. e
62. a	75. c	88. a	
63. a	76. d	89. d	

SUGGESTED READINGS

1. Aksoy EA, Ozden SU, Karaarslan E, et al. Reliability of high-pitch ultra-low-dose paranasal sinus computed tomography for evaluating paranasal sinus anatomy and sinus disease. *J Craniofac Surg.* 2014;25(5):1801-1804.

2. Al-Noury K, Lotfy A. Computed tomography and magnetic resonance imaging findings before and after treatment of patients with malignant external otitis. *Eur Arch Otorhinolaryngol.* 2011;268(12):1727-1734.

3. Calzada AP, Go JL, Tschirhart DL, et al. Cerebellopontine angle and intracanalicular masses mimicking vestibular schwannomas. *Otol Neurotol.* 2015;36(3):491-497.

4. Fitzek C, Mewes T, Fitzek S, et al. Diffusion-weighted MRI of cholesteatomas of the petrous bone. *J Magn Reson Imaging.* 2002;15(6):636-641.

5. Ho FC, Tham IW, Earnest A, et al. Patterns of regional lymph node metastasis of nasopharyngeal carcinoma: a meta-analysis of clinical evidence. *BMC Cancer.* 2012;12:98. doi:10.1186/1471-2407-12-98.

6. Katsura M, Mori H, Kunimatsu A, et al. Radiological features of IgG4-related disease in the head, neck, and brain. *Neuroradiology.* 2012;54(8):873-882.

7. La Fata V, McLean N, Wise SK, et al. CSF leaks: correlation of high-resolution CT and multiplanar reformations with intraoperative endoscopic findings. *AJNR Am J Neuroradiol.* 2008;29(3):536-541.

8. Minor LB, Solomon D, Zinreich JS, et al. Sound- and/or pressure-induced vertigo due to bone dehiscence of the superior semicircular canal. *Arch Otolaryngol Head Neck Surg.* 1998;124(3):249-258.

9. Prabhu RS, Magliocca KR, Hanasoge S, et al. Accuracy of computed tomography for predicting pathologic nodal extracapsular extension in patients with head-and-neck cancer undergoing initial surgical resection. *Int J Radiat Oncol Biol Phys.* 2014;88(1):122-129.

10. Razek AA, Huang BY. Lesions of the petrous apex: classification and findings at CT and MR imaging. *Radiographics.* 2012;32(1):151-173.

3 | History, Physical Examination, and the Preoperative Evaluation

Ericka King

TRUE OR FALSE QUESTIONS

T/F 1. The outer two-thirds of the external auditory canal is cartilaginous.

T/F 2. A positive Rinne test indicates the normal state in which air conduction is louder than bone conduction.

T/F 3. A white mass behind the anterosuperior quadrant of an intact tympanic membrane in a child is concerning for acquired cholesteatoma.

T/F 4. A negative Rinne test with a 512 Hertz (Hz) tuning fork suggests that a conductive hearing loss (HL) of at least 20 dB is present.

T/F 5. Vessels on the anterior nasal septum that cause the majority of nosebleeds are found in Woodruff's plexus.

T/F 6. Nasopharyngeal carcinoma most commonly presents in the fossa of Rosenmüller.

T/F 7. Aphthous ulcers most commonly present on mucosa that is tightly adherent to bone, particularly the hard palate and retromolar trigone.

T/F 8. In the Brodsky scale, tonsils that occupy 51% to 75% of the oropharyngeal width are considered 3+ in size.

T/F 9. Tonsillar asymmetry can be a sign of malignancy, most often Hodgkin lymphoma.

T/F 10. The subglottis begins 5 to 10 mm below the free edge of the true vocal fold and extends to the inferior margin of the cricoid cartilage.

T/F 11. When performing indirect laryngoscopy, it is important that the patient sits upright, leaning slightly forward from the waist and with the neck slightly extended.

T/F 12. Prompt imaging with computed tomography (CT) or magnetic resonance imaging (MRI) is warranted when a purplish, submucosal bulge is present in the postcricoid area in an otherwise asymptomatic patient.

T/F 13. Levels IIA and IIB are separated by the greater auricular nerve.

T/F 14. Lymph nodes are considered enlarged in adults when they are >1.5 cm in the greatest dimension.

T/F 15. A patient with a right-sided hypoglossal nerve lesion will have deviation of the tongue to the ipsilateral side on protrusion.

T/F 16. Approximately 50% of all perioperative deaths in the elderly are due to cardiovascular events.

T/F 17. All patients older than 35 should undergo routine electrocardiography prior to any surgical procedure.

T/F 18. Informed consent is a critical part of the preoperative evaluation and should be documented in the medical record.

T/F 19. The incidence of significant adverse reaction to penicillins is about 1%.

T/F 20. A patient who gets a rash with penicillin should never receive a cephalosporin, as there is a 10% to 15% chance of cross-reactivity.

T/F 21. At least 28% of children with spina bifida have a demonstrable reaction to latex proteins.

T/F 22. Patients with an egg allergy may be hypersensitive to propofol.

T/F 23. One dose of ampicillin given at the time of incision is considered adequate bacterial endocarditis prophylaxis by the American Heart Association.

T/F 24. Smokers have a threefold increased risk of pulmonary complications compared with nonsmokers.

T/F 25. There is an increased risk for postoperative pneumonia in cachectic patients.

T/F 26. Clubbing and cyanosis are specific indicators for pulmonary disease on physical examination.

T/F 27. Patients with $PaCO_2$ greater than 50 mmHg are at increased risk for postoperative pulmonary compromise.

T/F 28. A ratio of forced expiratory volume in 1 second (FEV1) to forced vital capacity (FVC) of 80% is considered abnormal and consistent with obstructive lung disease.

T/F 29. Preexisting renal disease increases the risk of perioperative acute tubular necrosis.

T/F 30. Chronic renal disease is an independent risk factor for cardiovascular disease.

T/F 31. Patients with chronic renal disease are predisposed to intraoperative hypotension.

T/F 32. Elective surgery should be delayed in a patient with an active urinary tract infection.

T/F 33. Patients with alcoholic cirrhosis and normal liver function tests are not at increased risk for perioperative liver failure.

T/F 34. Serum ammonia levels are directly proportional to the degree of hepatic encephalopathy.

T/F 35. Patients with moderate hypothyroidism are at increased risk for intraoperative bradycardia and hypotension.

T/F 36. The majority of patients with primary hyperparathyroidism present with kidney stones.

T/F 37. Facial nerve spasm elicited by tapping over the main trunk of the facial nerve is consistent with Trousseau sign and is a clinical indicator of hypocalcemia.

T/F 38. Diagnosis of adrenal insufficiency is typically made via a dexamethasone suppression test.

T/F 39. Patients with pheochromocytoma require preoperative treatment with alpha blockers prior to initiating beta-blocker therapy.

T/F 40. Perioperative hyperglycemia in diabetic patients is associated with increased risk of adverse outcomes.

T/F 41. Type I von Willebrand disease is associated with normal serum levels of factor VIII:C.

T/F 42. Anticoagulation due to warfarin can be reversed in approximately 6 hours by vitamin K administration.

T/F 43. Spontaneous bleeding is seen at levels below 50,000/μL.

T/F 44. In patients needing platelet transfusion, one unit per 10 g body weight is a typical starting dose.

T/F 45. Approximately 20% of African Americans are heterozygous for the gene for sickle cell anemia.

T/F 46. Patients with thalassemia major should undergo cardiac evaluation and echocardiogram prior to surgery.

T/F 47. Patients with degenerative neurological diseases such as amyotrophic lateral sclerosis (ALS) may be at increased risk for pulmonary complications following surgery.

T/F 48. Patients with autonomic dysfunction may be at risk for intraoperative hypotension and should be managed with preoperative glucocorticoids.

T/F 49. Fever can exacerbate the symptoms of multiple sclerosis.

T/F 50. The responsibility for an adequate preoperative evaluation lies with the surgeon.

SINGLE BEST ANSWER QUESTIONS

51. The oropharynx is bounded by:
    a. The soft palate superiorly and the epiglottis inferiorly
    b. The palatoglossal arch anteriorly and the posterior pharyngeal wall posteriorly
    c. The pharyngoepiglottic folds superiorly and cricopharyngeus inferiorly
    d. The circumvallate papillae superiorly and vallecula inferiorly
    e. The skull base superiorly and the level of the hyoid inferiorly

52. Which of the following blood vessels does *NOT* contribute a branch to the anterior nasal septum (Kiesselbach plexus)?
    a. Superior labial artery
    b. Greater palatine artery
    c. Anterior ethmoidal artery
    d. Posterior ethmoidal artery
    e. Posterior nasal artery

53. A 25-year-old female with a five-pack year smoking history presents with a history of a mass of the hard palate that has been slowly enlarging. On examination, there is a mucosally covered, lobulated, and very firm 6-mm mass in the midline of the hard palate. She is otherwise asymptomatic. Which of the following is the most appropriate next step in management?
    a. Observation
    b. Plain films
    c. Maxillofacial CT scan with contrast
    d. In-office biopsy
    e. Operative biopsy and panendoscopy

54. A 2-year-old male presents to your office with hoarseness and recurrent croup. He has a history of a repaired tetralogy of Fallot defect. On physical examination, a bifid uvula is present, and there is a small anterior laryngeal web present on fiberoptic laryngoscopy. Which of the following is the most likely underlying syndrome?
    a. CHARGE (coloboma, heart defect, atresia choanae, retarded growth and development, genital abnormality, and ear abnormality)
    b. VACTERL (vertebral, anal, cardiac, tracheal, esophageal, renal, and limb)
    c. 22q11.2 microdeletion
    d. Pallister-Hall
    e. Stickler

55. A 56-year-old male presents for excision of a T1N0 squamous cell carcinoma of the tongue. Preoperative cardiac evaluation demonstrates that he is at intermediate risk for myocardial ischemia, and the cardiologist has recommended initiating beta blockade. When is it best to initiate such therapy?
    a. 30 days before surgery
    b. 1 day before surgery
    c. 1 hour prior to incision
    d. Postoperative day 1
    e. Postoperative day 7

56. Which of the following is true regarding deep vein thrombosis (DVT) in head and neck surgical patients?
    a. Current or past malignancy, long surgical time, and advanced age are all risk factors for DVT.
    b. Heparin is not indicated in head and neck surgical patients because they ambulate early in the postoperative course.
    c. Heparin is not indicated in patients receiving antiplatelet agents such as aspirin after free tissue transfer.
    d. a and c
    e. All of the above

57. Which of the following is the most appropriate initial management of a patient with suspected anaphylaxis?
    a. Supplemental oxygen, intravenous (IV) access, and diphenhydramine and dexamethasone administration
    b. Remove exposure to trigger if possible, Trendelenburg positioning, and dexamethasone administration
    c. Supplemental oxygen, IV access, IV epinephrine bolus
    d. Supplemental oxygen, Trendelenburg positioning, and intramuscular epinephrine
    e. Remove exposure to trigger if possible, supplemental oxygen, transport to intensive care unit (ICU) setting

58. Which of the following contribute to intraoperative atelectasis?
    a. Supine positioning
    b. Impaired ciliary function

c. Reduced hypercarbic respiratory drive
d. Decreased ventilatory response to hypoxia
e. All of the above

59. Which of the following is *NOT* appropriate in the preoperative evaluation of a patient with chronic renal disease?
    a. Electrocardiogram
    b. Coagulation studies including prothrombin time (PT)/partial thromboplastin time (PTT), bleeding time, platelet counts
    c. Complete blood count
    d. Brain natriuretic peptide (BNP) level
    e. All of the above are appropriate studies

60. Propranolol is useful in the treatment of thyrotoxicosis because of:
    a. Reduction of symptomatic palpitations, tremulousness, and heat intolerance
    b. Decreased serum T3 levels due to reduction of thyroid hormone secretion
    c. Decreased serum T3 levels due to inhibition of peripheral conversion of T4 to T3
    d. a and c
    e. All of the above

61. A 47-year-old female with a history of poorly controlled Crohn disease and chronic sinusitis presents to the clinic with persistent symptoms following 4 weeks of medical management including nasal steroids, nasal saline, and 28 days of antibiotics. She is a good candidate for endoscopic sinus surgery and undergoes routine blood work, including coagulation studies. Her prothrombin time is elevated. Why?
    a. There is decreased absorption of dietary vitamin K due to Crohn disease.
    b. There is eradication of intestinal flora by antibiotics leading to reduced production of vitamin K.
    c. There is inadequate consumption of leafy green vegetables.
    d. a and b
    e. All of the above

62. Which of the following is most appropriate in preventing a vasoocclusive crisis in surgical patients with sickle cell disease?
    a. Pain control, supplemental oxygen, hydration, blood transfusion
    b. Warm room, hydration, cryoprecipitate
    c. Pain control, supplemental oxygen, hydroxyurea
    d. Warm room, supplemental oxygen, hydroxyurea
    e. Pain control, warm room, blood transfusion

63. A patient with long-standing epilepsy, well controlled by medication, presents with hyponatremia following parotidectomy for pleomorphic adenoma. Which of the following is the most likely explanation?
    a. Syndrome of inappropriate antidiuretic hormone secretion (SIADH)
    b. Seizures treated with carbamazepine
    c. Seizures treated with phenytoin
    d. Elevated prolactin levels
    e. Cerebral salt wasting syndrome

64. Which of the following medications should be withheld the morning of surgery for an elective procedure?
    a. Lamotrigine for seizures
    b. Risperidone for schizophrenia
    c. Fexofenadine for allergic rhinitis
    d. Theophylline for asthma
    e. All of these should be taken on the day of surgery

65. Which of the following symptoms describes neuroleptic malignant syndrome?
    a. Clonus, hyperthermia, diarrhea, agitation
    b. Severe muscle rigidity, hyperthermia, autonomic instability, changes in level of consciousness
    c. Tachycardia, hyperthermia, agitation, tremulousness
    d. Hyperthermia, tachycardia, hypertension
    e. Tachycardia, dyspnea, hypotension

66. A 15-year-old male presents with chronic fatigue, joint pain, and skin color changes. Preoperative laboratory results are significant for elevated liver function tests and serum glucose. Which of the following is the most likely cause?
    a. Addison disease
    b. Porphyria
    c. β-thalassemia major
    d. Hemochromatosis
    e. Polycythemia vera

67. A patient presents with incomplete eye closure, minimal forehead movement, and asymmetry of the smile. Which of the following is the House-Brackmann score?
    a. Grade I
    b. Grade II
    c. Grade III
    d. Grade IV
    e. Grade V

68. A patient with oropharyngeal squamous cell carcinoma is unable to work but able to perform all self cares. Which of the following is the Karnofsky performance status scale rating?
    a. 80%
    b. 70%
    c. 60%
    d. 50%
    e. 40%

69. Which of the following is the best description of a Battle sign?
    a. Proptosis of the ear, with fluctuance overlying the mastoid
    b. Abscess medial to the mastoid tip
    c. Deformity of the lobule seen following parotid surgery
    d. Ecchymosis overlying the mastoid
    e. Loss of definition of the folds of pinna

70. Which of the following is most consistent with a mucoid middle ear effusion on examination?
    a. Retracted tympanic membrane with fine radial blood vessels
    b. Air bubbles medial to the tympanic membrane
    c. Golden-colored fluid medial to the tympanic membrane
    d. Visible movement of the tympanic membrane when negative pressure is applied on pneumatic otoscopy
    e. White middle ear effusion and bulging of the tympanic membrane

71. Which of the following may be seen in otosclerosis?
    a. Blanching of an erythematous middle ear mass on pneumatic otoscopy
    b. White discoloration of the tympanic membrane
    c. Reddish discoloration of the promontory
    d. White mass medial to the tympanic membrane
    e. Vertigo on pneumatic otoscopy

72. On performing a tuning fork exam, a positive Rinne (air greater than bone conduction) is seen at 1024 Hz, but negative Rinne (bone greater than air conduction)

at 512 and 256 Hz. Which of the following degrees of hearing loss is suggested by this?
a. <15 dB HL
b. 15 to 30 dB HL
c. 30 to 45 dB HL
d. 45 to 60 dB HL
e. 60 to 85 dB HL

73. How long should an elective blepharoplasty be delayed following implantation of a drug-eluting cardiac stent?
a. 14 days
b. 30 days
c. 180 days
d. 365 days
e. Elective surgery is contraindicated.

74. Upper eyelid ptosis most likely indicates a defect in which of the following nerves?
a. Cervical sympathetics
b. Oculomotor nerve
c. Abducens nerve
d. Facial nerve
e. a or b

75. On examination of a middle-aged female in the clinic, a clicking sound is produced when applying lateral pressure to the larynx externally. What does this most likely indicate?
a. A normal examination finding
b. Thyroid cartilage fracture due to trauma
c. Pneumomediastinum
d. Calcification of the thyroid cartilage
e. Laryngeal carcinoma

76. When taking a pain history, one should ask about which of the following?
a. Pain onset
b. Aggravating or relieving factors
c. Quality of pain
d. Radiation
e. All of the above

77. Which of the following would be a cause for concern for melanoma arising within a nevus?
a. Irregular border
b. Heterogenous color
c. Increasing size
d. a and c
e. All of the above

78. The oral cavity is bounded by which of the following?
a. Vermillion border anteriorly, uvula posteriorly
b. Hard palate superiorly, floor of mouth inferiorly
c. Alveolar ridges anteriorly, retromolar trigone posteriorly
d. Incisive foramen anteriorly, junction of hard and soft palate posteriorly
e. Buccal mucosa laterally, soft palate posteriorly

79. Which of the following examination findings is most concerning for oral cavity carcinoma?
a. White patch on buccal mucosa
b. White patch on lateral tongue
c. Red patch on lateral tongue
d. Yellow patches on buccal mucosa
e. Ulcerative lesion on buccal mucosa with white base and erythematous rim

80. A 47-year-old male presents with a chief complaint of nasal obstruction, drainage, and headache. Which of the following endoscopic examination findings is most concerning and warrants further investigation?

a. Polypoid mucosa in middle meatus, purulent drainage in posterior nasal cavity
b. Turbinate hypertrophy with clear rhinorrhea
c. Asymmetric adenoid hypertrophy
d. Ectatic vessels on nasal septum
e. All of these findings warrant further investigation.

81. You decide to pursue further evaluation of your patient in the preceding question. Which of the following studies is most appropriate?
a. CT of sinuses and neck with contrast
b. Culture of middle meatus
c. Human immunodeficiency virus (HIV) serologies
d. a and b
e. a and c

82. Which of the following is consistent with a positive Tullio sign?
a. Nystagmus produced by pneumatic otoscopy
b. Dizziness induced by loud sounds
c. Sensitivity to normal, everyday sounds
d. Gaze-evoked tinnitus
e. Apparent movement of objects in the visual field

83. A patient reports that a 512K tuning fork is heard in the right side; when the same fork is applied to the mastoid bone, the sound is louder in front of the ear on both sides. What does this indicate?
a. Right conductive hearing loss
b. Left conductive hearing loss
c. Right sensorineural hearing loss
d. Left sensorineural hearing loss
e. Right mixed hearing loss

84. Which of the following is most appropriate in treating hypercalcemia?
a. Normal saline
b. IV furosemide
c. IV bisphosphonates
d. a and b
e. All of the above

85. Which of the following is an example of a clean-contaminated procedure?
a. Selective neck dissection
b. Bronchoscopy
c. Repair of a laceration of the face that does not enter the oral cavity
d. Thyroidectomy
e. Washout of a neck abscess that had previously undergone incision and drainage

86. Which of the following affects postoperative surgical site infection rates?
a. Age
b. Diabetes mellitus
c. Tobacco use
d. b and c
e. All of the above

87. Which of the following is the optimal timing for administration of preoperative prophylactic clindamycin?
a. At time of incision
b. Within 15 minutes of incision
c. Within 30 minutes of incision
d. Within 60 minutes of incision
e. Within 120 minutes of incision

88. What are Dennie-Morgan lines?
a. Folds in the infraorbital skin seen in allergy
b. Creases radiating from the lateral canthus seen in aging
c. Facial lines in children

d. A line that connects the notch above the tragus with the infraorbital rim

e. A line that connects the medial canthus to the angle of the mandible

89. Which of the following is independently associated with increased postoperative pulmonary complications?
a. Low serum albumin (<30 g/L)
b. Obesity
c. Emergency surgery
d. b and c
e. All of the above

90. Chronic renal failure is often associated with which of the following?
a. Polycythemia
b. Hyperkalemia
c. Postoperative infection
d. b and c
e. All of the above

91. A 36-year-old woman with a history of bipolar affective disorder treated with lithium and recurrent tonsillitis desires tonsillectomy. A review of her systems is positive for fatigue. What laboratory studies should be ordered before surgery?
a. Thyroid function studies
b. Complete blood count
c. Urine specific gravity and osmolality
d. a and b
e. All of the above

92. The submental lymph nodes are located in which cervical level?
a. IA
b. IB
c. IIA
d. IIB
e. III

93. Which of the following is important to note when describing a tympanic membrane perforation identified on examination?
a. Size
b. Location
c. Duration
d. a and b
e. All of the above

94. Which of the following statements regarding rigid nasal endoscopy is true?
a. All patients presenting with nasal and sinus complaints require endoscopic examination.
b. This examination is well tolerated by young children.
c. The true maxillary ostium is typically not visible with a zero degree telescope in an unoperated nose.
d. The endoscope is typically passed once through the nasal cavity, permitting visualization of the majority of the important nasal structures.
e. All of the above are true.

95. Obtaining informed consent is consistent with which of the following ethical principles?
a. Autonomy
b. Nonmaleficence
c. Justice
d. Beneficence
e. All of the above

96. Which of the following is important to the process of obtaining informed consent?
a. An assessment of the capacity of the patient to engage in discussion
b. A detailed discussion of the risks and benefits of the proposed procedure
c. A discussion of the alternatives to the proposed procedure, including nontreatment
d. b and c
e. All of the above

97. An asymptomatic 5-year-old female is referred urgently for an oropharyngeal mass. On examination, you see the smooth, curved top of what appears to be a mucosally covered mass in the midline of her oropharynx, just posterior to the base of tongue, that appears to be extending inferiorly. Which of the following is the most appropriate next step?
a. Observation
b. CT with contrast
c. MRI with contrast
d. Transoral ultrasound
e. Microdirect laryngoscopy with biopsy

98. Which of the following causes "cobblestoning" in the posterior oropharyngeal wall?
a. Visible submucosal sebaceous glands
b. Submucosal lymphoid hypertrophy
c. Eosinophilic infiltration of submucosal tissue
d. Chronic infection of pharyngeal mucosa
e. None of the above

99. What is the Schwabach test?
a. An examination that compares bone conduction in the patient with the examiner
b. An examination that compares air conduction in the patient with the examiner
c. An examination that compares bone conduction in the patient with a normal control
d. An examination that compares air conduction in the patient with a normal control
e. None of the above

100. Which of the following is the most prominent palpable landmark in a young child's larynx?
a. Hyoid bone
b. Thyroid cartilage
c. Cricothyroid membrane
d. Cricoid cartilage
e. Proximal tracheal rings

CORE KNOWLEDGE

OBTAINING THE HISTORY

- Review all available chart notes from the referring physician prior to the patient's visit, including radiographic images, operative notes, and pathology reports when available. Obtain the images for personal review, as well as pathologic slides for a second opinion when needed.

- Address the patient's primary concern first; this may or may not agree with the referring physician's reason for consultation.
- Take a thorough history of present illness, including a detailed account of the onset and disease course, aggravating and relieving factors, associated symptoms,

Table 3-1 American Academy of Otolaryngology Head and Neck Surgery Facial Nerve Grading System

Grade	Facial Movement	
I	Normal	Normal facial function at all times
II	Mild dysfunction	Forehead: moderate to good function Eye: complete closure Mouth: slight asymmetry
III	Moderate dysfunction	Forehead: slight to moderate movement Eye: complete closure with effort Mouth: slightly weak with maximum effort
IV	Moderately severe dysfunction	Forehead: no movement Eye: incomplete closure Mouth: asymmetric with maximum effort
V	Severe dysfunction	Forehead: no movement Eye: incomplete closure Mouth: slight movement
VI	Total paralysis	No movement

Table 3-2 Tuning Fork Assessment of Degree of Hearing Loss

Hearing Loss	256 Hz	512 Hz	1024 Hz
<15 dB	+	+	+
15-30 dB	−	+	+
30-45 dB	−	−	+
45-60 dB	−	−	−

+, Positive Rinne, air conduction > bone conduction.
−, Negative Rinne, bone conduction > air conduction.

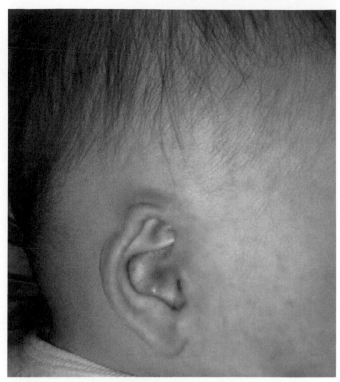

FIGURE 3-1 Right cryptotia.

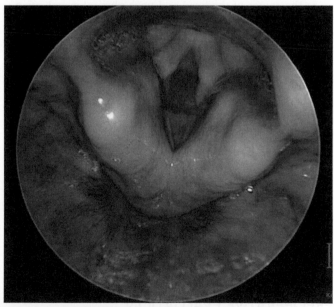

FIGURE 3-2 Subglottic hemangioma.

and response to prior therapy. Obtain a detailed pain history.
- Obtain a full past medical history including current medications, allergies, chronic conditions for which the patient is under a physician's care, previous hospitalizations and surgeries, and family and social history. A complete review of systems rounds out the history.

PHYSICAL EXAMINATION

- Assess the vital signs as well as general appearance, including any toxicity, affect, personal hygiene, and signs of substance use or abuse.
- Examine the head and face for shape, symmetry, signs of trauma, and facial motion (Table 3-1). The parotid gland is inspected externally and on bimanual palpation. The eyes are evaluated for placement, the presence of any discoloration or lesions of the conjunctiva and sclera, nystagmus, and motion.
- The pinnae are examined for placement and shape, definition of the helical cartilages, presence of pits/cysts in periauricular area, skin changes, and signs of infection (Figure 3-1). The external canals and tympanic membranes are then evaluated. Pneumatic otoscopy should be performed, observing for movement of tympanic membrane when positive and negative pressure are applied.
- A tuning fork examination should be carried out; a 512K tuning fork is used initially, with additional frequencies as needed. Weber and Rinne tests can be quite useful in delineating the degree of hearing loss (Table 3-2).

- Caution should be taken with rigid nasal endoscopy in uncooperative patients, and a flexible scope should be used to reduce the chance of laceration.
- The nasopharynx, hypopharynx, and larynx can be examined with a mirror and a headlight or with a flexible or rigid endoscope, depending on patient cooperation and gag reflex. The subglottis can occasionally be viewed when the vocal folds abduct, but frequently requires operative evaluation (Figure 3-2).
- The neck should be examined for normal laryngeal crepitus, as well as any masses or lymphadenopathy. The location of abnormal lymph nodes must be carefully

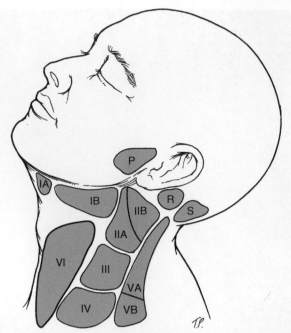

FIGURE 3-3 Lymph node regions of the neck. *Roman numerals* indicate neck level. *P,* Parotid; *R,* retroauricular; *S,* suboccipital.

described, as well as the size, palpation characteristics, and the presence of any matting (Figure 3-3).
- The skin including the scalp should be carefully inspected in the course of the head and neck physical examination.
- The cranial nerves must be carefully examined and any asymmetry noted.

SPECIAL POPULATIONS

- The stability and patency of the airway is of foremost concern in evaluating the trauma patient. Once secure, attention is then paid to respiration and cardiovascular assessment. Once stable, an abbreviated history including major medical comorbidities, current medications, and allergies is taken when possible.
- One must rely heavily on indirect history from caregivers and physical examination findings when treating young children.
- Surgery is very commonly undertaken in elderly patients, and due to comorbidities, physiologic changes due to aging, and polypharmacy, patients in this population are at increased risk for postoperative complications. Mitigating perioperative risk with appropriate evaluation and risk assessment is critical.

PREOPERATIVE EVALUATION

- Routine screening tests can include a complete blood count and electrolyte and coagulation studies. A chest radiograph and electrocardiogram are routinely performed in individuals over 40. A pregnancy test is routinely undertaken in women of childbearing age.
- Preoperative evaluations by the appropriate subspecialists as well as the anesthesia team is critical in the patient with complex disorders.
- Informed consent consists of a thorough explanation of the risks and benefits of surgery, as well as alternatives, including the risks of observation only. These must be documented in the medical record.
- A careful allergy history must be taken, particularly any history of antibiotic, latex, soybean, or egg allergy, as these can lead to intraoperative complications. Premedication

with steroids, antihistamines, and bronchodilators is necessary if the offending agent cannot be avoided.

COMPLICATIONS

Cardiovascular

- Perioperative myocardial infarction is associated with an almost 50% mortality rate.
- Risk factors for cardiovascular complications include jugular venous distension, previous myocardial infarction within 6 months, arrhythmia including frequent premature ventricular contractions, age >70 years, aortic stenosis, previous vascular or thoracic surgery, need for emergency surgery, and frailty/poor overall medical status.
- Suspicion of coronary artery disease, heart failure, uncontrolled hypertension, or peripheral vascular disease warrants anesthesia and/or cardiac clearance before surgery, including electrocardiography, exercise or chemical stress testing, and, in some patients, cardiac catheterization.
- Endocarditis prophylaxis should be planned in patients with prosthetic valves, history of endocarditis, unrepaired congenital heart defect, hypertrophic cardiomyopathy, or cardiac transplant. One dose of ampicillin (2 g in adults, 50 mg/kg in children) 30 to 60 minutes before incision is generally considered adequate.

Respiratory

- Postoperative respiratory complications are the second most common cause of perioperative mortality. Smokers and those with a history of chronic pulmonary disease are at increased risk. A history of hospitalizations and needed treatments for flares of these diseases should be taken. Comorbid cardiac and renal disease also impact pulmonary function and need to be detailed.
- Factors that affect postoperative ventilation include anesthetic agents, positive pressure ventilation, decreased ventilatory response to hypercarbia and hypoxia, impaired ciliary function related to intubation and lack of humidification, postoperative pain, and decreased coughing.
- On physical examination, obesity, kyphoscoliosis, pregnancy, and cachexia should be noted because these predispose to poor ventilation. Stridor, stertor, diaphoresis, increased work of breathing, clubbing, and cyanosis should all be noted. Abnormal lung sounds on auscultation should be documented.
- Preoperative evaluation of patients with chronic lung disease includes chest radiography as well as arterial blood gas testing. Spirometry can also be very useful.
- To minimize risk, smokers should quit at least 1 week before surgery, and chest physiotherapy can be instituted. Elective surgery should not be undertaken on patients in the midst of an acute flare of disease or active infection.

Renal

- Patients should be asked about symptoms of renal failure, including polyuria, polydipsia, fatigue, dyspnea, dysuria, hematuria, oliguria, and peripheral edema. Electrolyte abnormalities on preoperative screening should also prompt further evaluation of the renal system.
- Preexisting renal disease is a risk factor for developing acute tubular necrosis perioperatively. Additionally, chronic renal failure can be associated with anemia, platelet dysfunction, coagulopathy, hypernatremia, hypotensive episodes with anesthesia, postoperative infection, and increased risk for myocardial ischemia.
- Patients with renal disease may require changes in type, dosage, and intervals of medications, as well as careful fluid management.

- In dialyzed patients, it is imperative to work closely with the nephrologist, in both preoperative evaluation and management of postoperative dialysis needs.

Hepatic

- Liver failure should be considered in a patient with hepatotoxic drug therapy, jaundice, history of transfusion, and upper gastrointestinal bleeding history. Examination should include checking for hepatosplenomegaly, ascites, jaundice, and asterixis, as well as mental status changes consistent with encephalopathy.
- Laboratory tests include complete blood count, coagulation profile, electrolytes, serum albumin, serum aminotransferases, alkaline phosphatase, and lactate dehydrogenase. In patients with a suspected viral hepatitis, serologies can be ordered. Serum ammonia levels can be helpful in patients with suspected encephalopathy, although levels do not always correlate.
- Renal sequelae ranging from mild salt retention to acute renal failure can be seen in hepatorenal syndrome. Careful fluid management is necessary.

Endocrine

- Thyroid storm is a life-threatening exacerbation of hyperthyroidism that results in severe tachycardia and death. Hyperthyroidism should be treated before surgery to prevent this occurrence.
- Patients with mild to moderate hypothyroidism are not at increased anesthetic risk but should be treated before surgery when possible. Severe hypothyroidism is a medical emergency.
- Hypercalcemia, most commonly resulting from primary hyperparathyroidism, should be treated with loop diuretics, and hydration, as well as bisphosphonates, calcitonin, and hemodialysis when necessary.

- Positive Chvostek and Trousseau signs indicate clinically significant hypocalcemia.
- Stress-dose steroids may be needed for patients with >3 weeks of glucocorticoid use.
- Pheochromocytoma should be treated with alpha blockade prior to instituting beta blockade.
- In the diabetic patient, perioperative hyperglycemia is associated with an increased risk of complications and should be prevented.

Hematologic

- A history of easy bruising or excess bleeding should prompt laboratory studies including PT, PTT, and platelet counts. Measurement of bleeding time and fibrin split products can also be useful.
- Congenital deficiencies of hemostasis affect up to 1% of the population, the majority of which are mild.
- Warfarin should be stopped at least 3 days before surgery, and the patient bridged to heparin if needed.
- The platelet count should be at least 50,000/µL prior to surgery. Spontaneous bleeding is seen at levels <20,000/µL.
- Patients with sickle cell disease must be treated with aggressive oxygenation, hydration, pain control, and transfusion to prevent vasoocclusive crises.

Neurologic

- Chronic neurologic issues such as autonomic dysfunction, amyotrophic lateral sclerosis, Parkinsonism, and multiple sclerosis can predispose to pulmonary complications.
- Medications commonly used to treat seizures can cause electrolyte abnormalities, thrombocytopenia, and other laboratory abnormalities. Some anesthetic agents have the potential to lower the seizure threshold.

ANSWERS

TRUE OR FALSE QUESTIONS

1. F	14. F	27. T	40. T
2. T	15. T	28. F.	41. F
3. F	16. T	29. T	42. T
4. F	17. F	30. T	43. F
5. F	18. T	31. T	44. T
6. T	19. T	32. T	45. F
7. F	20. F	33. F	46. T
8. T	21. T	34. F	47. T
9. F	22. T	35. F	48. F
10. T	23. F	36. T	49. T
11. T	24. T	37. F	50. T
12. F	25. T	38. F	
13. F	26. F	39. T	

SINGLE BEST ANSWER QUESTIONS

51. b	64. c	77. e	90. d
52. e	65. b	78. b	91. e
53. a	66. c	79. c	92. a
54. c	67. d	80. c	93. d
55. a	68. b	81. c	94. c
56. a	69. d	82. b	95. a
57. d	70. a	83. d	96. e
58. e	71. c	84. e	97. a
59. e	72. c	85. b	98. b
60. d	73. d	86. e	99. a
61. d	74. e	87. d	100. a
62. a	75. a	88. a	
63. b	76. e	89. e	

SUGGESTED READINGS

1. Woodbury K, Ferguson BJ. Physical findings in allergy. *Otolaryngol Clin N Am.* 2011;44(3):603-610.
2. Grégoire V, et al. Delineation of the neck node levels for head and neck tumors: a 2013 update. *Radiother Oncol.* 2014;110(1):172-181.
3. Leclercq WK, et al. A review of surgical informed consent: past, present and future. *World J Surg.* 2010;34(7):1406-1415.
4. Garcia-Miguel FJ, Serrano-Aguilar PG, Lopez-Bastida J. Preoperative assessment. *Lancet.* 2003;362:1749-1757.
5. Fleisher LA, Fleischmann KE, Auerbach AD, et al. 2014 ACC/AHA guideline on perioperative cardiovascular evaluation and management of patients undergoing non-cardiac surgery. *J Am Coll Cardiol.* 2014;64(22):e77-e137.
6. Taylor A, DeBoard Z, Gauvin JM. Prevention of postoperative pulmonary complications. *Surg Clin N Am.* 2015;95(2):237-254.
7. Bratzler DW, et al. Clinical practice guidelines for antimicrobial prophylaxis in surgery. *Am J Health Syst Pharm.* 2013;70(3):195-283.
8. Bahl V, et al. Chemoprophylaxis for venous thromboembolism in otolaryngology. *JAMA Otolaryngol Head Neck Surg.* 2014;140(11):999-1005.
9. Schlitzkus LL, et al. Perioperative management of elderly patients. *Surg Clin N Am.* 2015;95(2):391-415.
10. American Academy of Pediatrics. Evaluation and preparation of pediatric patients undergoing anesthesia (RE 9633). *Pediatrics.* 1996;98(3 Pt 1):502-508.

Diagnostic Audiology | 4

Sameer Ahmed | Paul R. Kileny

TRUE OR FALSE QUESTIONS

T/F 1. On pure tone audiometry, a threshold is defined as the lowest signal intensity at which multiple presentations are detected 75% of the time.

T/F 2. On pure tone audiometry, the symbol > indicates unmasked bone conduction of the right ear.

T/F 3. Sound pressure level (SPL) is a sound pressure reference that has been calibrated to the hearing sensitivity of normal young adults under quiet test conditions.

T/F 4. The hearing level (HL) scale is used when discussing mild, moderate, moderate-severe, severe, and profound hearing loss.

T/F 5. The Hughson-Westlake "ascending method" is the most commonly used audiometric technique by which thresholds are obtained on a patient's audiogram.

T/F 6. If a patient has a 30 decibel (dB) HL threshold at 1000 Hertz (Hz), then a sound presented at 70 dB HL at that frequency will result in a 100 dB sensation level (SL).

T/F 7. In a normal patient, pure tone average (PTA) and speech reception threshold (SRT) should be within 5 to 10 dB of each other.

T/F 8. Crossover occurs when sounds are perceived by the better hearing ear when actually the poorer hearing ear is being tested.

T/F 9. Overmasking (i.e., when the masking signal exceeds intermural attenuation) the nontest ear may manifest in the artificial elevation of thresholds in the test ear.

T/F 10. The need for masking arises when air-conduction thresholds for the test ear are poorer than the bone-conduction thresholds for the nontest ear.

T/F 11. Narrow band noise is used as a masking signal on pure tone audiometry and speech audiometry.

T/F 12. A masking dilemma occurs when attempting to mask the nontest ear; overcoming the conductive component may involve masker levels that exceed interaural attenuation.

T/F 13. A type C tympanogram can be found in patients with a marginal tympanic membrane (TM) perforation.

T/F 14. A type As tympanogram is typically found in patients with an ossicular chain dislocation.

T/F 15. A type B tympanogram with large canal volume is typically seen in patients with a TM perforation.

T/F 16. A plugged pressure equalization tube results in a type B tympanogram.

T/F 17. A patient sustains an injury to the right facial nerve at the pes anserinus during parotidectomy. On a postoperative audiogram, his right stapedial reflex will remain intact.

T/F 18. A patient has bilateral severe sensorineural hearing loss without any conductive component of hearing loss. An acoustic reflex will be obtained bilaterally.

T/F 19. A patient has moderate-severe sensorineural hearing loss in the right ear. With a stimulating probe in the right ear, he obtains a stapedial reflex at 90 dB. He has right cochlear recruitment.

T/F 20. Patients with otosclerosis will have absent stapedial reflexes, while patients with superior semicircular canal dehiscence will have intact stapedial reflexes.

T/F 21. If the sensation level of the stimulus is 60 dB or lower and a stapedial reflex is obtained, this suggests cochlear recruitment.

T/F 22. Acoustic reflex decay is a sign of retrocochlear pathology.

T/F 23. Inner hair cells serve as amplifiers of the cochlear partition.

T/F 24. The acoustic by-products of cochlear hair cell amplification are otoacoustic emissions.

T/F 25. The presence of spontaneous otoacoustic emissions is abnormal and warrants further testing.

T/F 26. Otoacoustic emissions (OAEs) can be used to monitor noise-induced hearing loss and ototoxicity over time.

T/F 27. OAEs are absent/reduced in ears with hearing loss >80 dB.

T/F 28. In general, intact OAEs negatively influence the chance for hearing preservation in acoustic neuroma surgery.

T/F 29. Electrocochleography (ECOG) measures only the summating potential (SP) and the action potential (AP).

T/F 30. A summating potential/action potential (SP:AP) ratio >0.4 is abnormal.

T/F 31. ECOG must be done with a probe passing through the TM.

T/F 32. Given the presence of a third window lesion in superior semicircular canal dehiscence (SSCD), patients with this condition have absent stapedial reflexes.

T/F 33. The superior vestibular nerve is responsible for innervating the posterior semicircular canal.

T/F 34. The inferior vestibular nerve provides innervation to the saccule.

T/F 35. Cervical vestibular evoked myogenic potential (cVEMP) testing in SSCD patients results in elevated thresholds and reduced amplitudes.

T/F 36. Waves I and II on the auditory brainstem response (ABR) test correspond to the distal and proximal segments of the facial nerve.

T/F 37. Wave V on the ABR corresponds to the lateral lemniscus.

T/F 38. On ABR testing, the absence of wave V in the presence of waves I and III is a definitive indicator of retrocochlear pathology.

T/F 39. High-frequency sensorineural hearing loss does not influence the interpeak latency between waves I and V on ABR.

T/F 40. Hyperbilirubinemia and respiratory distress syndrome are two conditions associated with auditory neuropathy/auditory dyssynchrony.

T/F 41. Patients with auditory neuropathy who have no other cognitive or developmental disorders do well with cochlear implants.

T/F 42. Patients with auditory neuropathy do not have a cochlear microphonic on ABR.

T/F 43. Pseudohypacusis is more common in children than in adults.

T/F 44. A patient who claims bilateral significant hearing loss with normal voice level and articulation should be suspected of functional behavior.

T/F 45. When administering the Stenger test, the stimuli presented to each ear differ in intensity and in frequency.

T/F 46. Inadequate masking in unilateral moderate to severe sensorineural hearing loss may create a false air-bone gap and give the impression of a surgically correctable conductive hearing loss.

T/F 47. When an audiogram is available, the Weber and Rinne tests are not useful.

T/F 48. On an ABR, the interpeak latency for waves III to V is normally 2.1 milliseconds.

T/F 49. A hermetic seal needs to be obtained with the probe in the external auditory canal (EAC) in order to perform stapedial reflex testing.

T/F 50. Supranormal bone conduction thresholds are usually seen in otosclerosis.

SINGLE BEST ANSWER QUESTIONS

51. On pure tone audiometry, which of the following symbols reflect testing of the right ear?
    i.]
    ii. [
    iii. ▲
    iv. X
    v. ○

a. ii and v
b. i and v
c. ii, iii, and v
d. All of the above

52. How many decibels of SPL must be produced before a healthy human ear can perceive the sound at 250 Hz?
    a. 0 dB
    b. 12.5 dB
    c. 26.5 dB
    d. 40.5 dB

53. Severe hearing loss has thresholds that range between:
    a. 55 to 70 dB HL
    b. 70 to 90 dB HL
    c. 90 to 110 dB HL
    d. 110 to 130 dB HL

54. In bone conduction threshold testing, the bone oscillator is placed on which of the following?
    a. Mastoid process
    b. Zygomatic root
    c. External auditory meatus
    d. Temporomandibular joint

55. The pure tone average is the mean of the thresholds at which of the following frequencies?
    a. 1000 and 2000 Hz
    b. 250, 500, 1000, and 2000 Hz
    c. 250 and 500 Hz
    d. 500, 1000, and 2000 Hz

56. In speech audiometry, which type of speech material is used in identifying a patient's speech reception threshold?
    a. Phoneme
    b. Spondee
    c. Fricative
    d. Plosive

57. Relative to the SRT, how loud should be the testing for the word recognition score (WRS)?
    a. 0 to 10 dB louder
    b. 0 to 10 dB softer
    c. 40 to 50 dB louder
    d. 40 to 50 dB softer

58. Pediatric speech-recognition measures can be broken down into which of the following?
    i. Closed-set tests that measure prosodic cue, speech feature, and/or word perception
    ii. Open-set word and sentence tests that provide an estimate of the child's ability to communicate in the "real world"
    iii. Subjective report scale (e.g., Meaningful Auditory Integration Scale [MAIS])
    a. i and ii
    b. ii only
    c. ii and iii
    d. All of the above

59. Which of the following is the lower limit of interaural attenuation for bone conduction?
    a. 0 dB
    b. 10 dB
    c. 20 dB
    d. 30 dB

60. Which of the following is the lower limit of interaural attenuation for air conduction with standard headphones?
    a. 0 dB
    b. 20 dB
    c. 40 dB
    d. 60 dB

61. Which of the following is the lower limit of interaural attenuation for air conduction with insert earphones?
    a. 0 dB
    b. 20 dB
    c. 40 dB
    d. 60 dB

62. A masking dilemma occurs when a patient has bilateral air bone gaps of which of the following?
    i. 30 dB
    ii. 40 dB
    iii. 60 dB
    iv. 70 dB
    a. i and ii
    b. iii only
    c. ii only
    d. iii and iv

63. A type C tympanogram is typically seen in patient with which of the following?
    a. Patulous eustachian tube
    b. Chronic eustachian tube dysfunction
    c. Otosclerosis
    d. Malleus fixation

64. A normal adult's ear canal volume ranges between which of the following?
    a. 0.01 to 0.05 mL
    b. 0.1 to 0.5 mL
    c. 0.3 to 1.0 mL
    d. 0.6 to 2.0 mL

65. A normal child's ear canal volume ranges between which of the following?
    a. 0.01 to 0.05 mL
    b. 0.1 to 0.5 mL
    c. 0.5 to 1.0 mL
    d. 1.0 to 2.0 mL

66. An acoustic reflex is absent in all of the following conditions *EXCEPT*:
    i. Facial nerve injury at the midpoint of the internal auditory canal (IAC)
    ii. Facial nerve injury at the geniculate ganglion during a middle cranial fossa surgery
    iii. Facial nerve injury at the stylomastoid foramen during a temporal bone resection
    iv. Facial nerve injury during a submuscular aponeurotic system (SMAS) face lift
    a. i and iv
    b. i and ii
    c. iii and iv
    d. iv only

67. Which of the following conditions is associated with cochlear recruitment?
    a. Malleus fixation
    b. Stapedial footplate otosclerosis
    c. Connexin 26 mutation
    d. Meniere disease

68. A reduced dynamic range is seen in patients with cochlear recruitment and is demonstrated by a narrow range between which of the following two entities?
    a. Right stapedial reflex and left stapedial reflex
    b. Most comfortable listening (MCL) level and uncomfortable listening (UCL) level
    c. PTA and SRT
    d. SRT test and WRS

69. An acoustic reflex decay test is typically performed at which of the following?
    a. 500 Hz
    b. 500 or 1000 Hz

c. 2000 Hz
d. 2000 or 4000 Hz

70. An acoustic reflex decay test involves exposure to a loud stimulus and then measuring for changes in compliance of the TM for duration of which of the following?
    a. 3 seconds
    b. 5 seconds
    c. 7 seconds
    d. 10 seconds

71. Typically, the stimulating and recording probes are on opposite sides during an acoustic reflex decay test. A patient has retrocochlear pathology on the left side and has an abnormal acoustic reflex decay test with normal facial nerve function. To see this abnormality on the acoustic reflex decay test, the stimulus should be presented in which ear?
    a. Left ear
    b. Right ear

72. If a patient with normal hearing has a left facial nerve paralysis from a geniculate ganglion hemangioma and has an abnormal stapedial reflex pattern, which ear should the recording probe be placed in to detect this abnormality?
    a. Left ear
    b. Right ear

73. Which of the following is true of otoacoustic emissions?
    a. They reflect the motility status of the cochlea's inner hair cells.
    b. They indicate the presence of a working cochlear nerve.
    c. They are always abnormal.
    d. They reflect the motility status of the cochlea's outer hair cells.

74. When testing for transient evoked otoacoustic emissions (TE-OAEs) with a click stimulus (high-frequency stimulus), how long does one typically wait for a TE-OAE to appear after the stimulus has been delivered?
    a. 5 to 20 ms
    b. 20 to 40 ms
    c. 40 to 50 ms
    d. 40 to 60 ms

75. OAEs provide information about which of the following?
    a. Integrity of the distal segment of the cochlear nerve
    b. Integrity of the proximal segment of the cochlear nerve
    c. Frequency-specific regions of the cochlea
    d. Inferior colliculus

76. A patient with moderate-severe to severe sensorineural hearing loss is undergoing otoacoustic emission testing. His OAEs will be:
    a. Normal
    b. Absent
    c. Amplified/larger

77. A patient with auditory neuropathy/auditory dyssynchrony will have which of the following?
    a. Normal ABR and abnormal OAEs
    b. Abnormal/absent ABR and intact OAEs
    c. Abnormal/absent ABR and abnormal OAEs

78. ECOG provides which of the following?
    a. Information about cochlear inner hair cell motility
    b. Measurements of electrical events generated by the cochlea and auditory nerve
    c. Measurements of otolithic organ function
    d. None of the above

79. An elevated SP:AP ratio can be seen in which of the following?
    i. Endolymphatic hydrops
    ii. Cerebellar infarction
    iii. SSCD
    iv. Tensor tympani myoclonus
    a. i only
    b. i and iv
    c. ii and iii
    d. i and iii

80. Why is the summating potential higher in patients with SSCD?
    a. The basilar membrane is biased toward the scala tympani side.
    b. The basilar membrane is biased toward the scala vestibuli side.
    c. The stria vascularis is atrophic.
    d. The supporting hair cells of the organ of Corti are dysfunctional.

81. A patient with unilateral SSCD undergoes successful middle cranial fossa repair. Preoperatively, his SP:AP ratio was 0.70. After surgery, his SP:AP ratio should be which of the following?
    a. Greater than 0.70
    b. Less than 0.70 but greater than 0.40
    c. Less than 0.40
    d. The ratio should remain the same.

82. cVEMP testing is a(n):
    a. Contralateral excitatory response, which involves activation of the sternocleidomastoid (SCM) muscle mediated by the inferior vestibular nerve and saccule
    b. Contralateral inhibitory response, which involves relaxation of the SCM muscle mediated by the inferior vestibular nerve and saccule
    c. Ipsilateral excitatory response, which involves activation of the SCM muscle mediated by the inferior vestibular nerve and saccule
    d. Ipsilateral inhibitory response, which involves relaxation of the SCM muscle mediated by the inferior vestibular nerve and saccule

83. An ABR is which of the following?
    a. A surface-recorded response that measures the activity of primary auditory cortex
    b. A surface-recorded response that measures the distal auditory pathway
    c. A surface-recorded response that measures cochlear hair cell function

84. Wave IV on the ABR corresponds to which of the following?
    a. Proximal cochlear nerve
    b. Superior vestibular nerve
    c. Superior olivary complex
    d. Inferior colliculus

85. On ABR testing, the ipsilateral surface electrodes highlight which of the following?
    a. Wave I
    b. Wave III
    c. Waves IV and V
    d. None of the above

86. On ABR testing, the contralateral surface electrodes highlight which of the following?
    a. Wave I
    b. Wave III
    c. Waves IV and V
    d. None of the above

87. The ABR test is influenced by which of the following?
    a. Central nervous system depressants
    b. General anesthetics
    c. Sedatives
    d. None of the above

88. Which of the following waves is present on ABR in the context of significant hearing loss?
    a. Wave I
    b. Wave III
    c. Wave V
    d. All of the above

89. Which of the following waves on ABR testing is the most sensitive to hearing loss?
    a. Wave I
    b. Wave III
    c. Wave V
    d. All of the above

90. What is the normal duration for the interpeak latency between waves I and III?
    a. 2.8 sec
    b. 2.3 sec
    c. 2.8 ms
    d. 2.3 ms

91. What is the normal duration for the interpeak latency between waves I and V?
    a. 6.5 ms
    b. 5.3 ms
    c. 4.4 ms
    d. 1.0 ms

92. What is a normal absolute latency for wave V?
    a. 4.0 ms
    b. 1.0 ms
    c. 0.4 ms
    d. 0.04 ms

93. In the ABR diagram shown in Figure 4-1, which ear(s) is/are abnormal?
    a. Right ear
    b. Left ear
    c. Both ears
    d. Neither ear

94. A patient has intact otoacoustic emissions and the ABR shown in Figure 4-2. Which condition does this patient have?
    a. Usher syndrome
    b. Auditory neuropathy
    c. Pseudohypacusis
    d. Cochlear aplasia

95. A patient complains of hearing loss and has a negative Stenger test.
    a. This suggests that the patient is not exaggerating his/her hearing loss.
    b. This suggests that the patient is exaggerating his/her hearing loss.
    c. This test result is impossible to obtain in this clinical context.

96. A Stenger test should be routinely performed when:
    i. Suspecting pseudohypacusis
    ii. Evaluating unilateral hearing loss
    iii. Completing a newborn hearing screen
    a. i only
    b. ii only
    c. i and ii
    d. All of the above

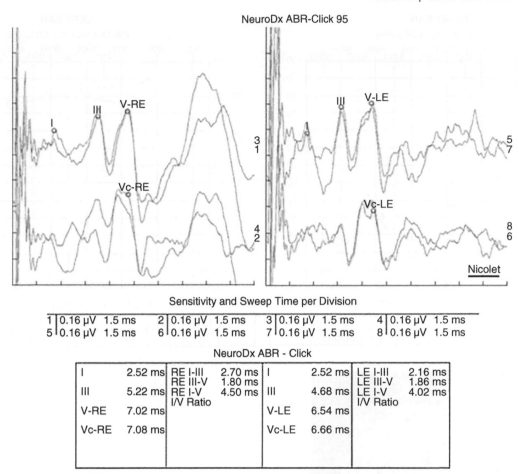

NeuroDx ABR-Click 95

Nicolet

Sensitivity and Sweep Time per Division

1	0.16 µV	1.5 ms	2	0.16 µV	1.5 ms	3	0.16 µV	1.5 ms	4	0.16 µV	1.5 ms
5	0.16 µV	1.5 ms	6	0.16 µV	1.5 ms	7	0.16 µV	1.5 ms	8	0.16 µV	1.5 ms

NeuroDx ABR - Click

I	2.52 ms	RE I-III	2.70 ms	I	2.52 ms	LE I-III	2.16 ms
		RE III-V	1.80 ms			LE III-V	1.86 ms
III	5.22 ms	RE I-V	4.50 ms	III	4.68 ms	LE I-V	4.02 ms
		I/V Ratio				I/V Ratio	
V-RE	7.02 ms			V-LE	6.54 ms		
Vc-RE	7.08 ms			Vc-LE	6.66 ms		

FIGURE 4-1 Auditory brainstem response (ABR) diagram. *LE,* Left ear; *RE,* right ear.

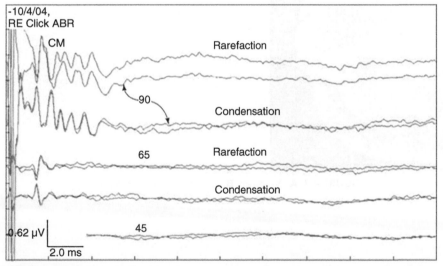

FIGURE 4-2 Auditory brainstem response (ABR) diagram. *CM,* Cochlear microphonic; *RE,* right ear.

97. A 29-year-old male patient presents with ataxia. He has a normal binocular otomicroscopic examination. How can you explain the supposedly low-frequency conductive hearing loss? (His audiogram and magnetic resonance imaging [MRI] scan are shown in Figure 4-3AB.)
    a. Middle ear effusion
    b. Ineffective masking
    c. Otosclerosis

98. On cVEMP testing, a patient has elevated thresholds and a reduced amplitude in response to click stimuli. Which condition does this patient have?
    a. SSCD
    b. Utricular paresis
    c. Saccular paresis
    d. Malingering

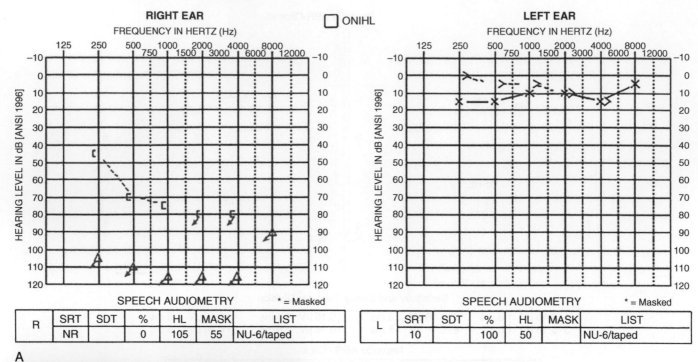

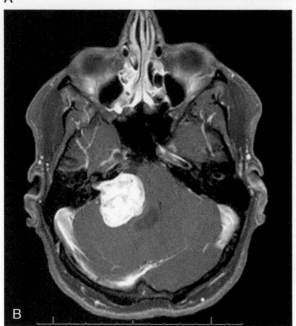

FIGURE 4-3 A, Audiogram. **B,** Magnetic resonance imaging scan.

99. Caloric testing reveals a 50% right vestibular weakness with normal caloric responses in the left ear. Which vestibular nerve is implicated in this weakness?
    a. Right superior
    b. Right inferior
    c. Left superior
    d. Left inferior

100. A 45-year-old man has decided to see the doctor for his hearing loss and bilateral tinnitus. He has a history of intermittent aural fullness in both ears that usually improved on its own after a cold but now it is persisting. (His audiogram is seen in Figure 4-4.) His acoustic reflexes are intact (not pictured). What is the next best step in management?
    a. MRI scan of his IAC
    b. Fluoride therapy
    c. Computed tomography (CT) scan of his temporal bones
    d. Left middle ear exploration with possible stapedectomy

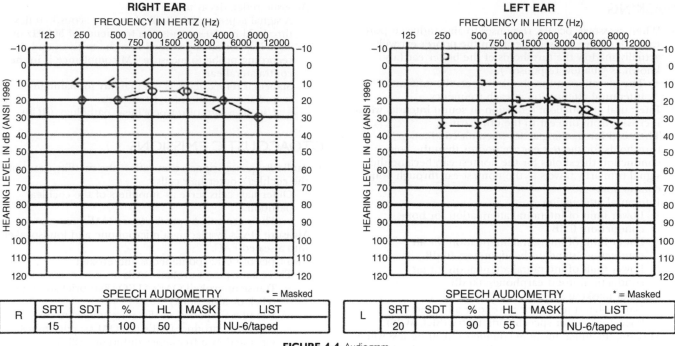

FIGURE 4-4 Audiogram.

CORE KNOWLEDGE

TESTS FOR HEARING SENSITIVITY

- Pure-tone audiometry is the most commonly used test for evaluating auditory sensitivity.
- Threshold is defined as the lowest signal intensity at which multiple presentations are detected 50% of the time.
- Audiometry legend
  - Symbol for masked air conduction in the right ear → Triangle
  - Symbol for unmasked air conduction in the right ear → Circle
  - Symbol for masked air conduction in the left ear → Square
  - Symbol for unmasked air conduction in the left ear → X
  - Color for the right ear → Red
- HL is calibrated to referent sound pressures that represent the hearing sensitivity of normal, young adults when tested under reasonably quiet test conditions.
- Hearing classification
  - Normal hearing: 0 to 25 dB HL
  - Mild hearing loss: 25 to 40 dB HL
  - Moderate hearing loss: 40 to 55 dB HL
  - Moderate-severe hearing loss: 55 to 70 dB HL
  - Severe hearing loss: 70 to 90 dB HL
  - Profound hearing loss: >90 dB HL
- Hughson-Westlake "Ascending Method"
  - This method obtains thresholds on pure tone audiometry.
  - Sounds are initially presented well above threshold and are then presented in decreasing steps of 10 to 15 dB, until the sound is inaudible.
  - The tone is then increased in steps that go up 5 dB, then down 10 dB, until the single hearing level at which a response is obtained three times is reached.
- In bone conduction threshold testing, the bone oscillator is placed on the mastoid process.

- Examples of clinical conditions associated with tympanometry
  - Type A: normal ear examination
  - Type As: ossicular chain fixation
  - Type Ad: ossicular chain dislocation, ossicular chain hypermobility, or atrophic TM
  - Type B, normal canal volume: middle ear effusion
  - Type B, large canal volume: TM perforation or patent pressure equalization tube
  - Type C: negative middle ear pressure from chronic eustachian tube dysfunction
- Ear canal volume (normal limits)
  - Adults: 0.6 to 2.0 mL
  - Children: 0.5 to 1.0 mL

SPEECH TESTING

- The PTA is the average of thresholds at 500, 1000, and 2000 Hz.
- The speech detection threshold (SDT) and PTA are typically 9 dB lower than the SRT.
- The spondee is a two-syllable word used in testing SRT.
- Phonemes (monosyllabic words) are used in testing WRS.
- When testing WRS, the speech stimulus intensity should be 50 dB louder than the SRT.
- Pediatric speech-recognition measures can be broken down into the following:
  - Closed-set tests that measure prosodic cue, speech feature, or word perception
  - Open-set word and sentence tests that provide an estimate of the child's ability to communicate in the "real world"
  - Subjective report scales, such as the Meaningful Auditory Integration Scale

MASKING

- When crossover occurs, responses to air-conducted pure tones that have crossed over from the poorer ear will actually shadow the thresholds of the better ear (also known as "shadow responses").
  - The elevation in thresholds reflects the amount of interaural attenuation at each frequency.
- Interaural attenuation: reduction in sound intensity when it crosses from one ear to the other ear
- The need for masking arises when air-conduction thresholds for the test ear are poorer than the bone-conduction thresholds for the nontest ear, because the signal primarily travels to the nontest ear through bone conduction.
- Interaural attenuation
  - Lower limit of interaural attenuation for bone conduction: 0 dB
  - Lower limit of interaural attenuation for air conduction, standard headphones: 40 dB
  - Lower limit of interaural attenuation for air conduction, insert earphones: 60 dB
- Types of masking signals
  - Narrow-band noises for pure tone audiometry
  - Speech noise for speech audiometry (SRT, WRS)
- Masking dilemma: bilateral conductive hearing loss when the air bone gaps are 55 to 60 dB or higher (this is a problem even if you use insert ear phones; if you use standard headphones, then the masking dilemma will appear around ~40 dB)
  - Occurs when attempting to mask the nontest ear; overcoming the conductive component may involve masker levels that exceed interaural attenuation; this can then cross over to the test ear and cause a falsely *elevated* threshold

ACOUSTIC/STAPEDIAL REFLEX

- Acoustic reflex pathway
  - Ipsilateral recording: cranial nerve (CN) VIII → ipsilateral ventral cochlear nucleus → trapezoid body → ipsilateral facial motor nucleus → ipsilateral facial nerve → ipsilateral stapedius muscle
  - Contralateral recording: CN VIII → ipsilateral ventral cochlear nucleus → contralateral medial superior olive → contralateral facial motor nucleus → contralateral facial nerve → contralateral stapedius
- Acoustic reflex will be absent if there is:
  - Conductive hearing loss or sensorineural hearing loss (SNHL) of 65 dB or greater in the stimulated ear
  - Significant conductive pathology in the recording/probe ear
- Acoustic reflex patterns in facial nerve paralysis
  - If nerve injury is proximally located (e.g., at the cerebellopontine angle), then the reflex should be absent because the branch to the stapedius muscle is distal to the injury.
  - If nerve injury is more distally located (e.g., near the stylomastoid foramen), then the reflex should be present.
- If the acoustic reflex is ~60 dB SL or lower, then recruitment is taking place.
  - Recruitment: cochlear hair cell dysfunction, which makes certain sounds seem much louder than they are. Patients with recruitment have some element of hearing loss, so their dynamic range (most comfortable listening level to uncomfortable listening level) can be narrow.

- Acoustic reflex decay test
  - A signal is presented 10 dB above the acoustic reflex threshold for 10 seconds at a frequency of 500 Hz or 1000 Hz. Sound is provided into the test ear, and the recording probe to measure TM compliance is in the contralateral ear.
  - Stapedial reflex decay is the inability to maintain stapedial contraction for 10 seconds.
    - Usually a sign of retrocochlear pathology (RCP)

OTOACOUSTIC EMISSIONS

- Audio frequency signals that reflect the motility status of the cochlea's outer hair cells
  - Outer hair cells serve as amplifiers of the cochlear partition.
    - Their acoustic by-products are OAEs.
- Measure OAEs by placing a microphone and loudspeaker into a sealed EAC.
- Two types of OAE: spontaneous and evoked
  - Three subtypes of evoked OAEs
    - Transient evoked OAEs (TEOAEs): brief stimulus (click or tone burst)
    - Stimulus-frequency OAEs: pure tone stimulus
    - Distortion product OAEs (DPOAEs): pure tones separated by a frequency difference (2f-f)
- TEOAEs: range between 400 Hz and 6 kHz
  - Latency is typically between 5 and 20 milliseconds after the stimulus is delivered.
- DPOAEs: two tones are presented (between 55 and 80 dB SPL), which are separated in frequency by 2f-f and are separated in amplitude by 10 to 15 dB.
- OAEs give information about frequency-specific regions of the cochlea.
  - Can monitor noise-induced hearing loss and ototoxicity over time
- OAEs are absent/reduced in ears with hearing loss >40 dB.
- Intact OAEs can support the notion of hearing preservation in acoustic neuroma surgery.
- Absent ABR but intact OAEs → auditory neuropathy/auditory dyssynchrony

ELECTROCOCHLEOGRAPHY

- Measurement of electrical events generated by the cochlea and auditory nerve
- Stimulus is an alternating click, typically at 85 dB.
- Measurements are cochlear microphonic (CM), summating potential (SP), and action potential (AP; cochlear nerve action potential).
- SP:AP ratio >0.4 is abnormal → seen in hydrops and SSCD.
  - In patients with SSCD, impedance is larger on the scala vestibuli side than at the scala tympani side.
    - Thus the basilar membrane is biased toward the scala tympani, which results in a higher SP amplitude.
    - SP:AP ratio normalizes (i.e., become <0.4) after successful repair of SSCD.

VESTIBULAR EVOKED MYOGENIC POTENTIAL TESTING

- Inferior vestibular nerve: posterior semicircular canal and saccule
- Superior vestibular nerve: superior semicircular canal, horizontal semicircular canal, utricle (and a small part of the saccule)

- cVEMP test: ipsilateral inhibitory response
  - Relaxation of the SCM muscle mediated by the inferior vestibular nerve and saccule
  - Unlike ocular VEMP, which is contralateral and excitatory; contralateral contraction of the inferior oblique muscle
- cVEMP testing in SSCD patients: low thresholds (65 dB or lower) and elevated amplitude

AUDITORY BRAINSTEM RESPONSE

- Surface recorded response that measures the distal auditory pathway
- Audiogram must be done before ABR to make sure that stimuli are within the dynamic range of the patient.
- Two types of stimuli
  - Clicks: 100 ms, brief rectangular pulses, at constant or alternating polarity; usually 2 kHz or 4 kHz
  - Tone pips: 1 to 2 cycles, short rise and fall times
- Waves I to V
  - Wave I: distal portion of cochlear nerve
  - Wave II: proximal portion of cochlear nerve
  - Wave III: cochlear nucleus
  - Wave IV: superior olivary complex
  - Wave V: lateral lemniscus (not the inferior colliculus, as initially thought)

NEURODIAGNOSIS WITH ABR

- Wave V is often present even in the presence of significant hearing loss.
  - Wave I is the most sensitive to hearing loss; 40 dB of hearing loss can make it difficult to see wave I at higher frequencies.
- The absence of wave V in the presence of waves I and III → think about RCP.
- Criteria
  - Normal: interpeak latencies of I to III (2.3 ms); III to V (2.1 ms); I to V (4.4 ms)
    - High-frequency SNHL causes latency of I to V to be increased.
  - Absolute latency of wave V (0.4 ms)
  - Interaural latency difference should be evaluated (ears should be symmetric).

AUDITORY NEUROPATHY (AUDITORY DYSSYNCHRONY)

- Not a problem with the cochlea/hair cells but more of a problem with the cochlear nerve
- Absent wave V on ABR and present OAEs
  - In auditory neuropathy, the cochlear microphonic should be present.

- In an electrically evoked ABR (with transtympanic stimulation), it is possible to see a wave V.
  - This indicates that with enough electrical stimulation, you can "resynchronize" the auditory pathway. This may explain why some auditory neuropathy patients perform well with cochlear implants (especially those with no other cognitive or developmental disorders).

FUNCTIONAL HEARING LOSS (PSEUDOHYPACUSIS)

- More common in adults than in children
- A patient who claims bilateral significant hearing loss with normal voice level and articulation should be suspected of functional hearing loss.
- PTA and SRT should be within 5 to 10 dB of each other.
- A positive Stenger test suggests that the patient is exaggerating his/her hearing loss.
- Stenger test
  - When two acoustic stimuli that are identical in every regard except intensity are introduced simultaneously into the left and right ears, the patient will perceive only the louder of the two stimuli.
- Example: The patient is lying about right-sided hearing loss. At 1000 Hz, the right ear threshold is supposedly 100 dB and left ear threshold is 20 dB. For the Stenger test, you provide a simultaneous stimulus to both ears. In the right ear, you'll give it at 90 dB and the left ear at 30 dB. The patient will hear the louder of the two stimuli (in this case, in his right ear). Because he is lying about his right ear, he will claim to have not heard anything. If he truly had a right hearing loss, then he would have heard the stimulus in his left ear and would have indicated this on the audiogram.

ERRORS IN CLINICAL JUDGMENT

- Stenger test is strongly recommended in all patients with a unilateral hearing loss.
- Inadequate masking in unilateral moderate to severe SNHL may create a false air-bone gap and give the impression of a surgically correctable conductive hearing loss.
  - This would occur because in the presence of inadequate masking, bone-conduction thresholds in the test ear with a true, severe SNHL will continue to reflect the shadow curve of the contralateral ear, thus exhibiting a false air-bone gap between the true air-conduction thresholds and the false bone-conduction thresholds.

ANSWERS

TRUE OR FALSE QUESTIONS

1. F	10. T	19. T	28. F
2. F	11. F	20. T	29. F
3. F	12. T	21. T	30. T
4. T	13. F	22. T	31. F
5. T	14. F	23. F	32. F
6. F	15. T	24. T	33. F
7. T	16. F	25. F	34. T
8. T	17. T	26. T	35. F
9. T	18. F	27. F	36. F

37.	T	41.	T	45.	F	49.	T
38.	T	42.	F	46.	T	50.	F
39.	F	43.	F	47.	F		
40.	T	44.	T	48.	T		

SINGLE BEST ANSWER QUESTIONS

51.	c	64.	d	77.	b	90.	d
52.	c	65.	c	78.	b	91.	c
53.	b	66.	c	79.	d	92.	a
54.	a	67.	d	80.	a	93.	a
55.	d	68.	b	81.	c	94.	b
56.	b	69.	b	82.	d	95.	a
57.	c	70.	d	83.	b	96.	c
58.	d	71.	a	84.	c	97.	b
59.	a	72.	a	85.	a	98.	c
60.	c	73.	d	86.	c	99.	a
61.	d	74.	a	87.	d	100.	c
62.	d	75.	c	88.	c		
63.	b	76.	b	89.	a		

SUGGESTED READINGS

1. Katz J. *Handbook of Clinical Audiology.* Philadelphia: Lippincott, Williams & Wilkins; 2002.

2. Kileny PR, Edwards BM. Objective measures of auditory function. In: Jackler RK, Brackmann DE, eds. *Textbook of Neurotology.* St Louis: Mosby-Year Book; 2004:287-305.

3. Kileny PR, Zwolan TA. Rehabilitation of the hearing impaired. In: DeLisa JA, Gans BM, eds. *Rehabilitation Medicine: Principles and Practice.* Philadelphia: Lippincott-Raven; 1998:1749-1758.

4. Burkard RF, Don M, Eggermont JJ. *Auditory Evoked Potentials: Basic Principles and Clinical Applications.* Philadelphia: Lippincott, Williams & Wilkins; 2007.

5. Ruben RJ, Elberling C, Salomon G. *Electrocochleography.* Baltimore: University Park Press; 1976.

6. Arts HA, Adams ME, Telian SA, et al. Reversible electrocochleographic abnormalities in superior canal dehiscence. *Otol Neurotol.* 2008;30:79-86.

7. Arts HA, Kileny PR, Telian SA. Diagnostic testing for endolymphatic hydrops. *Otolaryngol Clin North Am.* 1997;30: 987-1005.

8. El-Kashlan HK, Eisenmann D, Kileny PR. Auditory brainstem response in small acoustic neuromas. *Ear Hear.* 2000;21:257-262.

9. Gifford R. *Cochlear Implant Patient Assessment: Evaluation of Candidacy, Performance, and Outcomes.* San Diego: Plural Publishing; 2013.

10. Adams M, Edwards BM, Kileny PR. Different manifestations of auditory neuropathy. *Cochlear Implants Int.* 2010; 11:148-152.

Deafness | 5

François Cloutier | Douglas Backous

TRUE OR FALSE QUESTIONS

BASIC SCIENCE

T/F 1. The cochlea is organized tonopically so that the low frequencies are at the base.

T/F 2. Impedance is defined as the ratio between the acoustic pressure and the volume velocity generated by the acoustic pressure.

T/F 3. An increase in the middle ear stiffness causes a high-frequency hearing loss.

T/F 4. The primary auditory cortex is located on Heschl gyrus and is tonopically organized.

T/F 5. The auditory brainstem provides efferent input to the ear via two major descending systems: the middle ear muscle reflex pathways and the olivocochlear reflex pathways.

T/F 6. The cochlear aqueduct establishes a communication between the perilymphatic space and the subarachnoid space in the posterior fossa.

T/F 7. The area of the tympanic membrane is 20 times bigger than the area of the oval window.

T/F 8. The frequency resonance of the external auditory canal is approximately 3000 Hz.

T/F 9. The frequency range for human sound perception is between 10 Hz to 24 kHz.

T/F 10. For the impedance matching of the middle ear, one mechanism is called the *lever ratio*. It refers to the difference in length of the manubrium of the malleus and the long process of the incus.

CONGENITAL SENSORINEURAL HEARING LOSS

T/F 11. About 50% to 60% of congenital severe to profound hearing loss is caused by a genetic anomaly.

T/F 12. About 80% of nonsyndromic congenital deafness is autosomal dominant.

T/F 13. The most common cause of genetic congenital hearing loss is caused by mutation of the connexin 26 gene *(DFNB1)*.

T/F 14. The connexin 26 gene (on the chromosome 18) is a member of a large family of proteins involved in "gap junctions."

T/F 15. The carrier incidence in the population of mutation of the connexin 26 gene is 1 in 350.

T/F 16. The A1555G mutation in the 12S rRNA gene of human mitochondrial DNA causes an increased sensitivity to the toxic effect of cisplatin.

T/F 17. Immunoglobulin G (IgG) antibodies do not pass across the human placenta.

T/F 18. Ophthalmologic referral should be recommended for all children with hearing loss.

T/F 19. Cytomegalovirus (CMV) is the most common cause of nongenetic hearing loss and may represent up to 20% of nonsyndromic cases.

T/F 20. There is evidence that suggests that antiviral treatment of children with congenital CMV sensorineural hearing loss may stabilize or even improve hearing thresholds.

SENSORINEURAL HEARING LOSS

T/F 21. The difference between temporary threshold shift (TTS) and permanent threshold shift (PTS) is that TTS recovers within 7 days and PTS is permanent.

T/F 22. Noise-induced hearing loss (NIHL) begins to involve the midfrequency range, primarily 3 to 6 kHz.

T/F 23. Idiopathic sudden sensorineural hearing loss (ISSNHL) treated within the first 6 weeks with corticosteroids appears to offer the greatest recovery.

T/F 24. The rate of vestibular schwannomas for patients with sudden sensorineural hearing loss (SSNHL) ranges from 2.7% to 10.2%.

T/F 25. Current Quantitative Analyses of Normal Tissue Effect in the Clinic (QUANTEC) guidelines have suggested limiting the mean dose to the cochlea to ≤75 Gy to prevent sensorineural hearing loss (SNHL).

T/F 26. The frequencies most affected by presbycusis are those above 2 kHz.

T/F 27. Cisplatin and aminoglycoside antibiotics damage outer hair cells at the base of the cochlea, resulting in high-frequency SNHL that may later also involve lower frequencies.

T/F 28. Gentamicin and streptomycin are aminoglycoside antibiotics that are more vestibulotoxic than ototoxic.

T/F 29. Measurement of peak and trough serum levels of aminoglycosides provides rough guidelines for therapeutic efficacy but is not an absolute guarantee for prevention of ototoxicity, particularly vestibular ototoxicity.

T/F 30. A perilymphatic fistula consists of a pathologic communication between the perilymphatic spaces of the inner ear and middle ear.

CONDUCTIVE HEARING LOSS

T/F 31. Conductive hearing loss in the presence of normal acoustic reflexes and/or elevated bone thresholds should prompt investigation for superior semicircular canal dehiscence syndrome before middle ear exploration.

T/F 32. The Baha system is effective in treating conductive hearing loss by bypassing the damaged middle ear system, transmitting vibromechanical energy to the cochlea via direct bone conduction.

T/F 33. Tuning fork testing is not an effective method to screen for hearing loss, determine conductive versus sensorineural loss, and validate audiometric findings.

T/F 34. The expected hearing loss with ossicular interruption is worse with a perforated tympanic membrane than with an intact tympanic membrane.

T/F 35. The estimated conductive loss when the Rinne test is positive at 256 Hz and 512 Hz is 30 to 45 dB.

T/F 36. Narrowing of the external auditory canal (EAC) to <3-mm diameter results in high-frequency hearing loss.

T/F 37. Bony regrowth over the stapedotomy fenestration is the most common cause of failure of the surgery for otosclerosis.

T/F 38. Tympanosclerosis most commonly involves the tympanic membrane.

T/F 39. Otosclerosis is bilateral in 70% of cases.

T/F 40. Otosclerosis can also cause SNHL.

AUDITORY PROSTHETIC STIMULATION, DEVICES, AND REHABILITATIVE AUDIOLOGY

T/F 41. The diagnosis of auditory neuropathy/auditory dyssynchrony has been specified as a hearing disorder in which preserved outer hair cell function exists with abnormal auditory neural responses; it is a contraindication to cochlear implantation.

T/F 42. Patients who require revision implant surgery (reimplantation) generally do not perform as well with their second implant as with their first.

T/F 43. A second cochlear implant (implanted sequentially or simultaneously) improves sound localization and speech recognition in noise over a single implant.

T/F 44. For an auditory brainstem implant (ABI), the electrodes are placed over the cochlear nucleus within the lateral recess of the fourth ventricle.

T/F 45. The signal to noise ratio (SNR) is the difference between the level of sound you want to hear and the level of the background noise.

T/F 46. The Larsen effect is also known as acoustic feedback.

T/F 47. Contralateral routing of signal (CROS) hearing aids can be used when a patient has a deaf ear on one side and fairly normal hearing on the other.

T/F 48. The most common microorganism causing meningitis in patients with cochlear implants is *Streptococcus pneumoniae.*

T/F 49. Hearing aids with open-canal fittings are especially useful for low-frequency hearing loss.

T/F 50. Binaural fitting may not be successful in patients with large hearing asymmetries.

SINGLE BEST ANSWER QUESTIONS

BASIC SCIENCE

51. Which structure protects the round window and causes the "phase difference" so that the sound wave does not strike the oval and round windows simultaneously?
    a. Stapes
    b. Stapedial tendon
    c. Tympanic membrane
    d. Round window
    e. Promontory

52. Which part(s) of the inner ear is filled with perilymph?
    i.   Scala tympani
    ii. Scala vestibuli
    iii. Scala media
    a. i
    b. ii
    c. iii
    d. i and ii
    e. All of the above

53. Which scala(e) is/are just behind the stapes and the oval window?
    i.   Scala tympani
    ii. Scala vestibuli
    iii. Scala media
    a. i
    b. ii
    c. iii
    d. i and ii
    e. All of the above

54. There are a variety of decibel (dB) scales used in many applications of sound intensity measurements. Which decibel scale is normally used for pure tone audiograms?
    i.   dB sound pressure level (dBSPL)
    ii. dB hearing level (dBHL)
    iii. dB sensation level (dBSL)
    a. i
    b. ii
    c. iii
    d. i or ii
    e. Any of the above

55. What is the difference in decibels between the acoustic coupling (pathway of sound transmission to the inner ear in the absence of the ossicular system) and the ossicular coupling (pathway of sound transmission to the inner ear in the presence of the ossicular system)?
    a. 20 dB
    b. 30 dB
    c. 40 dB
    d. 50 dB
    e. 60 dB

56. In reality, what is the middle ear gain with the ossicular coupling?
    a. 5 dB
    b. 10 dB
    c. 15 dB
    d. 20 dB
    e. 25 dB

57. What are the mechanisms for impedance matching inside the middle ear?
    i. Area ratio
    ii. Lever ratio
    iii. Catenary lever
    a. i
    b. ii
    c. iii
    d. i and ii
    e. All of the above

58. What is the definition of a threshold of 40 dBHL at 1000 Hz?
    a. Four factors of 10 (i.e., 10,000 times) more intense than 0.0002 dynes/cm² (or 20 micropascals)
    b. Four factors of 10 (i.e., 10,000 times) more intense than 10^{-12} watts/m²
    c. Four factors of 10 (i.e., 10,000 times) more intense than a 1000-Hz tone that is barely audible to an average, normal-hearing listener

59. What is the velocity of sound propagation in dry air (at room temperature) and in water?
    a. 340 m/sec and 1500 m/sec
    b. 120 m/sec and 750 m/sec
    c. 120 m/sec and 5500 m/sec
    d. 340 m/sec and 10,000 m/sec
    e. 100 m/sec and 200 m/sec

60. The protection of the organ of Corti, provided by the acoustic reflex against excessive stimulation, is mainly useful for which frequencies?
    a. Low frequencies
    b. Mid frequencies
    c. High frequencies
    d. All frequencies
    e. There is no protection.

CONGENITAL SENSORINEURAL HEARING LOSS

61. Which milestones in language development are true?
    i. Birth: cries
    ii. 16 weeks: differentiates sound and responds to human sound
    iii. 20 weeks: makes vowel and consonant sounds
    iv. 18 months: utters 2 to 50 words
    v. 24 months: vocabulary 50+ words
    vi. 36 months: 1000-word vocabulary
    a. i, ii, and iii
    b. i and ii
    c. i, ii, iii, and iv
    d. i, ii, iii, iv, and v
    e. All of the above

62. What does the abbreviation of the gene *DFNB* stand for?
    a. Autosomal dominant transmission
    b. Autosomal recessive transmission
    c. X-linked
    d. Mitochondrial
    e. Nongenetic

63. What is the incidence of congenital deafness?
    a. 1 in 500 births
    b. 1 in 750 births
    c. 1 in 1000 births
    d. 1 in 10,000 births
    e. 1 in 20,000 births

64. Which statement about the nonsyndromic congenital X-linked deafness *DFN3* (X-linked gusher) is *INCORRECT*?
    a. Caused by mutation of *POU3F4*
    b. Congenital fixation of the stapes
    c. Absence of the bony partition between the fundus and the basal turn of the cochlea
    d. Females are principally affected.
    e. Dilation of the internal auditory canal

65. Which of the following is *NOT* a congenital deafness risk factor?
    a. Neonatal intensive care unit
    b. Male
    c. Perinatal infection (TORCH)
    d. Craniofacial anomaly
    e. Birth weight <1500 g
    f. Hyperbilirubilemia with treatment
    g. Ototoxic medication
    h. Bacterial meningitis
    i. APGAR between 0 and 4 at 1 minute and between 0 and 6 at 5 minutes
    j. Prolonged mechanical ventilation
    k. Other findings associated with syndromic congenital deafness

66. Mutation of the gene *SLC26A4* is associated with which of the following syndromes?
    a. Pendred
    b. Brachio-oto-renal
    c. CHARGE
    d. Treacher-Collins
    e. X-linked gusher

67. How can we confirm the diagnosis of CMV infection in the newborn within the first 3 weeks of life?
    i. Culture of the virus in urine
    ii. Culture of the virus in saliva
    iii. Polymerase chain reaction (PCR) testing for CMV DNA in urine
    iv. PCR testing for CMV DNA in serum
    a. i and ii
    b. iii and iv
    c. i and iii
    d. ii and iv
    e. All of the above

68. How can we confirm the diagnosis of CMV infection in the newborn after 3 weeks of life?
    a. Culture of the virus in urine
    b. Culture of the virus in saliva
    c. Detection of CMV DNA in the dried blood spots
    d. PCR testing for CMV DNA in urine
    e. PCR testing for CMV DNA in serum

69. Which of these selected syndromes are associated with autosomal recessive (AR) hearing loss?
    i. Usher syndrome
    ii. Pendred syndrome
    iii. Jervell and Lange-Nielsen syndrome
    iv. Neurofibromatosis type 2
    v. Stickler
    vi. Waardenburg
    a. i, ii, and iii
    b. ii, iii, and iv
    c. iv, v, and vi

d. i, iii, and v
e. i, ii, iii, and iv

70. Auditory neuropathy/dyssynchrony (AN/AD) is *NOT* associated with which of the following?
    a. Hearing loss
    b. Abnormal outer hair cell function (absent otoacoustic emission)
    c. Auditory nerve dysfunction (abnormal auditory brainstem response)
    d. Poor speech discrimination out of proportion to pure tone average

SENSORINEURAL HEARING LOSS

71. Which symptom or objective finding is *NOT* a characteristic present in NIHL?
    a. History of long-term exposure to dangerous noise levels (i.e., >85 dBA for 8 hours/day) sufficient to cause the degree and pattern of hearing loss
    b. Gradual loss of hearing over the first 5 to 10 years of exposure
    c. Speech-recognition scores consistent with the audiometric loss
    d. Hearing loss that gets worse even after the noise exposure is terminated
    e. Hearing loss is almost always bilateral.
    f. Loss is always greater at the frequencies 3000 to 6000 Hz than at 500 to 2000 Hz. Loss is usually greatest at 4000 Hz. The 4000-Hz notch is often preserved even in advanced stages.

72. In NIHL, which part of the cochlea is principally damaged?
    a. Outer hair cells (OHCs)
    b. Inner hair cells (IHCs)
    c. Reissner membrane
    d. Stria vascularis
    e. Basilar membrane

73. Which characteristics of sudden SNHL are distinctive from an autoimmune inner ear disease (AIED)?
    i. Occurs in 72 hours or less
    ii. Unilateral
    iii. Frequent
    iv. Occurs progressively over days to months
    v. Bilateral
    vi. Rare
        a. i, ii, and iii
        b. i, iii, and iv
        c. iii, iv, and v
        d. i, v, and vi
        e. All of the above

74. Which of the following are the characteristics of the primary AIED, as described by McCabe in 1979?
    i. Rapidly progressive (over a period of weeks to months)
    ii. Hearing loss frequently is associated with vestibular symptoms.
    iii. Bilateral SNHL
    iv. Good response to immunosuppressive drugs
        a. i, ii, and iii
        b. ii, iii, and iv
        c. iii and iv
        d. iv
        e. All of the above

75. Which of the following elements are present in Cogan syndrome?
    i. Acute nonsyphilitic interstitial keratitis
    ii. Vestibular dysfunction
    iii. SNHL
    iv. Anisocoria

a. i and ii
b. ii and iii
c. i, ii, and iii
d. i, iii, and iv
e. All of the above

76. Which of the following diseases is *NOT* in the differential diagnosis of both eye and inner ear disease?
    a. Sarcoidosis
    b. Congenital syphilis
    c. Vogt-Koyanagi-Harada syndrome
    d. Sjögren syndrome
    e. Rheumatoid arthritis
    f. Systemic lupus erythematosus
    g. Antiphospholipid antibody syndrome
    h. Polyarteritis nodosa
    i. Otosclerosis
    j. Granulomatosis with polyangiitis (Wegener)
    k. Relapsing polychondritis
    l. Behçet syndrome

77. The prognosis of recovery for patients with ISSNHL is dependent on which of the following?
    i. Patient age
    ii. Presence of vertigo at onset
    iii. Degree of hearing loss
    iv. Audiometric configuration
    v. Time between onset of hearing loss and treatment
        a. i, ii, and iii
        b. ii, iii, and iv
        c. iii, iv, and v
        d. i, ii, iii, and iv
        e. All of the above

78. Which audiological finding does not suggest a retrocochlear lesion?
    a. Asymmetric hearing loss
    b. Abnormally reduced or asymmetric speech discrimination
    c. Rollover
    d. Notch at 2 kHz
    e. Absence of acoustic reflexes

79. List the different histopathologic types of presbycusis as described by Gacek and Schuknecht.
    i. Sensory (hair cell loss)
    ii. Neural (loss of spiral ganglion)
    iii. Metabolic (strial atrophy)
    iv. Mechanical or conductive (stiffness of the basilar membrane)
        a. i and ii
        b. ii and iii
        c. i, ii, and iii
        d. All of the above

80. Which one is not a risk factor for cisplatin-induced hearing loss?
    a. Children younger than 5 years and older adults
    b. Renal insufficiency
    c. Preexisting hearing loss or noise exposure
    d. Genetic predisposition
    e. Exposition to sodium thiosulfate
    f. Cumulative dose

CONDUCTIVE HEARING LOSS

81. Which of the following is the most common cause of progressive conductive hearing loss in adults?
    a. Paget disease
    b. Otosclerosis
    c. Osteogenesis imperfecta

d. Tympanosclerosis

e. Keratosis obturans

82. The genetic transmission of otosclerosis is which of the following?
    a. Sporadic
    b. Autosomal recessive
    c. Autosomal dominant
    d. Autosomal dominant with variable penetrance
    e. X-linked

83. In which decade is the typical onset of noticeable hearing loss for otosclerosis?
    a. First decade
    b. Second decade
    c. Third decade
    d. Fourth decade
    e. Fifth decade

84. Early lesions of otosclerosis appear in which of the following regions first?
    a. Fissula ante fenestram
    b. Cochlea
    c. Annular ligament of the footplate
    d. Posterior footplate crus
    e. Anterior footplate crus

85. What is the usual distance between the lateral surface of the incus and the footplate?
    a. 3.0 mm
    b. 3.5 mm
    c. 4.0 mm
    d. 4.25 mm
    e. 4.5 mm

86. Which of the following is not a cause of conductive deafness with preserved stapedial reflexes?
    a. Superior semicircular canal dehiscence
    b. Other third-window fistulae
    c. Otosclerosis
    d. Fracture of the stapedial arch (below the attachment of the stapedius)
    e. Malingering

87. Where is the fissula ante fenestram located?
    a. Anterior to the posterior crura of the stapes
    b. Anterior to the round window
    c. Anterior to the cochleariform process
    d. Posterior to the oval window
    e. Anterior to the oval window and posterior to the cochleariform process

88. What are the possible postoperative complications of a stapedotomy?
    i. SNHL
    ii. Vertigo
    iii. Facial paralysis
    iv. Tinnitus
    v. Taste disturbance
    vi. Tympanic membrane perforation
    vii. Perilymphatic fistula
    a. i, ii, and iii
    b. ii, iii, and iv
    c. iii, iv, and v
    d. i and ii
    e. All of the above

89. What are the possible management options for otosclerosis?
    i. Stapes surgery (total stapedectomy, partial stapedectomy, stapedotomy)
    ii. Conventional hearing aids

    iii. Osseointegrated hearing device
    iv. Cochlear implant
    v. Follow-up
    a. i and ii
    b. i, ii, and iii
    c. i, ii, iii, and iv
    d. All of the above

90. After a temporal bone trauma, where is the most common injury site to the ossicular chain?
    a. Incudostapedial joint > dislocation of the incus > fracture of the stapes crura > fixation of the ossicles in the epitympanum > fracture of the malleus
    b. Dislocation of the incus > incudostapedial joint > fracture of the stapes crura > fixation of the ossicles in the epitympanum > fracture of the malleus
    c. Fracture of the stapes crura > incudostapedial joint > dislocation of the incus > fixation of the ossicles in the epitympanum > fracture of the malleus
    d. Incudostapedial joint > fracture of the malleus > dislocation of the incus > fracture of the stapes crura > fixation of the ossicles in the epitympanum

AUDITORY PROSTHETIC STIMULATION, DEVICES, AND REHABILITATIVE AUDIOLOGY

91. Labyrinthitis ossificans can occur after meningitis, particularly when which of the following microorganisms is present?
    a. *Streptococcus pneumoniae*
    b. *Staphylococcus aureus*
    c. *Haemophilus influenzae* type B
    d. *Neisseria meningitidis*
    e. *Listeria monocytogenes*

92. Which of the following is *NOT* a cause of secondary cochlear ossification?
    a. Purulent labyrinthitis
    b. Meningitis
    c. Advanced otosclerosis
    d. Autoimmune inner ear disease
    e. Vestibular neuritis
    f. Temporal bone trauma
    g. Surgery (labyrinthectomy)

93. Absolute contraindication to cochlear implantation includes which of the following?
    i. Michel aplasia
    ii. Absence of the cochlear nerve
    iii. Absence of the vestibular nerve
    iv. Mondini malformation
    v. Auditory neuropathy
    a. i and ii
    b. i, ii, and iii
    c. i, ii, iii, and v
    d. All of the above

94. In selected patients, the use of a cochlear implant with short/hybrid electrode has resulted in improved patient word understanding, particularly in noise, as well as improved music perception. Why?
    a. Low-frequency hearing may be preserved because the typical electrode does not extend into the distal apex of the cochlea, the frequency place of low tones.

b. High-frequency hearing may be preserved because the typical electrode does not extend into the distal apex of the cochlea, the frequency place of high tones.

95. Which part is *NOT* included in the external and internal component of a cochlear implant?
    a. Microphone
    b. Condensator
    c. Speech processor
    d. Transmittor
    e. Receiver and stimulator
    f. Array of electrodes

96. Which of the following is *NOT* a risk factor for the development of meningitis in cochlear implant recipients?
    a. Age >50 years
    b. Impaired immune status
    c. Presence of other neurologic prostheses such as ventricular shunts, a cerebrospinal fluid (CSF) leak
    d. Past history of meningitis
    e. Otitis media postimplantation
    f. Preexisting cochlear malformation (with or without a CSF fistula)
    g. Latent bacterial colonization as a result of local surgical trauma
    h. Inadequate packing of the cochleostomy (allowing bacteria to spread from the middle ear into the cochlea in the case of otitis media)

97. Which of the following is *NOT* a potential indication for an osseointegrated hearing device?
    a. Congenital atresia of the ear canal
    b. Chronic infection of the external or middle ear

c. Poor localization performance with regular hearing aids
d. Allergic reactions to standard hearing aids
e. Single-sided deafness

98. The advantages of digital and programmable hearing aids over conventional analog hearing aids include all of the following *EXCEPT:*
    a. Better sound quality
    b. Increased precision
    c. Improved speech recognition
    d. Low cost
    e. Flexibility of settings

99. List the causes of feedback with regular hearing aids.
    i. Poor fit of the hearing aid
    ii. Overamplification
    iii. External ear plugged
    iv. Microphone too close to the speaker
    v. Venting too large
    a. i and ii
    b. i, iii, and v
    c. i, ii, and iv
    d. i, ii, iii, and v
    e. All of the above

100. Choose the reason(s) why speech comprehension is improved in a binaural listening condition.
    i. Binaural redundancy effects due to summation
    ii. The squelch effect (ability to tune out unwanted noise)
    iii. Limitation of the head shadow effect
    a. i
    b. ii
    c. iii
    d. All of the above

CORE KNOWLEDGE

BASIC PHYSIOLOGY OF AUDITION

- The cochlea
  - Is organized tonotopically with low frequencies at the apex and high frequencies at the base
  - This tonotopic organization of the cochlea is reiterated throughout the central auditory system.
  - At the basal turn of the cochlea is the cochlear aqueduct, a bony channel that allows communication between the perilymphatic fluid and cerebrospinal fluid of the subarachnoid space in the posterior fossa.
- Impedance
  - Impedance can be thought of as the impediment to movement.
  - It is the measure of the opposition that a system presents to an acoustic flow when an acoustic pressure is applied to it.
  - In the study of acoustics, it is defined as the ratio of the acoustic pressure over the volume velocity generated by the acoustic pressure.
  - Stiffness varies inversely with frequency and dominates the acoustic impedance at low frequencies, whereas the impedance of a mass increases with frequency and dominates at high frequencies.
- Central auditory processing
  - The main auditory portion of the cerebral cortex resides in the temporal lobe, close to the sylvian fissure.
  - In this region, the two major centers for auditory processing are the primary auditory cortex and the auditory association cortex.

- The primary auditory cortex is located on the superior surface of the temporal lobe (Heschl gyrus).
  - This is also known as area A1, and corresponds to Brodmann area 41.
- The auditory association cortex is also known as area A2, and corresponds to Brodmann areas 22 and 42.
- It has been shown that the primary auditory cortex is tonotopically tuned, with high frequencies being represented more medially, and low frequencies being represented more laterally.
- The functions of the olivocochlear efferent pathways, especially the medial olivocochlear (MOC) pathway, are:
  - To protect the ears from acoustic trauma
  - To discriminate transient sounds from background noise
- The middle ear muscle reflex is another major feedback system to the auditory periphery.
  - The stapedius and tensor tympani muscles are the target organs of the middle ear muscle reflex.
  - This contraction exerts forces perpendicular to the stapes and malleus to increase the impedance of the ossicular chain.
- External ear
  - The external auditory canal, by virtue of being a blind-ended cylinder, increases the sound pressure at the tympanic membrane relative to that of the external field.
    - The magnitude of this amplification is maximum at a specific frequency, which is the resonance frequency.

- The pressure on a membrane is defined as the force pushing on it divided by the surface area of the membrane.
  - The human tympanic membrane has a surface area approximately 20 times larger than the stapes footplate (69 vs. 3.4 mm²).
    - If all the force applied to the tympanic membrane were to be transferred to the stapes footplate, the force per unit area would be 20 times larger (26 dB) on the footplate than on the tympanic membrane.
- It is the first mechanism for impedance matching (Figure 5-1).
- The second mechanism for impedance matching is called the *lever ratio,* which refers to the difference in length of the manubrium of the malleus and the long process of the incus.
  - In humans, the lever ratio is about 1.31:1 (2.3 dB).
- The human range is commonly given as 20 to 20,000 Hz, although there is considerable variation between individuals.

CONGENITAL HEARING LOSS

- Although autosomal recessive SNHL is heterogeneous, mutations in the connexin 26 *(GJB2)* gene at the DFNB1 (chromosome 13) locus contribute about half of all hereditary cases in Australia, the United States, Israel, and many European countries (Figure 5-2).
- High concentrations of aminoglycoside antibiotics interfere with the normal function of the cochlea. Individuals with an A1555G mutation in their mitochondrial 12S rRNA gene are more susceptible to the ototoxic effect of these drugs.
- Perilymphatic gusher X-linked mixed hearing loss is a disease caused by a mutation on the chromosome X that affects males.
  - It is a mutation in a DNA-binding regulatory gene known as *POU3F4.*
  - It is characterized by:
    - Profound SNHL, with or without a conductive element
    - Unique developmental abnormality of the inner ear
    - Congenital fixation of the stapes with perilymphatic gusher on attempted stapedectomy
- Congenital CMV
  - It is the most common intrauterine infection in humans as well as the leading infectious cause of congenital sensorineural deafness.
  - It may represent up to 20% of all nonsyndromic cases.
  - Eighty-five percent to 90% of newborns with congenital CMV infection present with asymptomatic infection.

- Of those, 6% to 25% will either present with or develop SNHL later in life.
- Diagnosis after 3 weeks of life is made by detection of CMV DNA in the dried blood spots used for newborn screening.

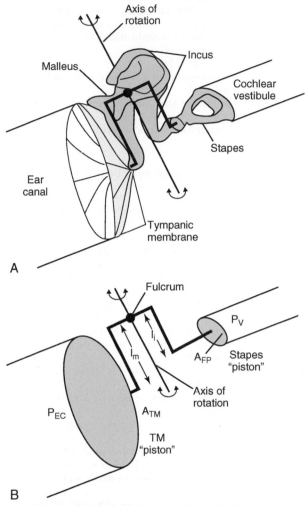

FIGURE 5-1 Schematic of the middle ear system. **A,** Motion of the ossicular chain along its axis of rotation. **B,** Area of the tympanic membrane (A_{TM}) divided by area of the footplate (A_{FP}) represents the *area ratio* (A_{TM}/A_{FP}). The length of the manubrium (l_m) divided by the length of the incus long process (l_i) is the *lever ratio* (l_m/l_i). P_{EC}, External canal sound pressure; P_V, sound pressure of the vestibule; *TM,* Tympanic membrane. (From Merchant SN, Rosowski JJ. *Auditory physiology.* In: Glasscock ME, Gulya AJ, eds. *Glasscock-Shambaugh Surgery of the Ear.* 5th ed. Ontario, Canada: Decker; 2003:64.)

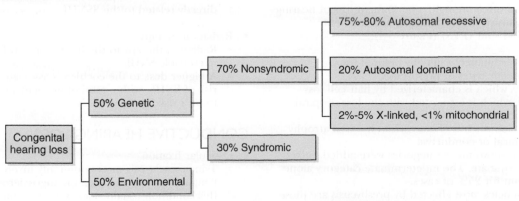

FIGURE 5-2 Incidence of different forms of congenital hearing loss.

- Before 3 weeks of life, the diagnosis can be made by:
  - Culture of the virus in urine or saliva
  - PCR detection of the CMV DNA in urine or serum of the newborn
- The prevalence of congenital SNHL among babies with low birth weight (>1500 g) is at least 51 per 10,000. This high rate of hearing loss has been linked to several factors, including administration of ototoxic drugs, such as aminoglycoside antibiotics; ambient noise produced by the incubator; and perinatal complications (e.g., hypoxia, acidosis, and hyperbilirubinemia).
- AN/AD is characterized by:
  - Detectable otoacoustic emissions and/or cochlear microphonics.
  - Abnormal or absent auditory brainstem responses and deficient speech understanding
  - Inconsistent cognitive responses with a behavioral tone audiogram

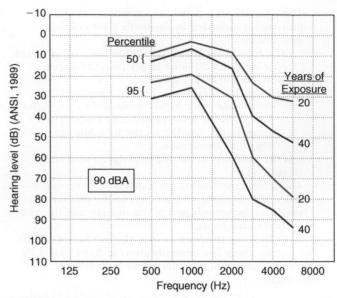

FIGURE 5-3 Predicted hearing thresholds (median and extreme values) after 20 years and 40 years of occupational noise exposure at 90 dBA. *ANSI,* American National Standards Institute. (From Dobie RA. *Medical-Legal Evaluation of Hearing Loss.* New York: Van Nostrand Reinhold; 1993.)

SENSORINEURAL HEARING LOSS

- NIHL
  - A permanent SNHL with damage principally to cochlear hair cells, primarily to outer hair cells (OHCs)
  - History of long-term exposure to dangerous noise levels (i.e., >85 dBA for 8 hours/day) is sufficient to cause the degree and pattern of hearing loss described by audiologic findings.
  - Gradual loss of hearing over the first 5 to 10 years of exposure
  - Hearing loss that involves initially the higher frequencies, from 3 to 8 kHz, before including frequencies of 2 kHz or less
  - The corresponding hearing loss is classically described as the "4-kHz notch."
  - Speech-recognition scores consistent with the audiometric loss
  - Hearing loss that stabilizes after the noise exposure is terminated
  - In the United States, the Occupational Safety and Health Administration (OSHA) has set standards and guidelines for noise exposure in order to protect workers.
    - All employees who are exposed to ≥85 dB on average must be enrolled in a hearing conservation program and provided with hearing protection equipment.
  - Most hazardous noise exposure produces a temporary SNHL that recovers over the next 24 to 48 hours.
    - This reversible loss is termed a temporary threshold shift (TTS).
    - If the noise is of high enough intensity or is repeated often enough, a permanent loss of hearing results, which is referred to as a permanent threshold shift (PTS) (Figure 5-3).
- Presbycusis
  - Gacek and Schuknecht initially defined four histopathologic types of presbycusis:
    - Sensory, which is characterized by hair cell loss
    - Neural, which is associated with the loss of spiral ganglion cells and axons
    - Metabolic, which is characterized by strial atrophy
    - Mechanical or conductive
  - Subsequently, two more categories were added: mixed and indeterminate. The indeterminate category alone may account for 25% of cases.
  - The frequencies most affected by presbycusis are those above 2 kHz.

- With progression of the disease, the high frequencies will continue to drop, and the middle and low frequencies (0.5 to 2 kHz), associated with human speech, also become progressively involved.
- The low to middle frequencies of human speech include most of the vowel information of words.
- It is the high frequencies, however, that carry the consonant sounds, and therefore the majority of speech information.
  - These consonant sounds become particularly difficult for patients with presbycusis to hear and understand.
- As a result of their hearing loss pattern, patients with high-frequency hearing loss will often report being able to hear when someone is speaking (from the louder, low-frequency vowels), but not being able to understand what is being said (due to the loss of consonant information).
- SSNHL
  - Magnetic resonance imaging (MRI) has the added advantage of identifying other causes of SSNHL (e.g., cochlear inflammation or multiple sclerosis) or findings that imply an underlying etiology for the SSNHL.
  - The overall rate of pathogenic MRI abnormalities directly related to the SSNHL ranges from 7% to 13.75%.
- Radiation therapy
  - Radiation therapy to the inner ear may lead to irreversible SNHL.
  - A higher dose to the cochlea is associated with a higher risk of SNHL, with a minimum cochlear dose reported to be a risk factor of 45 Gy.

CONDUCTIVE HEARING LOSS

- Ossicular fixation
  - Tympanosclerosis most commonly involves the tympanic membrane (i.e., myringosclerosis). However, this condition usually does not have much of an adverse effect on hearing.

Classification	Component	Disrupted Expected Loss
Table 5-1 Specific Lesions of the Conductive Apparatus and the Associated Hearing Loss		
Perforation of tympanic membrane	Loss of areal ratio, catenary lever	Proportional to size of perforation
Perforation of tympanic membrane with ossicular interruption	Hydraulic lever, areal ratio, catenary lever	38.3 dB
Total loss of tympanic membrane and ossicular chain	Hydraulic lever, areal ratio, catenary lever, phase cancellation	50 dB
Ossicular interruption with an intact tympanic membrane	Hydraulic lever, areal ratio, catenary lever, phase cancellation, reflection of sound energy away from middle ear at the tympanic membrane	55-60 dB
Ossicular interruption with an intact tympanic membrane and closure of the oval window (distinct congenital malformation)	Hydraulic lever, areal ratio, catenary lever, phase cancellation, reflection of sound energy away from middle ear at the tympanic membrane	55-60 dB

Data from Austin DF. Sound conduction of the diseased ear. *J Laryngol Otol.* 1978;92:367; and Austin DF. Acoustic mechanisms of middle ear sound transfer. *Otolaryngol Clin North Am.* 1994;27:641.

- Significant conductive hearing loss caused by tympanosclerosis is usually a result of the fixation of the ossicles in the middle ear or epitympanum.
- It can be suspected as the cause of conductive hearing loss when there is a history of chronic infections or when tympanosclerosis is seen on the tympanic membrane.
- Bony fixation of the ossicles can also occur as a result of infection, surgical trauma, or temporal bone fracture, or as a congenital anomaly.
- Otosclerosis
  - It is a disease of bone that is unique to the otic capsule.
  - It may cause a conductive hearing loss, a mixed conductive-SNHL, or occasionally a pure SNHL.
  - The most common area for stapedial fixation in otosclerosis is the fissula ante fenestram.
  - It is an autosomal-dominant hereditary disease with variable penetrance and expression.
  - Two-thirds of patients are women.
- Temporal bone trauma
  - Temporal bone trauma can cause conductive, sensorineural, or mixed hearing loss.
  - Otic capsule–sparing fractures extend along the roof of the EAC, often tearing the tympanic membrane in the region of the notch of Rivinus.
    - In 20% of patients, it disrupts the ossicular chain.
  - The most common injuries to the ossicular chain are separation of the incudostapedial joint (82%), dislocation of the incus (57%), and fracture of the stapes crura (30%).
  - Fixation of the ossicles in the epitympanum (25%) and fracture of the malleus (11%) occur less frequently.
- Specific lesions of the conductive apparatus and associated hearing loss (Table 5-1)
- Superior semicircular canal dehiscence (SSCD)
  - The key differences with otosclerosis are the conductive *hyperacusis* and the presence of acoustic stapedial reflex in patients with SSCD.
  - Key signs and symptoms are autophony, Tullio phenomenon, Hennebert sign.
  - Diagnostic evaluation includes a good history and physical examination, temporal bone computed tomography (formatted in the plane of the superior canal), and vestibular evoked myogenic potential (VEMP).

AUDITORY PROSTHETIC STIMULATION, DEVICES, AND REHABILITATIVE AUDIOLOGY

- Speech comprehension in quiet and in noise is improved in a binaural listening condition for three reasons:
  - Binaural redundancy effects due to summation
    - Brain receives some redundant information from each ear and can draw more meaningful acoustic information from those two sources than it could from a single ear's input.
  - The squelch effect
  - Reduction of the head shadow effect
    - Ability to help localize sound and also to eliminate background noise
  - In the context of bilateral cochlear implants, we note better speech comprehension in noise, better sound localization, and improved ease of listening.
- Cochlear implant
  - The selection criteria include severe to profound bilateral SNHL and little or no benefit from hearing aid use after 6 months.
  - Cochlear implant devices are approved by the US Food and Drug Administration (FDA) for use in children as young as 12 months, although off-label use has occurred for infants less than 12 months old. Criteria for candidacy for a cochlear implant device include (1) severe to profound bilateral SNHL; (2) medical clearance to undergo general anesthesia; (3) family support, motivation, and appropriate expectations; (4) rehabilitation and educational support for the development of aural language, speech, and hearing; and (5) expectation that the benefits of a cochlear implant will be greater than those of a hearing aid.
  - Low-frequency hearing may be preserved because the typical electrode does not extend into the distal apex of the cochlea, the frequency place of low tones.
  - Use of a short/hybrid electrode has resulted in improved patient word understanding, particularly in noise, as well as improved music perception.
  - Children with cochlear implants are at increased risk for meningitis, particularly pneumococcal meningitis.
- Hearing aid
  - Electronic circuitry of hearing aid can be analog, digital, or digitally programmable.
  - The advantages of digital and programmable hearing aids over conventional analog hearing aids include

better sound quality, increased precision, improved speech recognition, and flexibility of settings.
- Open-canal fittings are especially useful for high-frequency hearing loss.
  - Low-frequency sound is free to pass through the ear canal in an unobstructed manner, permitting natural hearing in the lower frequencies.

- Osseointegrated hearing device
  - Potential indications include:
    - Congenital atresia of the ear canal such that it does not exist or cannot accommodate a standard hearing aid (provided that the nerve is functional)
    - Chronic infection of the external or middle ear
    - Allergic reactions to standard hearing aids
    - Single-sided deafness

ANSWERS

TRUE OR FALSE QUESTIONS

1. F	14. F	27. T	40. T
2. T	15. F	28. T	41. F
3. F	16. F	29. T	42. F
4. T	17. F	30. T	43. T
5. T	18. T	31. T	44. T
6. T	19. T	32. T	45. T
7. T	20. T	33. F	46. T
8. T	21. F	34. F	47. T
9. T	22. T	35. F	48. T
10. T	23. F	36. T	49. F
11. T	24. T	37. F	50. T
12. F	25. F	38. T	
13. T	26. T	39. T	

SINGLE BEST ANSWER QUESTIONS

51. c	64. d	77. e	90. a
52. d	65. b	78. d	91. b
53. b	66. a	79. d	92. e
54. b	67. e	80. e	93. a
55. e	68. c	81. b	94. a
56. d	69. a	82. d	95. b
57. e	70. b	83. c	96. a
58. c	71. d	84. a	97. c
59. a	72. a	85. e	98. d
60. a	73. a	86. c	99. e
61. e	74. e	87. e	100. d
62. b	75. c	88. e	
63. c	76. j	89. d	

SUGGESTED READINGS

1. Guinan JJ Jr. Olivocochlear efferents: anatomy, physiology, function, and the measurement of efferent effects in humans. *Ear Hear.* 2006;27:589-607.
2. Brown MC, Santos-Sacchi J. Audition. In: Squire L, Bloom F, Spitzer N, eds. *Fundamental Neuroscience.* New York: Academic Press; 2008:609-636.
3. Dempster JH, Mackenzie K. The resonance frequency of the external auditory canal in children. *Ear Hear.* 1990; 11(4):296-298.
4. Chan DK, Chang KW. GJB2-associated hearing loss: systematic review of worldwide prevalence, genotype, and auditory phenotype. *Laryngoscope.* 2014;124(2):E34-E53.
5. Lammens F, Verhaert N, Devriendt K, Debruyne F, Desloovere C. Aetiology of congenital hearing loss. *Int J Pediatr Otorhinolaryngol.* 2013;77(9):1385-1391.
6. Duval M, Park AH. Congenital cytomegalovirus: what the otolaryngologist should know. *Curr Opin Otolaryngol Head Neck Surg.* 2014;22(6):495-500.
7. Kirchner DB, Evenson E, Dobie RA, et al. Occupational noise-induced hearing loss: ACOEM Task Force on Occupational Hearing Loss. *J Occup Environ Med.* 2012; 54(1):106-108.
8. Wegner I, Kamalski DM, Tange RA, et al. Laser versus conventional fenestration in stapedotomy for otosclerosis: a systematic review. *Laryngoscope.* 2014;124(7):1687-1693.
9. Yetiser S, Hidir Y, Karatas E, Karapinar U. Management of tympanosclerosis with ossicular fixation: review and presentation of long-term results of 30 new cases. *J Otolaryngol.* 2007;36(5):303-308.
10. Van Abel KM, Dunn CC, Sladen DP, et al. Hearing preservation among patients undergoing cochlear implantation. *Otol Neurotol.* 2015;36(3):416-421.

Cholesteatoma

6

Shawn M. Stevens | William W. Carroll

TRUE OR FALSE QUESTIONS

CLINICAL PRESENTATION AND RELEVANT ANATOMY

T/F 1. In a chronically infected ear with an aural polyp, the presence of cholesteatoma should be assumed until proven otherwise.

T/F 2. Males are three times more likely to have congenital cholesteatoma than females.

T/F 3. Laboratory testing provides little to no utility in making a diagnosis of cholesteatoma.

T/F 4. Both smoking and repeated microtrauma are risk factors for external auditory canal cholesteatoma.

T/F 5. Congenital cholesteatoma is usually diagnosed in late childhood or early adolescence.

T/F 6. The majority of attic retraction pockets will eventually develop clinical evidence of cholesteatoma based on their natural history.

T/F 7. If complicated by recalcitrant infections, a cholesteatoma may have developed an infectious colonization that is capable of quiescence and resistance to antibiotics.

T/F 8. A superinfected cholesteatoma may be more prone to aggressive bone erosion than a cholesteatoma that is not superinfected.

T/F 9. A cholesteatoma arising from a posterior pars tensa retraction pocket is capable of extending through the aditus ad antrum into the mastoid.

T/F 10. The anterior pouch of von Troeltsch is a route via which an attic cholesteatoma may extend to involve the sinus tympani.

T/F 11. An anterior epitympanic cholesteatoma may cause facial nerve dysfunction via compression of the second genu.

T/F 12. Persistent negative middle ear pressures would be most likely to cause a retraction of the posterior pars tensa as compared with other locations of the tympanic membrane.

T/F 13. Cholesteatoma has similar pathophysiologic behavior in both children and adults.

IMAGING

T/F 14. Dedicated temporal bone computed tomography (CT) is not indicated or necessary in cases of recidivistic cholesteatoma.

T/F 15. Diffusion-weighted magnetic resonance imaging (MRI) is more sensitive and specific than CT in the imaging of primary acquired cholesteatoma.

T/F 16. In many cases, diffusion-weighted MRI may replace second-look surgery in surveillance of recurrent cholesteatoma.

HISTOPATHOLOGY

T/F 17. Histopathologically, cholesteatoma has the appearance of grouped cholesterol crystals surrounded by thin, dense stroma and a pseudoepithelial rind.

T/F 18. Immunofluorescent staining of the squamous epithelium surrounding a cholesteatoma will demonstrate strong avidity for antibodies against epidermal growth factor receptor (EGFR).

T/F 19. Osteoclasts and fibroblasts found within a cholesteatoma-filled middle ear are phenotypically different from similar cells found in a healthy middle ear.

T/F 20. A finding of mixed anaerobic bacterial species within the keratin debris of a cholesteatoma would be unusual.

T/F 21. The histologic layer of cholesteatoma that directly borders adjacent bony structures within the middle ear and mastoid is termed the *matrix*.

PATHOPHYSIOLOGY AND THEORY

T/F 22. When a cholesteatoma becomes infected, the two most common organisms involved are *Staphylococcus aureus* and *Pseudomonas aeruginosa*.

T/F 23. A central tympanic membrane perforation is a common location for primary acquired cholesteatoma to form.

T/F 24. Both direct pressure as well as enzymatic activation of osteoclastic activity are thought to contribute to bony erosion secondary to cholesteatoma.

T/F 25. Secondary acquired cholesteatoma results from a retraction pocket.

T/F 26. The greater rate of recidivism in pediatric cholesteatoma is thought to be a result of increased eustachian tube dysfunction.

T/F 27. The natural migratory pathway for epidermal slough from the tympanic membrane is in a radial, outward direction from a point centered at the umbo.

T/F 28. Osteolytic enzymes have been shown to decrease when a cholesteatoma becomes secondarily infected.

T/F 29. Pressure-induced osteoclastic proliferation is the principal mechanism underlying the erosion of bone juxtaposed to cholesteatoma.

T/F 30. Primary acquired cholesteatoma may form medial to an intact tympanic membrane.

MANAGEMENT

T/F 31. A radical canal wall down (CWD) mastoidectomy is a procedure that preserves the middle ear space.

T/F 32. The primary goal of cholesteatoma surgery is to restore hearing to precholesteatoma thresholds.

T/F 33. Hearing outcomes are significantly better with canal wall up mastoidectomy versus CWD mastoidectomy.

T/F 34. Patients who refuse surgery for cholesteatoma should undergo regular cleaning in an effort to slow progression of disease.

T/F 35. In the event of a facial nerve injury in cholesteatoma surgery, the first step should be to decompress the nerve for a few millimeters on either side of the injury.

T/F 36. The major advantage of CWD surgery for cholesteatoma is the preservation of the normal anatomy of the external ear.

T/F 37. The choice of how to manage cholesteatoma surgically is dependent on many factors, including the extent of disease, patient reliability, hearing status of both ears, and experience of the surgeon.

T/F 38. The primary goal of cholesteatoma surgery is to create a safe, dry ear with complete eradication of disease.

T/F 39. After an intact canal wall (ICW) mastoidectomy for cholesteatoma, the purpose of a second-look procedure is primarily to restore hearing.

T/F 40. A CWD approach affords better visualization of the sinus tympani when compared with ICW mastoidectomy.

T/F 41. Hearing outcomes are generally the same following reconstruction regardless of whether an ICW or CWD approach is utilized.

T/F 42. Antibiotic coverage of superinfected cholesteatoma should include either a second-generation quinolone or a third-generation cephalosporin to cover both aerobic and anaerobic organisms.

T/F 43. Cholesteatoma discovered in an only hearing ear would best be treated with an ICW mastoidectomy so as to better preserve hearing in that ear.

T/F 44. The type of material utilized for ossicular chain reconstruction significantly affects hearing outcomes in ears damaged by cholesteatoma.

T/F 45. The ideal timing for a second-look procedure in surveillance of cholesteatoma and/or hearing restoration is 12 to 18 months.

T/F 46. Failure to lower the facial ridge will often result in surgical failure to obtain a dry ear and necessitate revision mastoidectomy following a CWD approach.

T/F 47. Radical mastoidectomy is synonymous with the Bondy procedure.

T/F 48. Otoendoscopy may be utilized during both primary and second-look procedures to prevent recurrent/residual disease.

CONGENITAL CHOLESTEATOMA

T/F 49. Congenital cholesteatomas are most commonly found in the posterior/superior epitympanum.

T/F 50. A 6-year-old boy presents with an opaque mass medial to the anterior 50% of an entirely intact tympanic membrane. He has never had otorrhea, otologic trauma, perforation, or surgery. He does have a history of six or seven cases of acute otitis media over the last 2 years treated with antibiotics. Assuming that this is not some other pathologic process, a clinical diagnosis of congenital cholesteatoma can be reached in this case.

SINGLE BEST ANSWER QUESTIONS

CLINICAL PRESENTATION AND RELEVANT ANATOMY

51. Labyrinthine fistulas secondary to cholesteatoma most commonly occur in which area?
    a. Cochlea
    b. Horizontal semicircular canal
    c. Oval window
    d. Superior semicircular canal

52. What structure(s) constitute the floor of Prussak space?
    a. Lateral process of the malleus and associated folds
    b. Chorda tympani
    c. Manubrium
    d. Space of von Troeltsch

53. Which of the following are the two most important tools in diagnosing cholesteatoma?
    a. Otoscopy and radiographic imaging
    b. History and culture data
    c. Audiometry and otoscopy
    d. Radiography and audiometry
    e. Physical examination and patient demographics

54. What is the most common presentation of an external auditory canal cholesteatoma?
    a. Unilateral otorrhea and otalgia
    b. Conductive hearing loss
    c. Conductive hearing loss with otorrhea
    d. Otalgia and aural fullness
    e. Otalgia and conductive hearing loss

55. The cog separates which of the following two structures?
    a. The scutum and the chorda tympani
    b. The sinus tympani and the pyramidal process
    c. Neck of the malleus and the pars flaccida
    d. Anterior epitympanum and posterior epitympanum
    e. None of the above

56. Vertigo and nystagmus in the setting of cholesteatoma are concerning for which of the following?
    a. Labyrinthine fistula
    b. Meningitis
    c. Brain abscess
    d. Sigmoid sinus thrombosis
    e. Superior semicircular canal dehiscence

57. An anterior epitympanic cholesteatoma would most likely threaten which of the following structures?
    a. Supratubal recess and scutum
    b. Second genu and sinus tympani
    c. Facial recess and sinus tympani
    d. Geniculate ganglion and supratubal recess
    e. None of the above

58. A middle ear filled with cholesteatoma via an attic retraction would mostly likely present with which of the following on tympanometry?
    a. Shallow pressure peak within the normal range, large volume
    b. Dynamic pressure peak within the normal range, normal volume
    c. Flat pressure curve, normal volume
    d. Flat pressure curve, restricted volume
    e. Tympanometry would be difficult to perform in a patient with extensive middle ear cholesteatoma.

59. All of the following are reasons that cholesteatoma should be managed surgically, even in early presentations of the disease, *EXCEPT:*
    a. Propensity of cholesteatoma to progressively erode structures within the middle ear space
    b. Propensity of cholesteatoma to form biofilms resistant to medical therapies
    c. Tendency of cholesteatoma to cause early cranial nerve VII palsy
    d. Risk of progressive hearing loss in unchecked disease
    e. All of the above are reasons for surgical management.

60. Which of the following structures within the middle ear does *NOT* play a significant role in limiting the predictable spread of cholesteatoma?
    a. Promontory
    b. Tympanic diaphragm
    c. Lateral mallear fold
    d. Incus body
    e. Malleus head

61. Which of the following is the second most common location for primary acquired cholesteatoma?
    a. Anterior pars tensa
    b. Inferior pars tensa
    c. Posterior pouch of von Troeltsch
    d. Anterior pouch of von Troeltsch
    e. Posterior pars tensa

62. The most common route for a posterior epitympanic cholesteatoma to reach the sinus tympani would be which of the following?
    a. Prussak space > posterior pouch of von Troeltsch > posterior mesotympanum > sinus tympani
    b. Prussak space > anterior pouch of von Troeltsch > anterior mesotympanum > sinus tympani
    c. Prussak space > superior incudal space > aditus ad antrum > sinus tympani
    d. Superior incudal space > posterior pouch of von Troeltsch > facial recess > sinus tympani

63. Shrapnell membrane is structurally distinct for which of the following reasons?
    a. As the only interossicular membrane in the middle ear, it has vibroelastic properties.
    b. Its pseudoepithelium is permeable to gas transfer.
    c. It is stabilized circumferentially by a thick, fibrous annulus.
    d. It lacks a central fibrous connective tissue layer.
    e. It is highly resistant to the propagation of cholesteatoma.

IMAGING

64. Which of the following best describes MRI imaging characteristics of cholesteatoma?
    a. Iso/hypointense on T1, intermediate/hyperintensity on T2, no contrast enhancement, no restriction on diffusion-weighted MRI
    b. Iso/hypointense on T1, hypointensity on T2, no contrast enhancement, no restriction on diffusion-weighted MRI
    c. Iso/hypointense on T1, hypointensity on T2, no contrast enhancement, restriction on diffusion-weighted MRI
    d. Hyperintensity on T1, intermediate/hyperintensity on T2, no contrast enhancement, no restriction on diffusion-weighted MRI
    e. Iso/hypointense on T1, intermediate/hyperintensity on T2, no contrast enhancement, restriction on diffusion-weighted MRI

65. In addition to cholesteatoma, diffusion-weighted MRI will also demonstrate increased signal intensity from which of the following?
    a. Cholesterol granuloma
    b. Mucoid secretions
    c. Granulation tissue
    d. Serous effusion
    e. None of the above

66. In the workup of primary acquired cholesteatoma, dedicated temporal bone CT provides the surgeon with excellent:
    a. Diagnostic sensitivity
    b. Diagnostic specificity
    c. Positive predictive value
    d. Negative predictive value
    e. None of the above

HISTOPATHOLOGY

67. Which of the following would *NOT* potentially be a histopathologic finding within a middle ear filled with cholesteatoma?
    a. Activated osteoclasts with evidence of bone erosion
    b. Keratin debris surrounded by a keratinizing pseudoepithelial matrix
    c. Bacterial biofilm formation harboring Gram-negative rods
    d. Papillary proliferation of epithelial cones through the basilar layers of the tympanic membrane
    e. Papillary proliferation of epithelial cones into the epineurium of the chorda tympani nerve

68. The most common organisms found to infect cholesteatomas are which of the following?
    a. Gram-negative cocci
    b. Gram-positive rods
    c. Acid-fast bacilli
    d. Gram-negative rods
    e. Yeast exhibiting septate hyphae branching at 45-degree angles

69. The histopathologic layers of a cholesteatoma, in order from innermost to outermost, are:
    a. Concentrically layered keratin debris, matrix, perimatrix, inflammatory infiltrate
    b. Concentrically layered keratin debris, perimatrix, matrix, inflammatory infiltrate
    c. Matrix, perimatrix, concentrically layered keratin debris, inflammatory infiltrate
    d. Matrix, perimatrix, inflammatory infiltrate, concentrically layered keratin debris

PATHOPHYSIOLOGY

70. Which of the following is *NOT* a theory describing the formation of cholesteatoma?
    a. Invagination of a retraction pocket of the tympanic membrane
    b. Basal cell hyperplasia
    c. Hypoxia-mediated fibrosis of keratin emboli
    d. Squamous metaplasia of middle ear epithelium
    e. Epithelial migration through a perforation

71. A retraction pocket arising from which of the following locations would be most likely to give rise to cholesteatoma involving the sinus tympani?
    a. Attic/Prussak space
    b. Anterior epitympanum
    c. Posterior mesotympanum
    d. Posterior, inferior external auditory canal

72. Which of the following is *NOT* a classification of cholesteatoma?
    a. Primary
    b. Secondary
    c. Tertiary
    d. Congenital
    e. Acquired

73. "Contact inhibition" refers to which of the following?
    a. The halting of epithelial migration in response to contacting another epithelial surface
    b. Inhibition of normal epithelial migration secondary to a tympanostomy tube
    c. The halting of epithelial migration in response to hypoxia
    d. Microangiopathic change secondary to smoking
    e. Facial nerve dysfunction secondary to cholesteatoma

74. Which of the following is an important feature that distinguishes cholesteatoma from neoplastic disease?
    a. Propensity for invasive growth and bone erosion
    b. Vulnerability to superinfection
    c. Lack of genetic instability
    d. Loss of response to cell-signaling mechanisms
    e. None of the above

75. Which combination of temporal bone subsite and ossification pattern is thought to be most resistant to the pressure-induced erosive effects of cholesteatoma?
    a. Petrous air cells, intramembranous ossification
    b. Otic capsule structures, intracartilaginous ossification
    c. Tympanic portion, intramembranous ossification
    d. Mastoid portion, intracartilaginous ossification
    e. Otic capsule structures, intramembranous ossification

76. Which pathoetiologic theory regarding primary acquired cholesteatoma formation is backed by the *LEAST* amount of clinical and histopathologic evidence?
    a. Retraction theory
    b. Papillary proliferation theory
    c. Immigration theory
    d. Metaplasia theory

77. Which of the following bacterial organisms have been shown to be capable of biofilm formation within cholesteatoma keratin debris?
    a. *Pseudomonas*
    b. *Staphylococcus*
    c. *Haemophilus*
    d. All of the above
    e. None of the above

MANAGEMENT

78. Which of the following is *NOT* a subclassification of mastoidectomy typically utilized in the removal of cholesteatoma?
    a. Retrograde mastoidectomy
    b. Modified radical mastoidectomy
    c. Firstenburg approach
    d. Bondy procedure

79. Which of the following is *NOT* a relative contraindication to canal wall up mastoidectomy?
    a. Labyrinthine fistula
    b. Operated ear is the only hearing ear.
    c. Significant posterior-superior canal wall defect
    d. Autoimmune disease

80. Removal of cholesteatoma from the stapes is often done last, and dissection should be parallel to which of the following structures?
    a. Tensor tympani tendon
    b. Stapedial tendon
    c. Tympanic segment of the facial nerve
    d. Sinus tympani

81. Intracranial complications, as well as death, are now uncommon complications of cholesteatoma due to all of the following *EXCEPT:*
    a. Earlier disease recognition
    b. Timely surgical intervention
    c. Increased antibiotic usage
    d. Decreasing patient comorbidities

82. Disadvantages of CWD mastoidectomy include all the following *EXCEPT:*
    a. Hearing aids may be difficult to fit postoperatively.
    b. Need for regular cleaning of defect created
    c. Higher rate of residual/recurrent disease
    d. Low tolerance for water exposure postoperatively

83. Where is the most common site of facial nerve injury in cholesteatoma surgery?
    a. At the second genu adjacent to the horizontal semicircular canal
    b. Tympanic segment above the oval window
    c. Distal vertical segment near the digastric ridge
    d. Perigeniculate region
    e. None of the above

84. A radical mastoidectomy involves which of the following?
    a. Reconstruction of the canal wall
    b. Reconstruction of the middle ear
    c. Plugging of the eustachian tube
    d. Preservation of the incus

85. Which of the following antibiotic choices would be the *LEAST* likely to adequately cover organisms known to superinfect cholesteatoma?
    a. Third-generation cephalosporin
    b. Second-generation macrolide
    c. Second-generation quinolone
    d. All of the above would provide adequate coverage.

86. Which of the following is a preoperative indication for performing CWD mastoidectomy during an initial procedure intended to eradicate cholesteatoma?
    a. Only hearing ear
    b. Child heavily active in water sports
    c. History of four to six bouts of acute otitis media in 1 year suggesting superinfection of the cholesteatoma
    d. Highly reliable patient with whom long-term follow-up is not a concern

87. Which of the following does *NOT* seem to influence hearing outcomes following surgery for removal of cholesteatoma?
    a. Integrity of the stapes suprastructure
    b. Depth of the middle ear cleft
    c. Choice of surgical approach
    d. Health of the middle ear mucosa

88. Which of the following intraoperative findings would *NOT* lead a surgeon to proceed with CWD mastoidectomy?
    a. Significant posterior canal erosion
    b. Cholesteatoma covering a large horizontal semicircular canal fistula
    c. Low tegmen and anterior sigmoid sinus
    d. Extensive mesotympanic disease

89. When performing a CWD mastoidectomy, which of the following is *NOT* a necessary step in order to obtain a successful outcome?
    a. Lowering the facial ridge
    b. Adequate meatoplasty
    c. Eradication of diseased air cells
    d. Contouring the canal to the mastoid bowl
    e. Occluding the eustachian tube

90. Which of the following would best distinguish a radical mastoidectomy procedure?
    a. Ossicular chain reconstruction using a total ossicular replacement prosthesis
    b. Creation of a wide meatoplasty
    c. Lowering of the facial ridge
    d. Canaloplasty
    e. Occlusion of the eustachian tube

91. All of the following are critical steps in a radical mastoidectomy *EXCEPT*:
    a. Removal of the ossicles
    b. Middle ear obliteration
    c. Plugging of the eustachian tube
    d. Removal of the tympanic membrane remnant
    e. CWD mastoidectomy

92. In which of the following cases would the Bondy procedure best be employed?
    a. Cholesteatoma in the posterior recesses
    b. Isolated cholesteatoma in the posterior meso-tympanum
    c. Isolated cholesteatoma in the epitympanum
    d. Anterior mesotympanic cholesteatoma
    e. Cases necessitating a CWD procedure

93. During an initial surgery for an extensive cholesteatoma that involved the ossicular chain and surrounding structures, you were able to clear all visible disease. At the time of a second-look procedure, where would be the most likely location you would expect to find recidivistic disease?
    a. Facial recess
    b. Stapes head
    c. Supratubal recess
    d. Sinus tympani
    e. Hypotympanic air cells

94. While peeling up cholesteatoma from a canal wall up mastoid cavity, you noticed a faint blue structure within the bone near the mastoid antrum. Which of the following is the next thing you should do?
    a. Abort the procedure.
    b. Determine the extent of what you are seeing before proceeding.
    c. Leave the cholesteatoma and convert to a CWD.
    d. Remove all cholesteatoma.
    e. All of the above would be reasonable next steps.

95. During a CWD procedure, you note that the patient has a very low tegmen and an anterior sigmoid sinus. Which of the following is most accurate regarding mastoid obliteration in such a patient?
    a. It would be a good idea, because this bowl would be difficult to clean.
    b. It would be necessary, because the facial ridge will likely be higher than normal.
    c. It would be easily achieved due to the small volume.
    d. It would be dangerous given the proximity of the sigmoid.

CONGENITAL CHOLESTEATOMA

96. By definition, a patient with congenital cholesteatoma meets all of the following criteria *EXCEPT*:
    a. Conductive hearing loss
    b. No prior otologic surgery
    c. No otorrhea
    d. An intact tympanic membrane

97. Congenital cholesteatoma is theorized to form secondary to failure to involute of which of the following structures?
    a. Squamoid formation
    b. Epidermoid formation
    c. Keratinoblast rest
    d. None of the above

98. What percentage of middle ear congenital cholesteatomas are found in the anterior superior quadrant?
    a. >60%
    b. 30% to 60%
    c. 15% to 30%
    d. <15%

99. All of the following support a diagnosis of congenital cholesteatoma *EXCEPT*:
    a. Whitish mass in anterior superior quadrant of mesotympanum
    b. Intact tympanic membrane
    c. No history of otorrhea
    d. An intact ossicular chain
    e. No prior otologic surgery

100. Which statement is *INCORRECT* with regard to congenital cholesteatoma?
    a. There is male predominance.
    b. It may involve the ossicular chain.
    c. It may extend to involve the mastoid.
    d. It may be associated with prior history of acute otitis media.
    e. Recurrence rates are typically higher than those seen with primary acquired cholesteatoma.

CORE KNOWLEDGE

CLINICAL PRESENTATION

- Cholesteatoma may develop in the middle ear, mastoid, and/or petrous apex.
- The exact incidence is unknown, but cholesteatoma is encountered frequently in both children and adults.
- Cholesteatomas are grouped into the following categories: (1) congenital and (2) acquired.
- Acquired cholesteatoma may be primary (Figure 6-1) or secondary.
- A number of theories exist regarding the origins of primary acquired cholesteatoma. These are discussed later.
- Secondary acquired cholesteatoma describes traumatically/iatrogenically introduced disease.
- Diagnosis of acquired cholesteatoma is made via direct otoscopic visualization, in either the clinic or surgical suite.
- Imaging plays an adjunct role but is not considered to be a definitive diagnostic modality. Temporal bone imaging is recommended in cases of recurrent cholesteatoma.
- Symptoms of cholesteatoma vary, ranging from asymptomatic to a painful, draining ear with hearing loss.
- Secondary infection of cholesteatoma typically leads to pain and malodorous otorrhea. For this reason, a misdiagnosis of otitis externa is sometimes made. Thorough examination including microscopic otoscopy and canal debridement are mandatory, because cholesteatoma may not be evident during an acute infectious flare-up.
- Cholesteatoma may cause extensive erosion and destruction of temporal bone structures if left unchecked. Symptoms of advanced cholesteatoma may include vertigo with hearing loss (labyrinthine fistula), facial nerve paralysis, and conductive hearing loss (ossicular chain disruption).
- Infection of cholesteatoma can lead to severe complications, including mastoiditis, abscess formation, suppurative labyrinthitis, sigmoid sinus thrombosis, meningitis, and/or intracranial abscess (Figure 6-2).

- Pediatric cholesteatoma is often associated with higher rates of infection and recidivism than cholesteatoma in adults, given a higher incidence of eustachian tube dysfunction. Deep air cell tracks often make disease eradication difficult.
- The phrase *recidivistic cholesteatoma* encompasses all recurrences (relapses) of the disease, regardless of the origin. Causes for recidivism include *residual cholesteatoma*, left either intentionally or unintentionally at the time of surgery, or *recurrent cholesteatoma*.

IMAGING

- Consensus has not been reached regarding the use of radiographic imaging in the workup of new cholesteatoma cases. Temporal bone imaging is recommended in recurrent cases.
- Temporal bone CT scan may provide useful information regarding the status of the ossicular chain, the facial nerve, tegmen, and semicircular canals (fistula vs. erosion).
- Though cholesteatoma cannot be diagnosed with CT, this imaging modality has a high negative predictive value in cases with a well-aerated middle ear and mastoid cavity devoid of soft tissue densities.
- Cholesteatoma presents on CT as a soft tissue density that does not enhance with contrast and cannot be differentiated from other middle ear/mastoid soft tissue entities.
- Diffusion-weighted MRI is more sensitive and specific than CT for imaging of cholesteatoma. This imaging modality may have difficulty detecting lesions smaller than 5 mm, however.
- Cholesteatoma will appear on diffusion-weighted MRI as a hyperintense mass (Figure 6-3).
- Silastic sheets may appear with increased signal intensity on diffusion-weighted MRI and may produce false-positive results.

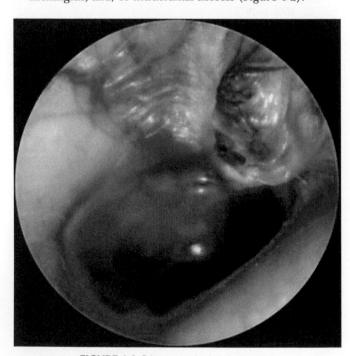

FIGURE 6-1 Primary acquired cholesteatoma.

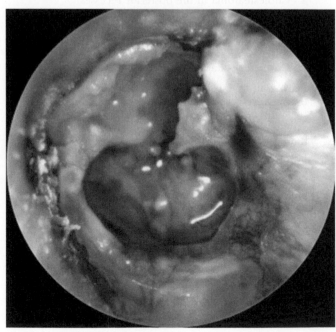

FIGURE 6-2 Primary cholesteatoma at perforation.

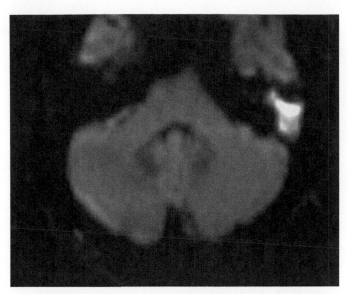

FIGURE 6-3 Diffusion-weighted magnetic resonance imaging (MRI).

- Diffusion-weighted MRI is more sensitive and specific in detecting novel cases of cholesteatoma. It is not as useful as a surveillance modality due to poor negative predictive value.

HISTOPATHOLOGY

- The histologic appearance of cholesteatoma is that of a cystic mass lined with keratin-producing squamous epithelium filled with concentrically layered desquamation debris.
- The lining of a cholesteatoma, which is also called the cholesteatoma matrix, consists of proliferating epidermal keratinocytes. An adjacent subepithelial region, termed the *perimatrix*, consists of fibroblasts, histiocytes (macrophages), and capillaries. An inflammatory infiltrate surrounds this and directly borders the surrounding ear anatomy.
- Many investigators believe that the cells in the perimatrix are responsible for the destructive characteristics of cholesteatomas.
- Superinfection of cholesteatoma is thought to enhance and/or alter the biologic profile of the cells within the perimatrix and inflammatory infiltrate, leading to more aggressive disease and bone erosion.

PATHOPHYSIOLOGY AND THEORY

- Multiple theories exist regarding the pathogenesis of primary acquired cholesteatoma.
  - The **retraction theory** suggests that cholesteatoma forms via trapping of desquamation debris within retraction pockets that form in various parts of the tympanic membrane due to chronic eustachian tube dysfunction and negative middle ear pressure.
  - The **papillary proliferation theory** states that cholesteatoma forms due to the formation of inward-boring epithelial cones (pinpoint papillary projections) through the basal layers of the tympanic membrane epithelial layer. The process is thought to be triggered by chronic middle ear inflammation.
  - The papillary proliferation theory may explain why cholesteatoma may present and/or expand within the middle ear and mastoid despite a seemingly intact tympanic membrane.

- The **immigration theory** suggests that cholesteatoma forms due to inward growth of keratinizing squamous epithelium through a preexisting perforation of the tympanic membrane. The perforation may later heal into an intact tympanic membrane.
  - The **metaplasia theory** suggests that cholesteatoma forms due to metaplasia of middle ear mucosal epithelium into keratinizing squamous epithelium when subjected to a chronic inflammatory environment.
- Cholesteatoma-mediated bone erosion is governed by a variety of factors. These may involve the secretion of matrix metalloproteinases, osteoclast activation, pH alterations, bacterial toxins, and pressure-mediated resorption.
- There is evidence that some parts of the temporal bone are more susceptible to bone resorption from the effects of cholesteatoma than others. In one study, intramembranous bone (origin of the mastoid portion of the temporal bone) was found to be more susceptible to bone erosion than intracartilaginous bone (otic capsule structures).
- Superinfection of cholesteatoma alters the inflammatory and secretory profile and may lead to more aggressive disease and bone erosion.
- Common aerobic bacteria known to cause superinfection of cholesteatoma include *Pseudomonas, Staphylococcus, Proteus, Escherichia,* and *Klebsiella.*
- Anaerobic bacteria are also common, including *Peptococcus, Peptostreptococcus, Bacteroides, Clostridium, Fusobacterium,* and *Propionobacterium.*
- There is evidence that most bacteria cultured from cholesteatoma are capable of biofilm formation, a possible explanation for the recalcitrant nature of some superinfections.
- The ideal antibacterial coverage for infected cholesteatoma includes a second-generation quinolone or third-generation cephalosporin to provide coverage for *Pseudomonas, Staphylococcus,* and anaerobes.

RELEVANT ANATOMY

- The most common locations from which primary acquired cholesteatoma may arise are the posterior epitympanum, posterior mesotympanum, and anterior epitympanum.
- Most cholesteatomas will grow in a relatively predictable fashion that is dictated by their site of origin and channeled along pathways by surrounding mucosal folds, ossicular suspensory ligaments, and the ossicles themselves (Figure 6-4).
- The middle ear cleft is separated into the epitympanum, mesotympanum, and hypotympanum.
- The floor of the epitympanum is at the level of the malleus lateral process. Its roof is the tegmen. It contains the malleus head, incus body, and associated ligaments and mucosal folds.
- The lateral entrance to the epitympanum is a fan-shaped dehiscence in the tympanic bone called the *notch of Rivinis.* This entrance is closed by the pars flaccida *(Shrapnell membrane).* The dense fibrous middle layer of the pars tensa is absent here, making it prone to retraction.
- *Prussak space* resides in the lateral epitympanum, medial to the pars flaccida and lateral to the neck of the malleus.
- Epitympanic cholesteatomas may break the confines of Prussak space via three potential routes (Figure 6-5):
  - Posterior route: enters the superior incudal space lateral to the body of the incus (most common). This provides access to the aditus ad antrum and mastoid.

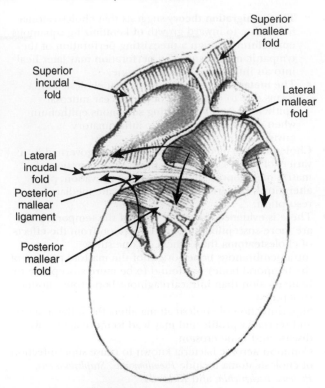

FIGURE 6-4 Middle ear membranes.

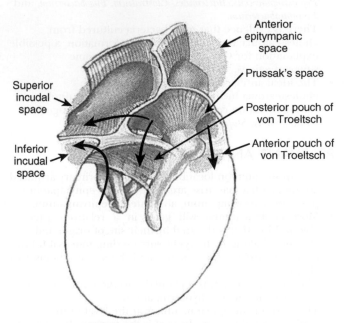

FIGURE 6-5 Pouches of von Troeltsch.

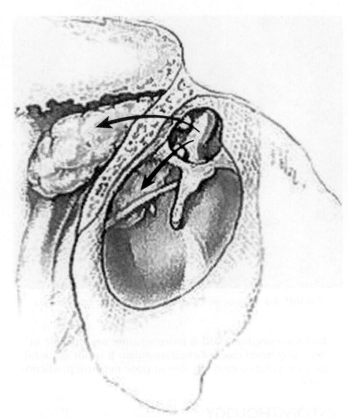

FIGURE 6-6 Routes of spread for posterior epitympanic cholesteatoma.

- Inferior route: enters the *posterior pouch of von Troeltsch.* This provides access to the posterior mesotympanum, stapes, round window, sinus tympani, and facial recess (Figure 6-6).
- Anterior route: leads anterior to the malleus head (less common). Provides access to the anterior epitympanum and supratubal recess. Downward growth into the anterior mesotympanum occurs via the *anterior pouch of von Troeltsch.*
- The epitympanum is almost completely separated from the mesotympanum by a structure called the *tympanic diaphragm* (dense mucosal folds and suspensory ligaments surrounding ossicles).

- The tympanic diaphragm is resistant to the spread of cholesteatoma between compartments.
- The mesotympanum contains the stapes, long processes of the malleus and incus, and both the oval and round windows. It opens anteriorly into the eustachian tube and posteriorly into two crescent-shaped recesses: the facial recess and sinus tympani.
- The vertical boundaries of the sinus tympani are the ponticulus superiorly and the subiculum inferiorly. The promontory lies anteriorly, while the facial nerve lies laterally. It is bounded medially by the medial wall of the tympanum.
- The second most common location for primary acquired cholesteatoma to arise is within a retraction of the posterior pars tensa (posterior mesotympanic cholesteatoma).
- Posterior mesotympanic cholesteatoma will commonly involve structures in that location, including the sinus tympani and facial recess. Posterior mesotympanic cholesteatoma can reach the mastoid.
- The *sinus tympani* often cannot be visualized directly via any surgical approach, and represents the most common site for recidivistic cholesteatoma to arise.
- The hypotympanum has its vertical boundary at the floor of the bony external auditory canal. Cholesteatoma rarely involves this compartment.
- The facial nerve is remarkably resistant to the effects of nearby cholesteatoma and inflammatory changes, as are the inner ear structures encased in the dense otic capsule.
- During cholesteatoma surgery, the facial nerve will most often be injured in the tympanic segment overlaying the oval window (common site of congenital and erosive bone loss).
- In rare cases, anterior epitympanic cholesteatomas can extend to and compress the geniculate ganglion, causing facial nerve dysfunction.

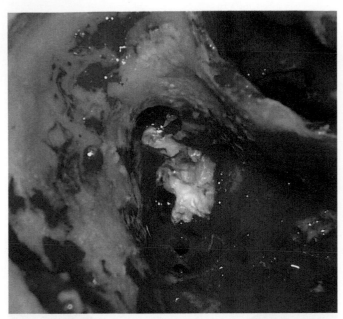

FIGURE 6-7 Cholesteatoma seen via mastoidectomy.

- Cholesteatoma is an exclusively surgical disease.
- The principal goals of cholesteatoma surgery, in order of greatest importance, are:
  1. Disease eradication
  2. Creation of a dry, safe ear
  3. Hearing preservation/restoration
- The surgical procedure for treatment of cholesteatoma is the tympanoplasty with mastoidectomy. In general, there are two types of surgical approaches to the mastoid: ICW mastoidectomy and CWD mastoidectomy.
- ICW mastoidectomy carries the following advantages: maintains the natural canal anatomy, allows for faster healing times, is less prone to infection, does not limit water activities, allows for better use of hearing aids, and avoids chronic maintenance (Figure 6-7).
- ICW mastoidectomy is associated with higher recidivism rates (residual and recurrent).
- ICW also provides the surgeon with less exposure.
- CWD mastoidectomy carries the following advantages: better operative exposure, easier detection of residual disease at second-look surgery, lower recidivism rates.
- CWD is associated with slower healing times, necessitates chronic postoperative bowl cleaning, is more susceptible to infection, and necessitates that the patient avoid water activities.
- The use of conventional hearing aids after CWD mastoidectomy may be problematic.
- The decision to proceed with ICW versus CWD mastoidectomy may be made during surgery based on the intraoperative extent of disease.
- Intraoperative findings that may lead a surgeon to consider CWD mastoidectomy include (1) low tegmen with anterior sigmoid sinus, (2) large horizontal semicircular canal fistula, and (3) extensive erosion of the scutum/posterior canal wall.
- In cases with extensive cholesteatoma and a large horizontal semicircular canal fistula, the safest approach may entail leaving cholesteatoma matrix over the fistula and performing CWD. The danger of removing the matrix in such cases is permanent sensorineural hearing loss.
- Cases in which a preoperative determination for CWD technique can be made include operating on an only hearing ear, a situation in which reliable follow-up would be a concern, comorbidities that increase risk from lengthy anesthesia times, and/or presence of extensive posterior external auditory canal erosion.
- Hearing outcomes are roughly the same regardless of the type of mastoidectomy. This has been demonstrated in both the pediatric and adult populations.
- Data seem to support the notion that hearing outcomes following cholesteatoma surgery are more dependent on the functional status of the native ossicular chain (especially the stapes suprastructure), health of the middle ear mucosa, and depth of the middle ear cleft.
- The material used for ossicular chain reconstruction is largely surgeon dependent and likely does not affect outcome.
- Regardless of the surgical approach, cholesteatoma may not be eradicated fully during an initial surgery. For this reason, most surgeons employ a second-look procedure.
- Recidivism rates following canal wall up procedures range widely between 6% and 57%.
- Second-look procedures are generally performed 6 to 9 months from the date of the initial surgery.
- The goals of a second-look procedure are to eradicate any remaining cholesteatoma and to reconstruct the hearing apparatus.
- Successful CWD mastoidectomy requires each of the following: removal of all diseased air cells, amputation of the mastoid tip, lowering the facial ridge to the mastoid segment of the facial nerve, contouring of the external canal floor to the mastoid bowl, and creation of an adequate meatoplasty.
- Mastoid obliteration is a safe and effective technique for producing a dry, low-maintenance, small mastoid cavity following CWD mastoidectomy.
- Radical mastoidectomy is a CWD procedure in which no attempt is made to restore middle ear space or function. The eustachian tube is occluded, the ossicles removed, and the tympanic membrane excised.
- "Modified radical mastoidectomy" can be a confusing terminology. This is typically used interchangeably with CWD mastoidectomy. In actuality, a modified radical mastoidectomy refers to the Bondy procedure. In such cases, cholesteatoma limited to the epitympanum is exteriorized by removing portions of the adjacent superior or posterior canal wall. The middle ear is not entered or manipulated. Cholesteatoma matrix is left in place at the lateral ossicular heads.
- Endoscopic visualization has been utilized successfully at the time of primary cholesteatoma surgery to ensure there is not residual disease in locations that are traditionally difficult to visualize (posterior recesses, supratubal recess). Outcomes data remain limited, but there may be a significant reduction in recurrent cholesteatoma rates.
- Another common utilization of otoendoscopy is at the time of a second-look procedure. Endoscopic-assisted removal of recidivistic disease is possible. Conversion to open surgery is also an option.

CONGENITAL CHOLESTEATOMA

- Congenital cholesteatoma accounts for 2% to 5% of all cholesteatomas.
- The incidence has been increasing steadily as access to microscopic visualization improves and more ear tubes are being placed.
- Congenital cholesteatoma presents in a male-predominant pattern with reported rates of 2.7:1.
- The typical age of presentation is between 1 and 5 years. The mean age in most studies is around 5.

- There does not appear to be a side predilection. Bilateral cases do occur but are rare.
- The most common presentation is that of an asymptomatic middle ear mass.
- There are distinct diagnostic criteria that must be met in order to reach a diagnosis of congenital cholesteatoma. The Levenson criteria include:
  - Presence of a whitish mass medial to an intact tympanic membrane
  - Normal pars flaccida and pars tensa
  - No prior history of prior perforation or otorrhea
  - No prior otologic surgery or procedures
  - Exclusion of aural atresia and intramembranous or giant cholesteatoma
- Previous history of acute otitis media does not exclude a diagnosis of congenital cholesteatoma.
- The embryonic cell rest theory is the favored pathoetiologic theory for the development of congenital cholesteatoma.
- When confined to one quadrant, the anterior superior quadrant most frequently harbors congenital cholesteatoma (up to 80% of cases; Figure 6-8). The posterior superior quadrant is the second most commonly involved.
- Nearly 50% of cases present with cholesteatoma in two or more quadrants.
- Definitive management is surgical. The goals of surgery should be total removal of the disease followed by restoration of hearing.
- At the time of surgery, many cases of congenital cholesteatoma are well circumscribed and enclosed within a membrane that readily separates from surrounding structures.
- Some cases of congenital cholesteatoma behave more like primary acquired cholesteatoma, with inflammatory middle ear changes and evidence of bone erosion.

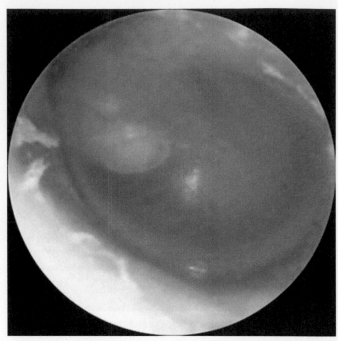

FIGURE 6-8 Congenital cholesteatoma.

- Congenital cholesteatoma may extend not infrequently to involve the ossicular chain and mastoid. A staging system exists based on involvement of multiple quadrants, the ossicular chain, and/or the mastoid cavity. Early stage cases tend to have an excellent surgical result and typically maintain preoperative hearing levels. Advanced stages are associated with high recidivism rates.

ANSWERS

TRUE OR FALSE QUESTIONS

1. T	14. F	27. T	40. F
2. T	15. T	28. F	41. T
3. T	16. F	29. F	42. T
4. T	17. F	30. T	43. F
5. F	18. F	31. F	44. F
6. F	19. T	32. F	45. F
7. T	20. F	33. F	46. T
8. T	21. F	34. T	47. F
9. T	22. T	35. T	48. T
10. F	23. F	36. F	49. F
11. F	24. T	37. T	50. T
12. F	25. F	38. T	
13. T	26. T	39. F	

SINGLE BEST ANSWER QUESTIONS

51. b	64. e	77. d	90. e
52. a	65. e	78. c	91. b
53. a	66. d	79. d	92. c
54. a	67. e	80. b	93. d
55. d	68. d	81. d	94. b
56. a	69. a	82. c	95. c
57. d	70. c	83. b	96. a
58. c	71. c	84. c	97. b
59. c	72. c	85. b	98. a
60. a	73. a	86. a	99. d
61. e	74. c	87. c	100. e
62. a	75. b	88. d	
63. d	76. d	89. e	

SUGGESTED READINGS

1. Evlice A, Tarkan Ö, Kiroğlu M, et al. Detection of recurrent and primary acquired cholesteatoma with echo-planar diffusion-weighted magnetic resonance imaging. *J Laryngol Otol.* 2012;126(7):670-676.
2. Sudhoff H, Tos M. Pathogenesis of attic cholesteatoma: clinical and immunohistochemical support for combination of retraction theory and proliferation theory. *Am J Otol.* 2000;21:786.
3. Chole RA. Differential osteoclast activation in endochondral and intramembranous bone. *Ann Otol Rhinol Laryngol.* 1993;102:616.
4. Chole RA, Faddis BT. Evidence for microbial biofilms in cholesteatomas. *Arch Otolaryngol Head Neck Surg.* 2002; 128:1129.
5. Ricciardiello F, Cavaliere M, Mesolella M, et al. Notes on the microbiology of cholesteatoma: clinical findings and treatment. *Acta Otorhinolaryngol Ital.* 2009;29:197.
6. Jackler RK. The surgical anatomy of cholesteatoma. *Otolaryngol Clin North Am.* 1989;22:883.
7. Dodson EE, Hashisaki GT, Hobgood TC, Lambert PR. Intact canal wall mastoidectomy with tympanoplasty for cholesteatoma in children. *Laryngoscope.* 1998;108(7): 977-983.
8. Sanna M, Zini C, Gamoletti R, et al. Prevention of recurrent cholesteatoma in closed tympanoplasty. *Ann Otol Rhinol Laryngol.* 1987;96:273-275.
9. Ayache S, Tramier B, Strunski V. Otoendoscopy in cholesteatoma surgery of the middle ear: what benefits can be expected? *Otol Neurotol.* 2008;29(8):1085-1090.
10. Potsic WP, Korman SB, Samadi DS, et al. Congenital cholesteatoma: 20 years' experience at The Children's Hospital of Philadelphia. *Otolaryngol Head Neck Surg.* 2002;126: 409.

7 | Otitis Media and Externa

Colleen Heffernan

TRUE OR FALSE QUESTIONS

T/F 1. Antihistamines, decongestants, antibiotics, and mucolytics, either oral or topical, are useful for the resolution of otitis media with effusion.

T/F 2. Adenoid size is directly proportional to the risk of developing otitis media with effusion.

T/F 3. Ciprofloxacin 750 mg twice daily (bid) by mouth (PO) has the same bioavailability as 400 mg three times a day (tid) intravenously (IV).

T/F 4. Labyrinthine fistulae as a complication of acute otitis media most commonly occur in the posterior semicircular canal.

T/F 5. A healed tympanic membrane perforation is often referred to as "dimeric" because it is missing the medial mucosal layer.

T/F 6. The maximum air–bone gap on a pure tone audiogram is 30 decibels (dB).

T/F 7. Posttympanostomy tube otorrhea should be treated with topical antibiotics.

T/F 8. *Streptococcus pneumoniae* is a Gram-positive, alpha-hemolytic, facultative anaerobe.

T/F 9. Presence of a middle ear effusion is necessary to diagnose acute otitis media.

T/F 10. Ninety percent of middle ear effusions resolve spontaneously.

T/F 11. Sixty percent of people have a congenital dehiscence of the horizontal portion of the facial nerve.

T/F 12. The term "central tympanic membrane perforation" refers to the position of the perforation in the tympanic membrane.

T/F 13. Autoinflation can be useful in the resolution of middle ear effusions.

T/F 14. The foramen tympanicum/foramen of Huschke is a defect in the anteroinferior bony external auditory canal, which allows the spread of infection and tumor between the canal and temporomandibular joint/infratemporal fossa.

T/F 15. Topical antimicrobials are delivered at such a high concentration to the middle ear and external ear as to render resistance inconsequential.

T/F 16. A type I tympanoplasty as described by HL Wullstein is the same as a myringoplasty.

T/F 17. The external auditory canal is composed of cartilage in its outer two-thirds and bone in its inner third.

T/F 18. Mirko Tos described a grading system for retraction pockets of the pars tensa.

T/F 19. Gentian violet is a dye that when used topically has antiseptic, antifungal, and antibacterial effects.

T/F 20. During aural toilet for otitis externa, it is important to pay particular attention to the posterosuperior portion of the medial external auditory canal.

T/F 21. A tympanic membrane perforation is necessary to diagnose chronic otitis media.

T/F 22. Otitis externa is more likely to result after irrigation of cerumen than microsuction.

T/F 23. Santorini fissures lie in the anteroinferior portion of the cartilaginous ear canal and allow spread of infection and tumor between the external auditory canal and the parotid gland.

T/F 24. Both the pars flaccida and the pars tensa are composed of three layers: squamous epithelium, a fibrous middle layer, and a mucous medial layer.

T/F 25. An infant's eustachian tube lies more horizontal and is narrower than an adult's.

T/F 26. The cog divides the hypotympanum into anterior and posterior portions.

T/F 27. There is gender preponderance to chronic otitis media.

T/F 28. Chronic otitis media is more common in Native Americans and Eskimos.

T/F 29. Griesinger sign is mastoid tenderness and edema secondary to thrombophlebitis of the mastoid emissary vein.

T/F 30. Sixty percent of children will have an episode of acute otitis media by age 1 and 80% by age 3.

T/F 31. Clindamycin is the antibiotic of choice for acute otitis media.

T/F 32. Pain is a common presenting feature of chronic otitis media.

T/F 33. A Bezold abscess presents as a fluctuant mass along the anterior border of the sternocleidomastoid.

T/F 34. Tympanostomy tube placement and traumatic perforations are risk factors for chronic otitis media.

T/F 35. A Citelli abscess spreads through the medial side of the mastoid into the digastric fossa.

T/F 36. Three percent of tympanic membranes will have a pars tensa retraction pocket, and 14% will have a pars flaccida retraction pocket post tympanostomy tube extrusion.

T/F 37. Chronic otitis media with and without cholesteatoma can cause bony erosion.

T/F 38. The main distinguishing factor between chronic otitis media and cholesteatoma is the presence of keratin.

T/F 39. Positive pressure in the middle ear predisposes a patient to acute otitis media and otitis media with effusion.

T/F 40. A child's eustachian tube lies at 45 degrees and an adult's lies at 10 degrees.

T/F 41. During tympanoplasty it is important to reconstruct the scutum to prevent future retraction pockets.

T/F 42. The skin of the outer third of the external auditory canal contains hair follicles and ceruminous, sweat, and sebaceous glands whose secretions keep it watertight and the pH neutral.

T/F 43. *Pseudomonas aeruginosa* is a Gram-positive, anaerobic, coccobacillus bacterium.

T/F 44. Systemic antibiotics should be routinely prescribed for diffuse acute otitis externa to prevent it from developing into necrotizing otitis externa.

T/F 45. Gentamicin is a very useful topical treatment for otitis media/externa in the presence of a tympanic membrane perforation.

T/F 46. Patients with human immunodeficiency virus (HIV) or hematologic malignancies are prone to fungal necrotizing otitis externa, such as caused by *Aspergillus*.

T/F 47. Debridement of involved bone is the most important initial step in managing necrotizing otitis externa.

T/F 48. A Carhart notch is seen only in otosclerosis.

T/F 49. Children with tympanostomy tubes should adhere to strict waterproofing of the ear canal.

T/F 50. At the time of tympanostomy tube insertion, it is imperative to suction all of the effusion out of the middle ear.

SINGLE BEST ANSWER QUESTIONS

51. Which of the following is the single most important initial investigation in an adult presenting with unilateral otitis media with effusion?
    a. Computed tomography (CT) of the temporal bones
    b. CT of the paranasal sinuses
    c. Immunoglobulin E (IgE) and radioallergosorbent test (RAST)
    d. Flexible nasoendoscopy

52. What is the attic portion of the middle ear also known as?
    a. Protympanum
    b. Mesotympanum
    c. Epitympanum
    d. Antrum

53. Which aspect of tympanostomy tube insertion affects how long the tube remains in the tympanic membrane?
    a. Diameter of the inner flange
    b. Part of the tympanic membrane into which the tube is inserted
    c. Material tube is made from
    d. Grade of surgeon who performs the procedure

54. What is the most common postoperative problem with tympanostomy tubes?
    a. Persistent perforation of the tympanic membrane
    b. Lack of resolution of conductive hearing loss
    c. Otorrhea
    d. Otalgia

55. The temporal line is the surface landmark for which important structure?
    a. Mastoid antrum
    b. Endolymphatic sac
    c. Sigmoid sinus
    d. Dura of the middle cranial fossa

56. Which portion of an ossicle is most commonly eroded by chronic/recurrent otitis media?
    a. Head of malleus
    b. Long process of incus
    c. Crura of stapes
    d. Stapes footplate

57. Which of the following is a useful landmark for the facial nerve during mastoid surgery?
    a. Horizontal semicircular canal
    b. Short process of the incus
    c. Posterior external auditory canal
    d. All of the above

58. Why might a mastoid cavity fail?
    a. High facial ridge
    b. Dependent mastoid tip
    c. No/inadequate meatoplasty
    d. All of the above

59. Which cranial nerve is most commonly involved in necrotizing otitis externa?
    a. Trigeminal
    b. Facial
    c. Vestibulocochlear
    d. Glossopharyngeal

60. Drops containing which of the following can be used to prevent otitis externa?
    a. Gentamicin
    b. Ichthammol
    c. Arachis oil
    d. Acetic acid

61. What is the mortality rate associated with necrotizing otitis externa?
    a. 5%
    b. 10%
    c. 50%
    d. 60%

62. Which organism most commonly causes acute otitis media?
    a. Influenza A virus
    b. *Moraxella catarrhalis*
    c. *Streptococcus pneumoniae*
    d. *Haemophilus influenzae*

63. What is the most common intracranial complication of acute/chronic otitis media?
    a. Sigmoid sinus thrombosis
    b. Meningitis

c. Temporal lobe abscess
d. Extradural abscess

64. Hyrtl fissure predisposes to which intracranial complication of acute/chronic otitis media?
    a. Meningitis
    b. Sigmoid sinus thrombosis
    c. Extradural abscess
    d. Temporal lobe abscess

65. Which organism is most commonly involved in chronic otitis media?
    a. *Haemophilus influenzae*
    b. *Staphylococcus aureus*
    c. *Bacteroides fragilis*
    d. *Pseudomonas aeruginosa*

66. Gradenigo syndrome is characterized by which of the following?
    a. Otorrhea, ipsilateral abducens palsy, and pain in trigeminal distribution
    b. Increased auriculocephalic angle
    c. Pyrexia and otalgia, followed by otorrhea
    d. Deafness, vertigo, and tinnitus

67. Which of the following is the most common constituent of topical medications to cause sensitization?
    a. Neomycin
    b. Hydrocortisone
    c. Ciprofloxacin
    d. Gentamicin

68. Which metal is most likely to cause sensitization?
    a. Platinum
    b. Copper
    c. Gold
    d. Nickel

69. Which of the following best describes the boundaries of Prussak space?
    a. Neck of the malleus medially, pars flaccida laterally, scutum superiorly, and lateral process of malleus inferiorly
    b. Anterior and posterior malleolar folds medially and tympanic membrane laterally
    c. Facial nerve medially, tympanic annulus and chorda tympani laterally, and incus buttress superiorly
    d. Posterior semicircular canal medially; pyramidal eminence, stapedius muscle, and facial nerve laterally; ponticulus superiorly; and subiculum inferiorly

70. Which of the following is the main risk factor for developing acute otitis media?
    a. Crowded living quarters
    b. Large number of siblings
    c. Attendance at day care
    d. All of the above

71. Which of the following best describes the boundaries of the facial recess?
    a. Neck of the malleus medially, pars flaccida laterally, scutum superiorly, and lateral process of malleus inferiorly
    b. Anterior and posterior malleolar folds medially and tympanic membrane laterally
    c. Facial nerve medially, tympanic annulus and chorda tympani laterally, and incus buttress superiorly
    d. Posterior semicircular canal medially; pyramidal eminence, stapedius muscle, and facial nerve laterally; ponticulus superiorly; and subiculum inferiorly

72. A type IV tympanoplasty is used when:
    a. The crura of the stapes are missing and the footplate is fixed.
    b. There is a perforation of the tympanic membrane, but the ossicles are intact.
    c. The crura of the stapes are missing, but the footplate is mobile.
    d. The incus and malleus are missing, but the stapes is intact and mobile.

73. A retracted tympanic membrane adherent to the promontory is described as:
    a. Tos I
    b. Tos IV
    c. Sade IV
    d. Sade III

74. Which of the following is the distinguishing feature of tuberculous otitis media?
    a. Subtotal perforation
    b. Pruritus
    c. Serosanguineous discharge
    d. Multiple small tympanic membrane perforations

75. What are the constituents of Sulzberger's powder?
    a. Iodine
    b. Boric acid
    c. Dexamethasone
    d. a and b

76. Characteristics of biofilms include:
    a. An extracellular polysaccharide matrix that adheres to organic and inorganic objects
    b. Resistance to host immune system and antimicrobials
    c. Cultures may be negative.
    d. All of the above

77. An area of enhancement with a low attenuation center seen in sigmoid sinus thrombosis on contrast-enhanced CT is called the:
    a. Delta sign
    b. Hitzelberger sign
    c. Hennebert sign
    d. Griesinger sign

78. Which of the following is most cochleotoxic?
    a. Amikacin
    b. Streptomycin
    c. Neomycin
    d. Gentamicin

79. Which of the following is the most constant bony landmark in the middle ear?
    a. Promontory
    b. Subiculum
    c. Processus cochleariformis
    d. Pyramidal eminence

80. What is the most appropriate treatment for facial nerve palsy secondary to acute otitis media?
    a. Observation
    b. IV antibiotics
    c. Tympanostomy tube
    d. b and c

81. With which muscle is a Luc's abscess associated?
    a. Sternocleidomastoid
    b. Digastric
    c. Temporalis
    d. Masseter

82. What percentage of children will still have a middle ear effusion after 3 months of watchful waiting?
    a. 90%
    b. 10%

c. 33%

d. 5%

83. A canal wall down mastoidectomy should be considered when:
    a. The patient presents with complications.
    b. The disease is in the only hearing ear.
    c. The mastoid is small.
    d. All of the above

84. What is the most common causative organism in otitis externa?
    a. *Aspergillus niger*
    b. *Aspergillus fumigatus*
    c. *Pseudomonas aeruginosa*
    d. *Staphylococcus aureus*

85. Which scan is most useful to assess for intracranial extension of necrotizing otitis externa?
    a. Technetium-99m
    b. Gallium-67 citrate
    c. Magnetic resonance imaging (MRI) with gadolinium enhancement and fat suppression
    d. CT

86. The triangle formed by the temporal line, posterior canal wall, and a tangential line between them is the surface marking of which of the following structures?
    a. Posterior cranial fossa
    b. Endolymphatic sac
    c. Mastoid antrum
    d. Sigmoid sinus

87. Which scan is most useful to stage the extent of disease in necrotizing otitis externa?
    a. Technetium-99m
    b. Gallium-67 citrate
    c. MRI with gadolinium enhancement and fat suppression
    d. CT

88. Which scan is most useful in determining treatment endpoint in necrotizing otitis externa?
    a. Technetium-99m
    b. Gallium-67 citrate
    c. MRI with gadolinium enhancement and fat suppression
    d. CT

89. Which scan is most useful for an early diagnosis of necrotizing otitis externa?
    a. Technetium-99m
    b. Gallium-67 citrate
    c. MRI with gadolinium enhancement and fat suppression
    d. CT

90. Cortisporin Otic contains:
    a. Acetic acid 2% and hydrocortisone 1%
    b. Framycetin 0.5%, gramicidin 0.005%, and dexamethasone 0.05%
    c. Neomycin, polymyxin B, and hydrocortisone
    d. Triamcinolone, neomycin, gramicidin, and nystatin

91. Körner septum represents the suture line between which parts of the temporal bone?
    a. Squamous and mastoid
    b. Tympanic and mastoid

c. Petrous and squamous

d. Petrous and tympanic

92. Which statement is *INCORRECT* regarding cerumen?
    a. It is bactericidal.
    b. It needs to be cleared regularly.
    c. It contains secretions from sebaceous and apocrine glands.
    d. It is slightly acidic.

93. All of the following are true regarding acute otitis media *EXCEPT:*
    a. It is more common in lower socioeconomic groups.
    b. It is more common in bottle-fed children.
    c. It is more common if child lives in a crowded environment.
    d. It is more common in children cared for at home.

94. A child less than 2 years of age with otalgia and otorrhea is most likely to have which of the following?
    a. Otitis externa
    b. Otitis media with effusion
    c. Acute otitis media
    d. Congenital cholesteatoma

95. An elderly diabetic with otalgia and otorrhea should be suspected of having which of the following?
    a. Otitis externa
    b. Necrotizing otitis externa
    c. Acute otitis media
    d. Congenital cholesteatoma

96. Features of acute mastoiditis in a child include:
    a. Otalgia
    b. Fever
    c. Lateral displacement of the pinna
    d. All of the above

97. Which of the following is *NOT* a landmark used for planning a postauricular incision?
    a. Temporal line
    b. Zygomatic arch
    c. Mastoid tip
    d. Postauricular sulcus

98. Where is a tympanic membrane graft most likely to fail?
    a. Anterior
    b. Posterior
    c. Superior
    d. Inferior

99. Anaphylaxis occurs in what percentage of patients given penicillin?
    a. 0.01%
    b. 0.1%
    c. 1%
    d. 10%

100. A type B tympanogram may suggest:
    a. A middle ear effusion
    b. A tympanic membrane perforation
    c. A patent ventilation tube
    d. All of the above

CORE KNOWLEDGE

ACUTE OTITIS MEDIA

- Acute otitis media is defined as inflammation and infection (viral/bacterial) of the mucosa of the middle ear with or without eustachian tube and mastoid air cells associated with an effusion.
- The risk factors for developing middle ear disease are eustachian tube dysfunction, poor immune response, and exposure to otopathogenic organisms (Figure 7-1).
- All children have immature eustachian tubes; children with craniofacial anomalies including cleft palate and Down syndrome are particularly at risk.
- Poor immune response may be due to immaturity, exposure to passive smoke, bottle feeding, malnutrition, and known immunodeficiency states.
- Exposure to otopathogenic organisms increases with the number of siblings, attendance at day care, and chronic upper respiratory tract infections.
- Always consider mucociliary disorders such as cystic fibrosis.
- The organisms most commonly implicated are *Streptococcus pneumoniae* (40%), *Haemophilus influenzae* (20%-30%), *Moraxella catarrhalis* (10%-15%), respiratory syncytial virus, influenza A virus, parainfluenza virus, human rhinovirus, and adenoviruses.
- Mucosal edema secondary to infection leads to obstruction of the eustachian tube. Oxygen is absorbed from the middle ear, leading to negative pressure and the production of an effusion that contains inflammatory cells and mucoproteins.
- Pressure necrosis of the tympanic membrane may lead to perforation.
- Occurs between ages 3 and 7, most common in the second 6 months of life
- Sixty percent of children will have had an episode of acute otitis media by age 1 and 80% by age 3.
- Presents in a child with a preceding upper respiratory tract infection who now becomes irritable and pyretic with progressive otalgia. Child may pull at ears. Otalgia settles with the onset of otorrhea. Parents may note decreased hearing.

- Tympanic membrane is initially retracted due to negative middle ear pressure, then bulges as middle ear effusion develops.
- Similar presentations can occur with otitis externa, external auditory canal foreign body, teething, and tonsillitis.
- Pneumatic otoscopy is the gold standard for diagnosing acute otitis media.
- Consider sending cultures if the child is less than 6 weeks of age.
- CT scan should be performed if there is suspicion of disease extension beyond middle ear.
- MRI with gadolinium should be performed if intracranial complications are suspected.
- Treatment is initially supportive (i.e., analgesia).
- If the child is less than 2 years of age or does not improve after 48 hours, then give oral amoxicillin or co-amoxiclav (if resistant organism suspected) for 1 week.
- Administer second- or third-generation cephalosporins, macrolides, or clindamycin if allergic to penicillin.
- If child has three episodes in 6 months or four in 12 months, consider tympanostomy tubes or long-term antibiotics.
- Complications of acute and chronic otitis media can be divided into intracranial and extracranial.
  - Extracranial are further divided into intratemporal (mastoiditis [Figures 7-2 and 7-3], labyrinthitis, Gradenigo syndrome, facial nerve palsy, tympanic membrane perforation, middle ear effusion, sensorineural hearing loss, retraction pockets, perilymphatic fistula, cholesteatoma, tympanosclerosis, and ossicular chain erosion) and extratemporal (subperiosteal abscess, Bezold abscess, Luc's abscess, and Citelli abscess).
  - Intracranial complications include extradural/subdural abscess, sigmoid sinus thrombosis, cerebral abscess, otitic hydrocephalus, and meningitis.

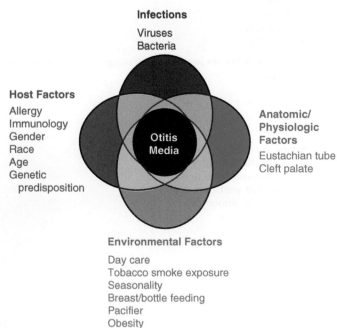

Infections

Viruses
Bacteria

Host Factors

Allergy
Immunology
Gender
Race
Age
Genetic
predisposition

Otitis
Media

Anatomic/Physiologic Factors

Eustachian tube
Cleft palate

Environmental Factors

Day care
Tobacco smoke exposure
Seasonality
Breast/bottle feeding
Pacifier
Obesity

FIGURE 7-1 Various factors interact in the pathogenesis of otitis media.

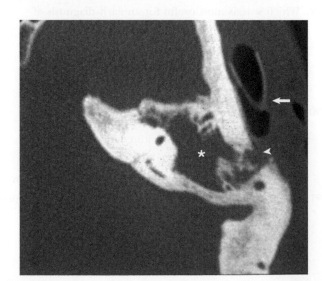

FIGURE 7-2 Axial temporal bone computed tomography (CT) scan (soft tissue) shows abscess cavity with gas *(arrow)*. Note cortical defect *(arrowhead)*, mastoid opacification, and loss of bony septa *(asterisk)*.

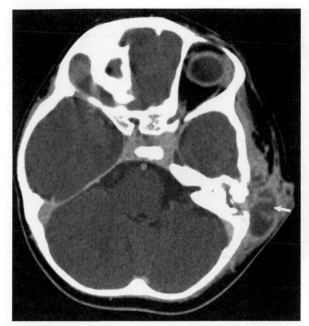

FIGURE 7-3 Axial temporal bone CT scan (soft tissue) with contrast enhancement. Note postauricular abscess with enhancing capsule (*arrow*).

OTITIS MEDIA WITH EFFUSION

- Otitis media with effusion is defined as chronic accumulation of mucus in the middle ear with or without mastoid.
- Risk factors and pathogenesis are similar to acute otitis media. Also consider allergies, nasopharyngeal malignancy, recurrent sinus infections, and autoimmune problems (e.g., granulomatosis with polyangiitis and polyarteritis nodosa).
- Adenoid tissue is a source of pathologic bacteria.
- Eighty percent of children will have otitis media with effusion at some stage in their lives.
- Bimodal peak: age 2 at the start of daycare and age 5 at the start of school
- Present with decreased hearing, behavioral problems, imbalance, or speech delay as noted by parents and/or school personnel. May have a history of recurrent ear infections.
- Otoscopy may reveal a tympanic membrane that is dull or yellow and it may be bulging or retracted. Air bubbles, a fluid level, or a neoannulus may be visible. Pneumatic otoscopy will show an immobile tympanic membrane.
- The child will have an air–bone gap on pure tone audiometry and a type B tympanogram.
- Examine postnasal space in an adult.
- Consider IgE and RAST.
- Initial management is watchful waiting for 3 months and Valsalva maneuvers if tolerated.
- After 3 months the child is a candidate for tympanostomy tubes if there is a persistent 20 dB loss in the better hearing ear.
- Consider adenoidectomy if having a second set of tympanostomy tubes or if symptomatic. Adjuvant adenoidectomy improves hearing and decreases the need for reinsertion.
- Tympanostomy tubes should be placed anteroinferiorly to prevent damage to the ossicular chain and to increase their longevity.
- Grommet shaped and 'T' shaped tympanostomy tubes have a 2% and 50% persistent perforation rate,

respectively. If a tympanostomy tube has been left in situ for greater than 2 years, its persistent perforation rate rises to 50%.
- Other long-term sequelae of tympanostomy tubes include otorrhea, atrophy and retraction of the tympanic membrane, tympanosclerosis, and need for reinsertion (25% of children and 50% of adults).
- Hearing aids are a reasonable nonsurgical option.

CHRONIC OTITIS MEDIA

- Chronic otitis media is a tympanic membrane perforation with persistent inflammation of the middle ear and mastoid.
- Risk factors are similar to acute and chronic otitis media, and these two conditions may also be predisposing factors. Traumatic perforations and tympanostomy tube placement are also risk factors.
- Presents with malodorous discharge and hearing loss and potentially with complications of otitis media
- Binocular microscopy will reveal a perforation with myringitis and inflammation of middle ear mucosa. Polyps may be seen, and these represent underlying osteitis.
- Chronic mucoid discharge is associated with goblet cell hyperplasia, metaplasia of middle ear mucosa, and poor mucociliary function.
- Bacteria associated with chronic otitis media include aerobes (*Pseudomonas aeruginosa, Staphylococcus aureus, Klebsiella pneumonia*) and anaerobes (*Bacteroides* spp.).
- Infection leads to the release of inflammatory mediators that activate osteoclasts and lead to bony erosion.
- Beware deep ear pain because it may signal carcinoma of the middle ear, tympanic membrane, or ear canal.
- Diagnosis is by binocular microscopy. Examine the cranial nerves. Consider cultures; remember methicillin-resistant *Staphylococcus aureus* (MRSA) and fungal causes. Make an audiologic assessment. Send polyps for histology; query carcinoma. Consider high resolution CT (≤1 mm coronal and axial cuts) and/or diffusion-weighted MRI.
- Treatment options include debridement and topical treatments, myringoplasty, and/or cortical mastoidectomy.
- Ideally the patient should be infection-free for 3 months preoperatively.
- Surgery aims
  - Eradicate disease
  - Make the ear safe
  - Aerate the middle ear
  - Reconstruct the tympanic membrane, ossicles, and scutum
- Topical treatment: antibiotics/steroids. Reduce secondary infection and granulation tissue. Use tragal pumping to deliver drops.
- Dry ear precautions

OTITIS EXTERNA

- Otitis externa is an acute or chronic inflammatory process of the skin of the external auditory canal (Figure 7-4).
- Otitis externa caused by fungal infections is called otomycosis.
- The colloquial name for otitis externa is "swimmer's ear" or "tropical ear."
- Causes include trauma to the external auditory canal, moisture, skin conditions (eczema, psoriasis, and seborrheic dermatitis), and obstruction to keratin migration (foreign body, hearing aid, exostoses, osteoma, congenital/iatrogenic canal stenosis, and hirsute canal).

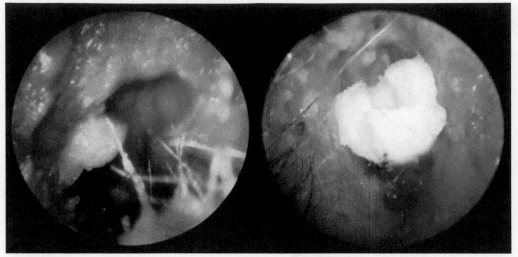

FIGURE 7-4 Acute otitis externa. Erythema, edema, and copious purulent debris are seen *(left),* and in some cases, an edematous canal with granulation tissue *(right)* necessitates placement of an ear wick to facilitate topical drug delivery in the acute setting. (Courtesy John House, MD.)

- Chronic otitis externa may be due to irritants and allergens such as cosmetics, ear molds, topical medications, and metal.
- Prolonged use of ototopic drops can predispose to developing otomycosis.
- In 90% of cases it is a bacterial infection, with the most common bacteria being *Pseudomonas aeruginosa.* In the remaining 10% of cases it is a fungal infection, with the most common fungi being *Aspergillus niger* and *Aspergillus fumigatus.*
- Retained moisture from swimming/showering will alkalize the canal, making it prone to bacterial infection.
- Due to the rich lymphatic drainage of the external auditory canal, lymphadenopathy can occur, and otitis externa can progress to auricular cellulitis or perichondritis.
- The most common symptoms are itching, followed by malodorous otorrhea and otalgia with a sensation of a blocked ear and muffled hearing.
- Mucopus may fill the external auditory canal. The canal skin will be erythematous and edematous. It may be difficult to see the tympanic membrane.
- Pressing on the tragus or pulling the pinna may lead to significant pain.
- In otomycosis, pruritus is marked and the mucopus may resemble wet newspaper. Sometimes fungal hyphae are visible under the microscope.
- Culture of the debris for bacteria, fungi, and acid-fast bacilli is useful in recalcitrant cases.
- Measurements of blood glucose and HbA_1C are useful if patient is a known diabetic or suspected diabetic.
- If there is a polyp, granulation tissue, a nonresolving otitis externa, or persistent pain, then biopsy is imperative.
- Meticulous aural toilet, paying particular attention to the anteroinferior external auditory canal, followed by topical medications is curative in uncomplicated cases.
- Systemic therapy is required if the infection spreads out of the confines of the canal or if the patient is immunocompromised or a poorly controlled diabetic.
- A range of topical medications is available: antibiotics, antifungals, hygroscopic drops, antiseptics, and steroids.
- Ideally, treatment should continue for 7 days after resolution of otitis externa.
- Placement of a wick (sponge or gauze) to carry drops medially may be required if the external auditory canal is

very swollen. The wick should be removed or changed in 48 hours.
- Consider consulting a dermatologist.
- Analgesics or even narcotics may be needed. Nonsteroidal antiinflammatory drugs (NSAIDs) work very well.
- Otitis externa due to a foreign body will usually settle with removal of the foreign body.
- Topical preparations are superior to systemic medications in cost, lower rate of side effects, lower resistance, and higher concentration of the medication at the site of infection.
- Currently, US Food and Drug Administration (FDA)-approved preparations for middle ear exposure are ofloxacin and ciprofloxacin/dexamethasone.
- In some cases of chronic otitis externa with canal stenosis, a canaloplasty, meatoplasty, and skin grafting may be necessary; if surgery is not an option, then a bone-anchored hearing aid may be necessary.
- Chronic or recurrent otomycosis warrants an investigation into underlying causes such as a compromised immune system.
- Most cases resolve within 7 to 10 days of treatment.
- Patients should keep the ears dry for 7 to 10 days.
- Swimmers can return to swimming in 3 days if they use earplugs.
- Hearing aids can be replaced after pain and discharge resolve.
- Prevention: acetic acid drops.

MALIGNANT/NECROTIZING OTITIS EXTERNA

- Malignant/necrotizing otitis externa is defined as otitis externa that progresses to cellulitis, chondritis, periostitis, osteitis, and osteomyelitis of the skull base. It is potentially life threatening but at the very least can lead to serious sequelae.
- Traditionally called malignant otitis externa, not because it is a neoplastic process but due to a high incidence of morbidity and mortality
- Common in elderly diabetics and the immunocompromised (HIV, leukemia, alcoholism)
- Ninety-five percent of cases are caused by *Pseudomonas aeruginosa.*

- Patients present with purulent or bloody otorrhea, hearing loss, severe pain out of proportion to the clinical appearance, and possibly a facial nerve palsy.
- The classic finding is granulation tissue in the floor of the ear canal at the junction of the bony and cartilaginous portions with an intact tympanic membrane.
- Cranial nerves may be affected if the infection reaches the petrous apex.
- Admit patient for assessment. Examine cranial nerves. Perform aural toilet with binocular microscopy. Check complete blood count, erythrocyte sedimentation rate, C-reactive protein, blood glucose, and HbA$_1$C. Send a swab

- for microscopy, culture, and sensitivity. Obtain a baseline audiogram.
- Consider technetium-99m, gallium-67 citrate, CT, and MRI with gadolinium enhancement/fat suppression for diagnosis and follow-up.
- Ciprofloxacin topically and orally/intravenously is useful but be aware that monotherapy may lead to resistance. Consider adding aminoglycoside.
- Involve the infectious disease team, microbiology, and endocrinology.
- Continue drug therapy for 6 to 12 weeks.
- Complications are similar to acute/chronic otitis media.

ANSWERS

TRUE OR FALSE QUESTIONS

1. F	14. T	27. F	40. F
2. F	15. T	28. T	41. T
3. T	16. T	29. T	42. F
4. F	17. F	30. T	43. F
5. F	18. F	31. F	44. F
6. F	19. T	32. F	45. F
7. T	20. F	33. T	46. T
8. T	21. T	34. T	47. F
9. T	22. T	35. T	48. F
10. T	23. T	36. T	49. F
11. F	24. F	37. T	50. F
12. F	25. T	38. T	
13. T	26. F	39. F	

SINGLE BEST ANSWER QUESTIONS

51. d	64. a	77. a	90. c
52. c	65. d	78. c	91. c
53. a	66. a	79. c	92. b
54. c	67. a	80. d	93. d
55. d	68. d	81. c	94. c
56. b	69. a	82. c	95. b
57. d	70. d	83. d	96. d
58. d	71. c	84. c	97. b
59. b	72. c	85. c	98. a
60. d	73. c	86. c	99. a
61. b	74. d	87. d	100. d
62. c	75. d	88. b	
63. b	76. d	89. a	

SUGGESTED READINGS

1. American Academy of Pediatrics Subcommittee on Management of Acute Otitis Media. Diagnosis and management of acute otitis media. *Pediatrics.* 2004;113(5):1451-1465.
2. Dewey C, Midgeley E, Maw R, et al. The relationship between otitis media with effusion and contact with other children in a British cohort studied from 8 months to 3.5 years of age. *Int J Pediatr Otorhinolaryngol.* 2000;55:33-45.
3. Rosenfeld RM, Schwartz SR, Pynnonen MA, et al. Clinical practice guidelines: Tympanostomy tubes in children. *Otolaryngol Head Neck Surg.* 2013;149(1 suppl):S1-S35.
4. Wullstein H. Theory and practice of tympanoplasty. *Laryngoscope.* 1956;66:1076-1093.
5. Persaud R, Hajioff D, Trinidade A, et al. Evidence-based review of aetiopathogenic theories of congenital and acquired cholesteatoma. *J Laryngol Otol.* 2007;121(11):1013-1019.
6. Wilde WR. *Practical Observation on Aural Surgery and the Nature and Treatment of Diseases of the Ear.* Philadelphia: Blanchard and Lea; 1853 <www.archive.org>.
7. Roland PS, Belcher BP, Bettis R, et al. A single topical agent is clinically equivalent to the combination of topical and oral antibiotic treatment for otitis externa. *Am J Otolaryngol.* 2008;29(4):255-261.
8. Rosenfeld RM, Schwartz SR, Cannon CR, et al. Clinical practice guideline: acute otitis externa executive summary. *Otolaryngol Head Neck Surg.* 2014;150(2):161-168.
9. Grandis JR, Curtin HD, Yu VL. Necrotizing (malignant) external otitis: prospective comparison of CT and MR imaging in diagnosis and follow-up. *Radiology.* 1995;196(2):499-504.
10. Phillips JS, Jones SE. Hyperbaric oxygen as an adjuvant treatment for malignant otitis externa. *Cochrane Database Syst Rev.* 2013;(5):CD004617.

Facial Nerve Disorders

Esther Vivas | Douglas Mattox

TRUE OR FALSE QUESTIONS

T / F 1. Most patients with Bell palsy completely recover 3 to 4 months after onset of symptoms.

T / F 2. Pregnancy and severe preeclampsia are known risk factors for Bell palsy.

T / F 3. Antiviral monotherapy is recommended for Bell palsy patients.

T / F 4. The facial nerve exits the brainstem at the pontomedullary junction, cranial to cranial nerve (CN) V.

T / F 5. The cochlear nerve lies inferior to the facial nerve in the internal auditory canal (IAC).

T / F 6. The length of the IAC component of the facial nerve is approximately 8 to 10 mm.

T / F 7. Vascular supply to the facial nerve is provided by the posterior inferior cerebellar artery.

T / F 8. Wallerian degeneration peaks at 48 hours after injury.

T / F 9. Electroneurography (ENOG) is most useful in the first 48 hours after facial nerve injury.

T / F 10. Voluntary electromyogram (EMG) testing is performed in conjunction with ENOG when there is >90% neural degeneration.

T / F 11. Intratemporal facial nerve schwannomas may involve multiple segments of the facial nerve and appear as "beads on a string" on enhanced magnetic resonance imaging (MRI).

T / F 12. There is no gender predilection for Bell palsy.

T / F 13. Transverse fractures make up the majority of temporal bone fractures.

T / F 14. Sensorineural hearing loss (SNHL) and vestibular dysfunction may be a sign of otic capsule or IAC involvement in temporal bone trauma.

T / F 15. The most common malignancy to affect the facial nerve is squamous cell carcinoma.

T / F 16. Möbius syndrome can present with unilateral or bilateral facial palsy.

T / F 17. The facial nerve's embryologic origin is the otic placode.

T / F 18. At the meatal foramen, the facial nerve occupies 83% of the fallopian canal, as opposed to 23% in the tympanic portion.

T / F 19. The facial nerve branches to the stapedius muscle and the chorda tympani nerve emerge from the vertical segment.

T / F 20. An aberrant facial nerve is generally associated with other embryologic abnormalities, most often abnormal development of the stapes.

T / F 21. Within a nerve fiber, the perineurium represents the primary barrier to the spread of infection.

T / F 22. Schwann cells produce collagen in response to injury, which promotes axonal growth during the regenerative period.

T / F 23. The retrosigmoid approach provides nearly an identical view of the facial nerve as that from the translabyrinthine approach for the cerebellopontine angle (CPA) and medial IAC segments.

T / F 24. The arcuate eminence represents the bulge of the posterior semicircular canal.

T / F 25. EMG fibrillation can be seen within a week after nerve injury.

T / F 26. With facial nerve injuries, electrical recovery accompanies spontaneous potentials.

T / F 27. Melkersson-Rosenthal syndrome is associated with migraine headaches and megacolon.

T / F 28. A pathognomonic sign of necrotizing otitis externa is evidence of granulation tissue at the bony-cartilaginous junction most commonly caused by infection with *Staphylococcus aureus*.

T / F 29. Acyclovir is a synthetic purine nucleoside analog.

T / F 30. Neurofibromas arise intrinsically in nerves, and their removal requires nerve resection.

T / F 31. A common presentation of neurofibromatosis type 2 is bilateral facial schwannomas.

T / F 32. Facial paralysis may be the presenting symptom of childhood leukemia.

T / F 33. Single branch facial paralysis may be indicative of an underlying facial schwannoma.

T / F 34. Hearing loss is an expected finding in patients with Bell palsy.

T / F 35. For patients with facial nerve tumors undergoing resection and grafting, the most important determinant of postoperative facial nerve function is the duration of the preoperative paralysis.

T / F 36. Bifid and trifid facial nerves have been described.

T / F 37. The vertical crest of the fundus of the IAC separates the superior vestibular nerve and the cochlear nerve.

T / F 38. Injury to the nervus intermedius during acoustic neuroma surgery can result in postoperative dysgeusia.

T / F 39. During cochlear implant surgery, the most likely site of facial nerve injury is adjacent to the round window.

T / F 40. Facial nerve stimulation is an unavoidable effect of cochlear implant activation.

T / F 41. The stapedius muscle is absent in 1% of patients.

T / F 42. Facial paralysis in chronic otitis occurs from direct extension of infection or by compression from a cholesteatoma.

T / F 43. Cholesteatoma limited to the petrous apex is likely secondarily acquired in origin.

T / F 44. Basal cell carcinoma is the most common primary temporal bone malignancy to affect the facial nerve.

T / F 45. Facial paralysis is a complication of malignant otitis externa.

T / F 46. Facial paralysis secondary to malignant otitis externa requires surgical decompression of the facial canal.

T / F 47. Recurrent Bell palsy can occur in up to 10% of patients.

T / F 48. The incidence of facial nerve paralysis in gunshot wounds to the temporal bone is at least 50%.

T / F 49. Voluntary motor units and polyphasic potentials indicate nerve regeneration.

T / F 50. Patients with immediate onset complete facial nerve paralysis after a penetrating injury should be offered surgery as soon as stable due to the high likelihood of facial nerve transection and the need for repair.

SINGLE BEST ANSWER QUESTIONS

51. The facial nerve origina tes from the facial motor nucleus, which lies in the:
    a. Anterior pons
    b. Posterior pons
    c. Lateral portion of anterior pons
    d. Lateral portion of posterior pons

52. The nervus intermedius carries:
    a. Afferent fibers for taste from the anterior two-thirds of the tongue and conveys sensation from the anterior wall of external auditory canal (EAC)
    b. Afferent fibers for taste from the anterior two-thirds of the tongue and conveys sensation to the posterior EAC
    c. Afferent fibers for taste from the anterior two-thirds of the tongue and conveys sensation to the posterior EAC, as well as secretory fibers to the lacrimal, sublingual, and submaxillary glands
    d. Only afferent fibers conveying sensation to the posterior wall of the EAC

53. The chorda tympani carries:
    a. Preganglionic, parasympathetic fibers that synapse at the submandibular ganglion
    b. Preganglionic, sympathetic fibers that synapse at the submandibular ganglion
    c. Postganglionic, parasympathetic fibers that innervate only the submandibular gland
    d. Postganglionic, sympathetic fibers that innervate only the sublingual gland

54. Transverse fractures:
    a. Are less common than longitudinal fractures but more likely to cause facial nerve damage, occurring in up to 50% of fractures
    b. Are more common than longitudinal fractures but more likely to cause facial nerve damage, occurring in up to 50% of fractures
    c. Are more common than longitudinal fractures but less likely to cause facial nerve damage
    d. Are a result of trauma to the temporal and parietal region of the skull

55. Facial nerve schwannomas are typically:
    a. Extratemporal and most often involve the tympanic segment and geniculate ganglion
    b. Extratemporal and most often involve the labyrinthine segment and geniculate ganglion
    c. Intratemporal and most often involve the labyrinthine segment and geniculate ganglion
    d. Intratemporal and most often involve the tympanic segment and geniculate ganglion

56. The most common neurologic manifestation of Lyme disease is:
    a. Sensorineural hearing loss (SNHL)
    b. Facial nerve paralysis
    c. Neuralgia
    d. Hypesthesia

57. Which is the most accurate statement regarding the etiology and management of Ramsay Hunt syndrome (RHS)?
    a. Herpes simplex virus (HSV) reactivation at the geniculate ganglion and is treated with antivirals only
    b. Varicella-zoster virus (VZV) reactivation at the geniculate ganglion and is treated with corticosteroids only
    c. VZV reactivation at the geniculate ganglion and is treated with antivirals only and is treated with corticosteroids only
    d. VZV reactivation at the geniculate ganglion and is treated with antivirals and corticosteroids

58. Neonatal facial palsy is most likely caused by which of the following?
    a. Möbius syndrome
    b. Maternal transmission of HSV
    c. Melkersson-Rosenthal syndrome
    d. Birth trauma

59. Beginning at Bill bar and ending in the stylomastoid foramen, the facial canal is approximately how long?
    a. 30 mm
    b. 50 mm
    c. 60 mm
    d. 10 cm

60. The greater superficial petrosal nerve:
    a. Supplies taste fibers to the anterior palate
    b. Contains taste fibers and preganglionic parasympathetic fibers
    c. Contains sympathetic fibers that supply the nasal and palatine mucosal glands
    d. Does not carry any sensory or parasympathetic fibers

61. The digastric ridge and tendon is:
    a. Anterior, inferior, and superficial to the facial nerve
    b. Anterior, superior, and superficial to the facial nerve
    c. Posterior, inferior, and superficial to the facial nerve
    d. Posterior, superior, and superficial to the facial nerve

62. The most common abnormality within the vertical segment of the facial nerve is:
    a. Anterior medial displacement
    b. Anterior lateral displacement
    c. Posterior medial displacement
    d. Posterior lateral displacement

63. Synkinesis:
    a. Refers to mass movement of the face
    b. Results from adequate facial nerve regeneration
    c. Results from abnormal facial nerve regeneration
    d. a and c

64. On EMG, fibrillation potentials or denervation potentials:
    a. Occur as part of normal nerve regeneration
    b. Occur 14 to 21 days after wallerian degeneration occurs
    c. Occur immediately after nerve injury
    d. Occur only if the nerve does not undergo wallerian degeneration

65. Recurrent facial palsy, furrowed tongue, and faciolabial edema are seen in which of the following?
    a. Melkersson-Rosenthal syndrome
    b. Familial Bell palsy
    c. Möbius syndrome
    d. Millard-Gubler syndrome

66. Bilateral facial palsies can be encountered with all listed *EXCEPT*:
    a. Bell palsy
    b. Syphilis
    c. Melkersson-Rosenthal syndrome
    d. Multiple sclerosis

67. The following are considered typical presentations for Bell palsy *EXCEPT*:
    a. Pain or numbness of the ear or midface
    b. Progressive facial paralysis occurring over 3 weeks or longer
    c. Taste disturbances
    d. Acute onset facial paralysis or paresis

68. Herpes zoster oticus:
    a. Can affect the ear canal, external ear, and soft palate
    b. Is referred to as Ramsay Hunt syndrome when there is concurrent facial palsy
    c. Presents with otalgia and varicelliform lesions
    d. All of the above

69. With House-Brackmann grade IV dysfunction, there is:
    a. Complete eye closure with maximal effort
    b. Incomplete eye closure with maximal effort
    c. Perceptible forehead movement
    d. Barely perceptible motion

70. Histopathology studies of patients with Bell palsy have shown:
    a. Intraneural vascular congestion of the facial nerve
    b. Hemorrhage in the labyrinthine segment of the facial nerve
    c. Leukocytic infiltration of the facial nerve
    d. All of the above

71. In adults, Lyme disease is promptly treated with which of the following?
    a. 3 weeks of Keflex
    b. 3 weeks of amoxicillin
    c. 3 weeks of doxycycline
    d. 1 million units of penicillin G intramuscularly × 1

72. Facial palsy with concurrent acute otitis media is treated with which of the following?
    a. Systemic antibiotics
    b. Wide myringotomy and systemic antibiotics
    c. Cortical mastoidectomy only if antibiotics and myringotomy fail
    d. Facial nerve decompression

73. Contrast-enhanced MRI in patients with Bell palsy may show:
    a. Diffuse enhancement of the ipsilateral facial nerve
    b. Focal enhancement of the ipsilateral facial nerve
    c. Diffuse enhancement of bilateral facial nerves
    d. No enhancement of the facial nerve

74. The trigeminofacial (blink) reflex:
    a. Assesses facial nerve conduction via activation of the facial nucleus centrally
    b. Records action potentials reflexively generated in the orbicularis oculi muscle in response to an electrical stimulus to the supraorbital area
    c. Is not relevant to facial nerve function
    d. a and b

75. Facial neuromas in the temporal bone exhibit a distinct predilection for which of the following?
    a. The labyrinthine segment
    b. The geniculate ganglion
    c. The tympanic segment
    d. The vertical segment at the stylomastoid foramen

76. On Sunderland's description of the pathophysiology of nerve compression, stage 2 refers to which of the following?
    a. Compromised arterial supply with subsequent fibrosis and permanent damage
    b. Venous congestion with reversible damage
    c. Endothelial damage, intrafascicular edema with subsequent ischemia, and segmental demyelination
    d. None of the above

77. Traumatic neuromas are:
    a. Nonneoplastic proliferations of peripheral nerves
    b. Composed of disrupted axons, Schwann cells, and fibroblastic cells
    c. Caused by relatively trivial injuries to the head/face
    d. All of the above

78. Facial nerve hemangiomas have a predilection for:
    a. Geniculate ganglion
    b. Scarpa ganglion
    c. a only
    d. a and b

79. Granular cell tumors:
    a. Are derived from Schwann cells
    b. Are seen predominantly in Caucasian men
    c. Develop in the second and third decades of life
    d. Are commonly found in the breast

80. Typical presentations of facial nerve tumors include which of the following?
    a. Gradually progressive facial paralysis
    b. Twitching of the facial musculature
    c. Recurrent facial paralysis
    d. All of the above

81. The presence of a stapedial reflex in a patient with facial paralysis:
    a. Is consistent with a parotid gland tumor
    b. Is an expected finding

c. Is consistent with an intratemporal tumor

d. Is irrelevant in the workup of facial paralysis

82. Treatment of facial schwannomas includes:
    a. Watchful waiting when there is underlying good facial function
    b. Radiosurgery immediately on diagnosis
    c. Surgical resection immediately on diagnosis
    d. Partial debulking to help prevent dysfunction

83. Facial schwannomas are seen in patients with which of the following?
    a. Neurofibromatosis type 1
    b. Neurofibromatosis type 2
    c. Schwannomatosis
    d. All of the above

84. Patients with a complete transection of the facial nerve can achieve eye closure by:
    a. Contralateral innervation of the facial nerve
    b. Relaxing the superior levator palpebrae muscle
    c. Motor innervation by CN V
    d. None of the above

85. The paralytic effect of injectable lidocaine wears off:
    a. 15 minutes after injection
    b. 90 minutes after injection
    c. 2 to 3 hours after injection
    d. 5 to 6 hours after injection

86. The rationale for prompt exploration of iatrogenic facial nerve injury lies in:
    a. Preventing the accumulation of granulation tissue at the site of nerve injury, which would make later repair more difficult
    b. Evacuation of a possible expanding hematoma within the nerve sheath
    c. Grafting or direct repair if complete transection is found
    d. All of the above

87. Anatomic preservation of the facial nerve in acoustic neuroma surgery:
    a. Translates to intact facial nerve function postoperatively
    b. Results in immediate postoperative paresis in more than 50% of cases
    c. Results in immediate postoperative paralysis in up to 13.5% of cases
    d. b and c

88. Facial nerve injury during middle fossa surgery:
    a. May occur with elevation of the dura over a dehiscent geniculate ganglion
    b. May be avoided by elevating dura off the middle fossa floor in anterior to posterior fashion
    c. Is reduced by making skin cuts and staying in the fascial plane between the subdermal fat and temporalis muscle at the level of the superficial muscular aponeurotic system
    d. May occur only when drilling directly over the IAC

89. In congenital atresia surgery, the facial nerve most commonly lies:
    a. Inferiorly and anteriorly to the atretic bone
    b. Inferiorly and posteriorly to the atretic bone
    c. Superiorly and anteriorly to the atretic bone
    d. Superiorly and posteriorly to the atretic bone

90. The most common site for dehiscence of the facial canal is:
    a. Vertical segment
    b. Horizontal segment
    c. Labyrinthine segment
    d. Meatal foramen

91. Primary temporal bone carcinoma is predominantly:
    a. Squamous cell carcinoma
    b. Adenoid cystic carcinoma
    c. Basal cell carcinoma
    d. Melanoma

92. According to the revised Pittsburgh staging system for primary temporal bone squamous cell cancer (SCCA), facial nerve involvement confers:
    a. Stage 2
    b. Stage 3
    c. Stage 4
    d. The facial nerve is not taken into account for staging criteria.

93. Facial paralysis with ear canal edema and underlying deep facial pain in an elderly diabetic patient is due to:
    a. *Pseudomonas aeruginosa* infection
    b. Basal cell cancer of the ear canal
    c. A parotid malignancy
    d. SCCA of the ear canal

94. Metastasis to the temporal bone:
    a. Originates in the prostate
    b. Occurs by hematogenous spread to the marrow of the petrous apex
    c. Occurs by extension up the eustachian tube
    d. Is seen mostly in the pediatric population

95. Facial paralysis can be the result of collagen vascular diseases, which include all of the following *EXCEPT*:
    a. Scleroderma
    b. Periarteritis nodosa
    c. Sarcoidosis
    d. Systemic lupus erythematosus

96. Iridocyclitis, parotid enlargement, and facial palsy are seen in which of the following?
    a. Heerfordt syndrome
    b. Leprosy
    c. Poliomyelitis
    d. Wegener granulomatosis

97. The procedure of choice to restore facial function after discontinuity of the facial nerve is:
    a. Cable graft with sural nerve
    b. Cable graft with great auricular nerve
    c. Primary anastomosis
    d. Hypoglossal-facial anastomosis

98. Gunshot wounds to the temporal bone are most likely to injure the:
    a. Tympanic segment
    b. Mastoid segment
    c. Labyrinthine segment
    d. Main trunk distal for the stylomastoid foramen

99. A regenerating nerve will have which of the following characteristics on EMG?
    a. Fibrillation potentials
    b. Absent volitional compound muscle action potentials (CMAPs)
    c. Denervation potentials
    d. Polyphasic potentials

100. Facial reanimation for patients who are not candidates for primary repair includes:
    a. Cross facial nerve graft
    b. Hypoglossal-facial jump graft
    c. Free muscle transfer
    d. All of the above

CORE KNOWLEDGE

- The facial motor nucleus contains approximately 7000 neurons and lies within the reticular formation of the lower third of the pons.
- The superior portion of the facial nucleus receives bilateral cortical input, while the inferior portion receives only contralateral cortical input and is responsible for innervation of the lower facial musculature. This is basis for the "forehead sparing" in central nerve palsies.
- The relative position of the facial nerve to the cochleovestibular complex changes as it leaves the brainstem and progresses through the IAC by rotating 90 degrees.
- The course of the nerve from the brainstem to the facial musculature is divided into three segments: intracranial, intratemporal (Figure 8-1), and extratemporal.
- The meatal segment of the facial nerve is a transition zone between the lateral portion of the IAC and the proximal fallopian canal.

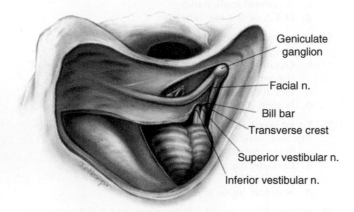

FIGURE 8-1 Intratemporal course of the facial nerve.

- The facial canal is formed by contributions from Reichert cartilage of the second arch and the cartilaginous otic capsule.
- The transverse crest divides the IAC into superior and inferior portions.
- The superior portion houses the facial nerve anteriorly and the superior vestibular nerve posteriorly, while the inferior portion contains the cochlear nerve anteriorly and the inferior vestibular nerve posteriorly (Figure 8-2).
- Bill bar is a surgical landmark and separates the superior compartment of the IAC into anterior and posterior segments. The anterosuperior compartment carries the facial nerve, while the posterosuperior compartment is filled by the superior vestibular nerve.
- The geniculate ganglion and nervus intermedius (second branchial arch) form independently of the motor division of the seventh nerve.
- The geniculate ganglion carries sensory functions for the nervus intermedius and gives rise to the greater superficial petrosal nerve (GSPN), which enters the middle fossa floor through the facial hiatus.
- The GSPN contains secretory fibers to the lacrimal gland. These synapse in the pterygopalatine ganglion.
- The most narrow portion of the fallopian canal is found at the labyrinthine segment, where the diameter is <0.7 mm.
- The labyrinthine segment of the facial nerve is 4 mm in length, whereas the tympanic segment is 11 mm in length, and the vertical or mastoid segment is approximately 13 mm in length.
- The five landmarks used to identify the tympanic segment of the facial nerve are the cochleariform process, oval window, pyramidal process, lateral semicircular canal, and the cog.
- The angle between the chorda tympani nerve and the vertical portion of the facial nerve is approximately 30 degrees, an area also known as the facial recess.

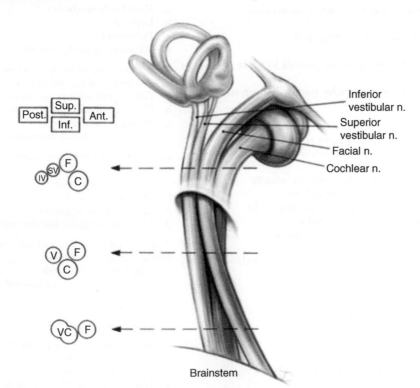

FIGURE 8-2 Relationship of the facial nerve to the cochlear and vestibular nerves from the cerebellopontine angle through the external auditory canal. *C,* Cochlear nerve; *F,* facial nerve; *IV,* inferior vestibular nerve; *SV,* superior vestibular nerve; *V,* vestibular. (Reproduced with permission from Adour KK. Facial nerve electrical testing. In: Jackler RK, Brackmann DE, eds. Neurotology. St Louis: Mosby; 1994:1287.)

- The extratemporal portion of the facial nerve divides into the temporal, zygomatic, buccal, marginal, mandibular, and cervical branches.
- The blood supply to the facial nerve is segmented and derived from branches of the anterior inferior cerebellar artery, middle meningeal artery, and postauricular artery.
- The most common anatomic variation of the facial nerve is dehiscence of the fallopian canal at the tympanic segment.
- On physical examination, unilateral corneal irritation produces *bilateral* orbicularis oculi contraction because of the corneal reflex arc, which is composed of afferents from the cornea via V_1 into the brainstem that synapse with interneurons and connect to the facial nuclei to produce muscular contraction of the orbicularis oculi muscles.
- In cases with complete paralysis, the examiner should press his/her thumbs on the midline of the patient's face to prevent the unopposed normal side from distorting the examination of the paralyzed side.
- Single branch facial paralysis is caused by a tumor unless proved otherwise.
- Bell palsy refers to an idiopathic facial paralysis.
- Bell palsy is the most common cause of unilateral facial palsy and is characterized by an abrupt onset of unilateral paresis that develops over 24 to 48 hours and can progress to complete paralysis over a 7-day period.
- Incidence of Bell palsy is estimated at 15 to 40 per 100,000 individuals in the general population.
- Inflammation and ischemia appear to dominate the early events in Bell palsy, followed by neural blockade, degeneration, and subsequent fibroblastic response.
- HSV-1 has been repeatedly isolated from patients with Bell palsy.
- Serologic tests for Lyme disease (immunoglobulin G, immunoglobulin M) are an important part of the workup for unexplained facial paralysis, particularly in endemic areas.
- Preeclampsia was found to be six times more prevalent among women with pregnancy-associated facial palsy than in the general population of gravid women.
- Immunodeficiency confers a risk of acute facial palsy.
- In treating patients with Bell palsy, the use of an antiviral agent in addition to corticosteroid treatment has been shown to improve the recovery of facial function when compared with corticosteroid treatment alone.
- Accepted doses include oral prednisone 1 mg/kg × 7 days and oral valacyclovir 500 mg three times a day × 10 days.
- The antiinflammatory effect of glucocorticoids is attributed to effects on vascular tone, permeability and suppression of leukocytes, and collagen biosynthesis.
- Bilateral facial palsy occurs in <2% of patients who present with acute facial nerve dysfunction and typically reflects a systemic disorder.
- Twitching of the facial nerve in association with facial palsy is not seen in Bell palsy and should raise suspicion for an underlying neoplasm.
- In cases of Bell palsy with >90% degeneration on ENOG and absence of CMAP on EMG, middle fossa craniotomy with decompression of the labyrinthine, geniculate, and proximal tympanic segments of the nerve should be offered.
- RHS is associated with VZV and accounts for 10% to 15% of acute facial palsy cases (second to Bell palsy).
- RHS has an active phase that persists for a longer period of time than that of Bell palsy, therefore requiring an extended 3-week course of corticosteroid and antiviral therapy.

- High-resolution thin-cut computed tomography (CT) with bone algorithms and enhanced MRI are complementary in the evaluation of patients with a facial paralysis.
- Compressive nerve injury is progressive and ranges from neuropraxia to axonotmesis and eventually to neurotmesis. Distal wallerian degeneration occurs in the last two.
- Seddon described progressive degrees of nerve injury as neuropraxia, axonotmesis, and neurotmesis, but Sunderland then expanded this classification to five degrees of injury (Figure 8-3).
- Wallerian degeneration begins 12 to 24 hours following injury and is at a peak within 72 hours.
- The rate of axon regeneration is approximately 1 mm/day.
- An evoked electric stimulus generates synchronous facial muscle movement that can be recorded from the skin surface (CMAP).
- Voluntary facial contractions also generate CMAPs, which are graded on a scale ranging from 1 to 4 (4 is normal).
- The amplitude of the biphasic CMAP has been found to correlate with the number of blocked or neuropraxic nerve fibers.
- As the percentage of degenerated fibers within the nerve increases, the amplitude of the CMAP decreases compared with the normal side of the face.
- In ENOG, the nerve is stimulated with a supramaximal stimulus, and the functional status is assessed on the basis of the CMAP recorded amplitude.
- The time interval between nerve stimulation and initiation of CMAP is represented as the facial nerve latency and considered an indication of nerve function.
- Selection for surgical decompression of the facial nerve is based on ENOG comparison of the CMAP on the affected and unaffected sides of the face.
- When the CMAP on the affected side is 90% less than on the unaffected side within 2 weeks after onset of paresis, decompression is advised.
- ENOG is most useful between 4 and 21 days after onset of complete paralysis.
- The House-Brackmann nerve grading system is the most commonly used system by otolaryngologists, with function ranging from normal (HB I) to complete paralysis (HB VI).
- One of the important features of the House-Brackmann grading scale is its use of eye closure as an indicator of severity.
- Complete mobilization of the facial nerve from the brainstem to the pes anserinus leads to a House-Brackmann grade III to IV function at best.
- Faulty myelination and shunting of electrical activity is thought to be responsible for synkinesis in regenerating nerves.
- Frey syndrome or gustatory sweating occurs when postganglionic parasympathetic fibers of CN IX, normally targeted for the parotid gland, innervate sweat glands normally supplied by postganglionic sympathetic fibers. This can occur after parotid surgery.
- The Schwann cell is the parent cell of both schwannomas and neurofibromas.
- The Schwann cell is a sheath cell, not a nerve cell.
- Schwannomas have a predilection for sensory nerves and affect the facial nerve much less frequently than the cochleovestibular nerve.
- Schwannomas are rarely if ever associated with malignant degeneration.
- Histologically, there two patterns seen in schwannomas: Antoni type A (densely cellular areas with cohesive cells arranged in regular patterns) and Antoni type B (areas of vacuolation between cells due to accumulation of extracellular matrix).

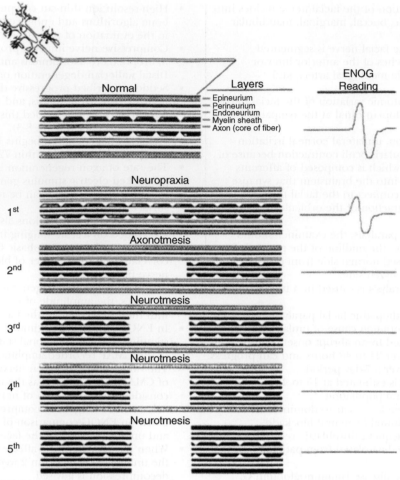

FIGURE 8-3 Schematic drawing of Sunderland's five degrees of nerve injury and resultant effect on summation compound muscle action potential (CMAP). *ENOG*, Electroneurography. (Reproduced with permission from Adour KK. Facial nerve electrical testing. In: Jackler RK, Brackmann DE, eds. *Neurotology*. St Louis: Mosby; 1994:1287.)

- Facial schwannomas have been historically referred to as facial neuromas, neurilomas, neurinoma, neurilemmoma, neurolemmoma, or perineural fibroblastoma.
- Neurofibromatosis type 1, neurofibromatosis type 2, and schwannomatosis predispose patients to facial schwannomas.
- Facial nerve schwannomas can arise at any point along the course of the facial nerve and can be multicentric (Figure 8-4).
- The majority of facial schwannomas originate in the region of the geniculate ganglion, followed by the labyrinthine and tympanic segments of the facial canal.
- As many as 50% of facial nerve fibers may have degenerated before clinical signs of facial nerve dysfunction appear.
- Facial neuromas usually do not cause symptoms until advanced and may manifest with hearing symptoms.
- In patients with benign facial nerve tumors, bony decompression of the nerve may be a compromise, with definitive surgery postponed until the paralysis progresses.
- Watchful waiting is an acceptable strategy for patients with facial neuromas and good facial nerve function.
- Facial nerve schwannomas can erode into the otic capsule bone, causing hearing loss and/or vestibular dysfunction.
- Unlike schwannomas, hemangiomas can produce facial paralysis even when they are only a few millimeters in diameter, suggesting a vascular steal phenomenon with nerve ischemia.

- Hemangiomas are extraneural and can cause paralysis by compression.
- A rich vascular plexus at the geniculate ganglion may explain its predilection for benign vascular tumors.
- Facial function after a facial nerve graft is typically House-Brackmann grade IV, rarely III in the most experienced hands.
- Facial hemangiomas at the geniculate ganglion exhibit characteristic bony changes, termed "honeycomb bone" on CT (Figure 8-5).
- Facial nerve hemangiomas can be removed with preservation of facial nerve function; early surgery offers the best outcome.
- A "pseudotumor" of the facial nerve consists of an inflammatory swelling of the nerve sheath caused by trauma from a previous surgery and active inflammation.
- Iatrogenic injury of the intracranial and intracanalicular components of the facial nerve is easier secondary to the lack of perineural and epineural connective tissue found in the distal segments.
- The absence of an overlying mastoid tip in neonates places the vertical segment of the facial nerve at risk for birth trauma injury.
- With iatrogenic facial nerve injury, if disruption to the nerve is 50% or less than the total cross-sectional area, adequate function should return and the surgeon should avoid further intervention. However, if >50% of the nerve is traumatized, formal repair is warranted.

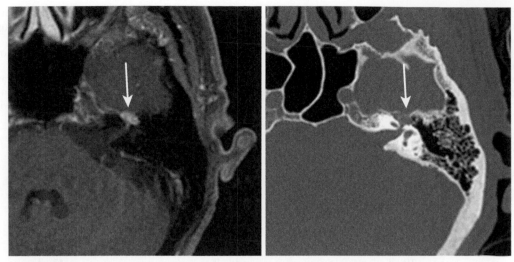

FIGURE 8-4 Facial hemangioma: Enhancing mass centered at the geniculate ganglion *(arrow)* on contrast enhanced magnetic resonance imaging, with permeative bone matrix *(arrow)* on computed tomography. (From Kwan PF, Thomas R: Pathology of the facial nerve: a pictorial review. 2014 Combined Scientific Meeting. http://dx.doi.org/10.1594/ranzcr2014/R-0215.)

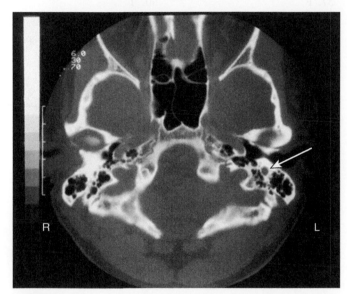

FIGURE 8-5 Temporal bone computed tomographic image showing facial neuroma in the mastoid portion of the facial nerve *(arrow)*. (Reproduced with permission from Adour KK. Facial nerve electrical testing. In: Jackler RK, Brackmann DE, eds. *Neurotology.* St Louis: Mosby; 1994:1287.)

- Within the temporal bone, if enough of the fallopian canal remains as a trough, placement of a graft in approximation to the nerve end may be sufficient, followed by microfibrillar collagen (Avitene), which forms a clot over the anastomosis.
- Primary anastomosis may be achievable by removing the facial nerve from the fallopian canal and rerouting to gain extra length.
- Postoperative cerebrospinal fluid leaks occur in <10% of patients undergoing facial neuroma surgery.
- Regardless of the extent of facial nerve injury, eye care is paramount. Even with minor injuries, blink reflexes can be diminished, increasing the likelihood of corneal injury.
- Temporal bone fractures are classified as either longitudinal (along the long axis of the petrous pyramid), transverse (at right angles to the petrous pyramid), or mixed.

- It has recently been advocated to reclassify temporal bone fractures as either affecting or sparing the otic capsule rather than only referencing its relation to the petrous apex/pyramid.
- Transverse fractures can have up to a 50% incidence of facial paralysis, whereas in longitudinal fractures the incidence is 20%.
- A transverse temporal bone fracture can be suspected with SNHL, vertigo, and facial paralysis. The external canal is frequently intact with no hemotympanum.
- Longitudinal fractures account for 80% of temporal bone fracture.
- A longitudinal fracture often extends to the foramen ovale.
- The ossicles are most often damaged in longitudinal temporal bone fractures.
- Gunshot wounds of the temporal bone frequently result in loss of a segment of the nerve, requiring cable grafting for repair.
- Residual bullet fragments can remain lodged in the temporal bone and become nidus for infection. A canal wall down or radical mastoidectomy has been advocated as the approach of choice.
- In congenital facial paralysis, the sensory contributions of the facial nerve can function normally in the presence of a complete motor paralysis.
- Melkersson-Rosenthal syndrome is usually sporadic, but familial occurrence has been described. Pathophysiology is unknown.
- Albers-Schönberg disease refers to osteopetrosis, a generalized bone disorder that can present with unilateral or bilateral recurrent facial paralysis and other cranial nerve neuropathies.
- Autism and mental retardation can be seen in up to one-third of patients with Möbius syndrome.
- In hypothyroidism with myxedema, the cochlear nerve is the most frequently involved cranial nerve, whereas the facial nerve is one of the least affected.
- Malignant otitis externa reaches the facial nerve through the fissures of Santorini or by exiting through the junction of the bony-cartilaginous canal and into the parotid gland.
- Surgical decompression of the facial nerve in patients with Wegener granulomatosis or periarteritis should not

be performed because this may aggravate the underlying pathophysiology.
- Squamous cell carcinoma is the most common primary temporal bone malignancy, followed by basal cell carcinoma. Involvement of the facial nerve confers advanced stage disease with poor prognosis (stage 4 on the Pittsburgh staging system).

- Hematogenous spread to the temporal bone occurs from primary sites such as the breast, kidney, lung, and stomach and occasionally from skin and prostate.
- Facial paralysis caused by tumors may respond to steroids, causing delay in diagnosis.
- Hemifacial spasm is caused by arterial irritation of the facial nerve at the brainstem root entry zone and is relieved by microvascular decompression with Teflon.

ANSWERS

TRUE OR FALSE QUESTIONS

1. T	14. T	27. T	40. F
2. T	15. T	28. F	41. T
3. F	16. T	29. T	42. T
4. F	17. F	30. T	43. F
5. T	18. T	31. F	44. F
6. T	19. T	32. T	45. T
7. F	20. T	33. T	46. F
8. F	21. T	34. F	47. T
9. F	22. F	35. T	48. T
10. T	23. T	36. T	49. T
11. T	24. F	37. F	50. T
12. T	25. F	38. T	
13. F	26. F	39. F	

SINGLE BEST ANSWER QUESTIONS

51. c	64. b	77. d	90. b
52. c	65. a	78. d	91. a
53. a	66. c	79. a	92. c
54. a	67. b	80. d	93. a
55. c	68. d	81. a	94. b
56. b	69. b	82. a	95. c
57. d	70. d	83. d	96. a
58. d	71. c	84. b	97. c
59. a	72. c	85. c	98. b
60. b	73. a	86. d	99. d
61. c	74. d	87. d	100. d
62. d	75. b	88. a	
63. d	76. c	89. b	

SUGGESTED READINGS

1. Peitersen E. The natural history of Bell's palsy. *Am J Otol.* 1982;4:107-111.
2. House JW, Brackmann DE. Facial nerve grading system. *Otolaryngol Head Neck Surg.* 1985;93:146-147.
3. Grogan PM, Gronseth GS. Practice parameter: steroids, acyclovir and surgery for Bell's palsy (an evidence-based review): Report of the Quality Standards Subcommittee of the American Academy of Neurology. *Neurology.* 2001;56(7): 830-836.
4. Gantz J, Rubinstein JT, Gidley P, Woodworth GG. Surgical management of Bell's palsy. *Laryngoscope.* 1999;109(8): 1177-1188.
5. Angeli SI, Brackmann DE. Is surgical excision of facial nerve schwannomas always indicated? *Otolaryngol Head Neck Surg.* 1997;117:S144-S147.
6. Liu R, Fagan P. Facial nerve schwannoma: surgical excision versus conservative management. *Ann Otol Rhinol Laryngol.* 2001;110:1025-1029.
7. Conley J, Selfe RW. Occult neoplasms in facial paralysis. *Laryngoscope.* 1981;91:205-210.
8. Balkany TJ, Fradis M, Jafek BW, Rucker NC. Hemangioma of the facial nerve: role of the geniculate capillary plexus. *Skull Base Surg.* 1991;1:59-63.
9. May M, Blumenthal F, Klein SR. Acute Bell's palsy: prognostic value of evoked electromyography, maximal stimulation, and other electrical tests. *Am J Otol.* 1983;5:1-7.
10. Baugh RF, Basura GJ, Ishii LE, et al. Clinical practice guideline: Bell's palsy. *Otolaryngol Head Neck Surg.* 2013;149(3 suppl):S1-S27. doi:10.1177/0194599813505967.

Hearing Aids | 9

Chelsea Conrad | Brad A. Stach | Virginia Ramachandran

TRUE OR FALSE QUESTIONS

HEARING LOSS

T/F   1. Nature, degree, and configuration of hearing sensitivity alone determine success of hearing aid use.

T/F   2. Hearing aids are predominantly fit on ears with sensorineural or mixed hearing loss.

T/F   3. Conductive hearing loss is generally fit with amplification if surgical options have been exhausted or are contraindicated.

T/F   4. A patient with a mild hearing loss should not be considered a candidate for amplification because it would provide limited benefit.

T/F   5. Patients who lack recognition of their hearing loss will likely have a limited positive prognosis regarding hearing aid use.

T/F   6. Patient motivation is a key indicator of hearing aid success.

T/F   7. Cognitive ability may influence amplification options for a patient or may preclude an individual from candidacy.

T/F   8. Central auditory nervous system function influences an individual's success with amplification, and that success may change over time.

T/F   9. Hearing sensitivity does not influence style options for a patient; any hearing loss can be fit with any style hearing aid.

T/F   10. A patient's perception of communication impairment is a more significant influence on motivation for amplification than hearing sensitivity.

SIGNAL PROCESSING

T/F   11. Dynamic range describes the decibel difference in the level of a person's threshold of minimum hearing sensitivity and maximum hearing sensitivity.

T/F   12. Linear amplification uses compression to provide amplification across a wide range of inputs.

T/F   13. In some hearing aids, compression can be adjusted independently in multiple frequency bands.

T/F   14. Use of hearing aids relies on microphones located away from the tympanic membrane. This disrupts an individual's normal ability to hear in background noise.

T/F   15. Digital noise reduction circuitry is limited in capability because both speech and nonspeech noise always have similar variations in frequency and intensity over time.

T/F   16. Acoustic feedback is managed with both physical modifications and digital feedback suppression technology.

T/F   17. A telecoil is an input transducer that can bypass the microphone of a hearing aid to communicate electromagnetically with telephones and assistive listening devices (ALDs).

T/F   18. Modern hearing aids may be able to receive Bluetooth or other wirelessly transmitted signals from personal audio devices, televisions, computers, phones, or ALDs.

T/F   19. The frequency response of a hearing aid is influenced by both the microphone and the speaker through which the sound is transduced.

T/F   20. Many patients with sensorineural hearing loss have normal detection of loud sounds, but soft sounds are inaudible. For these patients, linear amplification is most appropriate.

T/F   21. Most hearing aids have some form of output limiting to avoid adding excessive gain to loud sounds.

T/F   22. Hearing aids may be capable of processing sound appropriately for different acoustic environments, but they all require the user of the device to manually select the correct program or memory.

T/F   23. Use of a hearing aid may disrupt the unique resonance characteristics of the ear, but these properties can be accurately simulated with use of digital signal processing to correct an individual's ability to localize sound sources.

T/F   24. Alternative input transducers such as telecoils can deliver a signal to both hearing aids at once and may eliminate the detrimental impact of noise, reverberation, and distance in an acoustic environment.

T/F   25. The amplifier of a hearing aid may be able to apply gain independently to different input frequencies but is unable to apply gain independently to different input intensities.

T/F   26. Individuals with flat, moderate hearing losses are most likely to benefit from frequency-transposition or frequency-lowering technology.

HEARING AID STYLES

T/F   27. The term *open-fit hearing aid* refers to a device that does not occlude the ear canal.

T/F 28. In general, acoustic feedback is least likely to occur in a properly fit behind-the-ear (BTE) hearing aid.

T/F 29. In-the-ear (ITE) hearing aids range in style from those that completely fill the concha to those that are inserted deeply into the ear canal.

T/F 30. BTE hearing aids with custom earmolds are the most suitable option for children, given cost concerns, durability, and anatomical changes of the child over time.

T/F 31. Venting and use of an open-style hearing aid may assist in reduction of acoustic feedback.

T/F 32. Individuals with significant cerumen or perspiration should consider ITE hearing aids rather than BTE hearing aids due to durability of the devices.

T/F 33. BTE hearing aid styles have many benefits compared with ITE hearing aid styles with the exception of increased risk of acoustic feedback.

T/F 34. Earmolds are made in many different styles and of different materials to accommodate patient preference but have limited influence on the acoustics of the amplified sounds.

T/F 35. A receiver-in-the-canal (RIC) hearing aid is the same as a BTE hearing aid in appearance, but the microphone of the device is housed in the ear canal.

T/F 36. Individuals at risk for external otitis would likely benefit from a large vent in a hearing aid or earmold or an open-fit device to allow aeration of the ear canal.

SELECTION AND FITTING

T/F 37. Prescribed target gain of a hearing aid is based on an individual's hearing sensitivity alone according to National Acoustic Laboratory NL2 and Desired Sensation Level version 5.0 fitting strategies.

T/F 38. The response of a hearing aid is unique to the acoustics of the ear into which it is fit.

T/F 39. In general, an individual with hearing loss bilaterally should be fit with bilateral amplification to take advantage of binaural hearing benefits.

T/F 40. A unilateral fitting of a hearing aid for an individual with symmetric hearing loss may be degrading to the speech perception ability of the unaided ear over time.

T/F 41. A contralateral routing of signals (CROS) or bilateral CROS (BiCROS) device will afford a patient the same binaural benefits as a bilateral fitting of traditional amplification.

T/F 42. Hearing aids are initially programmed and generally require little or no adjustment due to sophisticated fitting methods and intensive research into patient preference.

T/F 43. Smaller ear canals of infants and children require higher sound pressure levels (SPLs) to be delivered from the hearing aid for sound audibility.

T/F 44. Functional gain assessment is more commonly used with pediatric patients.

T/F 45. Probe microphone measurements are made near the tympanic membrane and allow the clinician to assess the influence of the resonance of the pinna, concha, and ear canal on the amplified signal of a hearing aid.

T/F 46. The fitting range of a hearing aid helps to determine whether or not a specific hearing aid is appropriate for a patient's hearing loss.

T/F 47. The Baha, Ponto, and Alpha 2 are surgically anchored devices that may be used in the treatment of unilateral deafness.

T/F 48. For ITE hearing aids, an impression of the ear canal must be made using a powder and liquid mix, silicon material, or 3D digital scanner.

T/F 49. Individuals with tinnitus should always use amplification with incorporated sound generators because amplification alone cannot alleviate tinnitus.

T/F 50. Electroacoustic analysis of a hearing aid provides information about the hearing aid's gain, maximum output, and battery drain.

SINGLE BEST ANSWER QUESTIONS

51. Physical components of a hearing aid must include which of the following?
    a. A noise damper
    b. A receiver
    c. A compressor
    d. An earmold

52. Which of the following is the greatest advantage of an open-fit hearing aid for an appropriate hearing aid candidate relative to other amplification styles?
    a. It is easier to remove.
    b. It is more durable.
    c. The thicker tubing requires less maintenance.
    d. It allows low-frequency sound to pass through naturally.

53. Limiting acoustic feedback may be accomplished by all of the following *EXCEPT*:
    a. Tightly occluding the ear canal with a well fit hearing aid or earmold
    b. Increasing the distance between the microphone and the loudspeaker
    c. Applying digital feedback reduction controls in the device software
    d. Increasing vent size of the hearing aid or earmold

54. Most modern hearing aids are programmed to each individual patient via which of the following?
    a. Use of a hearing aid analyzer to adjust the maximum output
    b. Manual adjustment of the frequency response of the microphone
    c. Controls in software specific to the manufacturer of each hearing aid
    d. Electroacoustic verification of the device

55. In situ hearing aid verification measurements are generally performed using which of the following?
    a. A sound level meter
    b. A 2-cc coupler
    c. A probe microphone
    d. Insert earphones

56. Which of the following statements is true about specific prescriptive measurements developed for pediatric populations?
    a. They are available only in specific pediatric hearing instruments.

b. They are designed to incorporate the resonance characteristics of the child's ear.

c. They are designed for patient comfort rather than audibility.

d. They can be used only until a child reaches age 9.

57. Frequency transposition technology may be of greatest benefit to individuals with which of the following?
a. Cochlear dead regions
b. A rising audiogram
c. Hyperacusis
d. Mixed hearing loss

58. All of the following statements are true *EXCEPT:*
a. Hearing aids are predominantly fit on ears with sensorineural or mixed hearing loss.
b. Hearing aid users tend to have hearing loss that is at least moderate in degree.
c. Most patients with mild to moderate hearing loss do not pursue hearing aid use.
d. Patients with minimal hearing loss cannot benefit from mild gain hearing aids.

59. Which of the following statements is true regarding patients with anatomical abnormalities of the ear such as microtia or stenosis?
a. They would most likely benefit from an ITE style hearing aid.
b. They will generally not have issues with device retention.
c. They may require use of a bone conducted hearing device.
d. They are generally able to use conventional amplification.

60. Which of the following statements is true regarding patients with external ear canal concerns such as excessive moisture or otitis externa?
a. They are unable to use amplification without resolution of their symptoms.
b. They would likely benefit from a traditional BTE rather than ITE or RIC.
c. They would likely benefit from an ITE rather than a RIC or traditional BTE.
d. They would likely benefit from a RIC rather than an ITE or traditional BTE.

61. Which of the following statements regarding hearing aid style decisions is *INCORRECT?*
a. They are made individually for each patient.
b. They are affected by the anatomy of the external auditory canal and pinna.
c. They are made without regard for durability of the devices.
d. They are limited by the patient's visual status and dexterity.

62. Which of the following statements is true of the telecoil of a hearing aid?
a. It is a standard feature in every device.
b. It communicates via Bluetooth technology.
c. It is an ALD that creates a visual stimulus.
d. It interacts with external inputs electromagnetically.

63. Patients with significant cognitive impairment may require consideration of which of the following?
a. A CROS system
b. Unilateral fitting of a device
c. A personal sound amplifier
d. Written communication

64. Digital signal processing does all of the following *EXCEPT:*

a. Always provides more natural sound quality
b. Converts an analog signal to digital and back to analog
c. Uses an amplifier to shape different frequencies independently
d. May control acoustic feedback better than analog technology

65. The membrane of a microphone vibrates to capture all of the following *EXCEPT:*
a. The amplitude of an acoustic signal
b. The frequency of an acoustic signal
c. The phase of an acoustic signal
d. The resistance of an acoustic signal

66. Alternative input transducers (such as telecoils or FM signals) reduce degradation of a signal by removing the effects of all of the following *EXCEPT:*
a. Distance
b. Flat frequency response
c. Noise
d. Reverberation

67. Gain is adjusted to vary as a function of which of the following?
a. Frequency depending on the user's hearing loss
b. Phase depending on the user's hearing loss
c. Resistance depending on the user's hearing loss
d. Impedance depending on the user's hearing loss

68. The input-output function of a hearing aid describes the relationship of which of the following?
a. Input and output frequency
b. Input and output intensity
c. Input and output phase
d. Input and output resistance

69. Linear amplification is typically best applied to which of the following?
a. Sensorineural hearing loss
b. Auditory processing disorder
c. Conductive hearing loss
d. Mixed hearing loss

70. Abnormal loudness growth (or recruitment) refers to the phenomenon in which:
a. Individuals with conductive hearing loss hear high-intensity sounds normally
b. Individuals with conductive hearing loss hear high-intensity sounds normally only if amplified
c. Individuals with sensorineural hearing loss hear high-intensity sounds normally
d. Individuals with sensorineural hearing loss hear high-intensity sounds normally only if amplified

71. Which of the following statements is true of nonlinear amplification?
a. Gain is applied uniformly to low- and high-intensity inputs.
b. The same amount of gain is added regardless of input intensity.
c. Gain is applied only to low-intensity inputs.
d. The amount of gain applied is dependent on the input signal intensity.

72. Nonlinear amplification is designed to do all of the following *EXCEPT:*
a. Make soft sounds audible
b. Maintain loudness of high-intensity sounds but not overamplify the signal
c. Address the altered loudness growth of an ear with sensorineural hearing loss
d. Address the increased dynamic range of an ear with sensorineural hearing loss

73. Which of the following statements regarding wide dynamic range compression circuitry is *INCORRECT*?
    a. It allows the entire frequency bandwidth of an input acoustic signal to be processed by a hearing aid.
    b. It limits the maximum output of a hearing aid.
    c. It provides nonlinear amplification across a wide range of acoustic inputs.
    d. It diminishes gain near the maximum output level.

74. Hearing aids may adversely affect a patient's ability to hear in background noise largely because:
    a. The normal spatial cues provided by the resonance of the pinna and ear canal are altered when a hearing aid is placed in the ear canal.
    b. Sound delivered by a hearing aid has poor low-frequency sound fidelity.
    c. Expansion maximizes gain for very low-intensity inputs.
    d. Noise is louder than amplified speech sounds, effectively masking the listener's target signal.

75. Which of the following statements is true of BTE hearing aids?
    a. They have the shortest distance between the microphone and ear canal.
    b. They offer limited flexibility in terms of fitting range.
    c. They are not compatible with telecoils.
    d. They house the receiver in the ear canal or in the case behind the ear.

76. Open-fit hearing aids are most appropriate for individuals with which of the following?
    a. Low-frequency hearing loss
    b. High-frequency hearing loss
    c. Severe hearing loss
    d. Profound hearing loss

77. Microphone directionality is generally available in all of the following *EXCEPT*:
    a. BTE hearing aids
    b. Completely-in-the-canal (CIC) hearing aids
    c. Full-shell hearing aids
    d. RIC hearing aids

78. Which of the following statements is true of occlusion of the ear canal?
    a. It results in a sensation of increased volume of the patient's own voice.
    b. It results in a sensation of decreased volume of the patient's own voice.
    c. It reduces the echo quality of external sounds.
    d. It reduces the echo quality of the patient's own voice.

79. Which of the following statements is true of venting of hearing aids or earmolds?
    a. It is important for patients with profound hearing loss.
    b. It increases the occlusion effect.
    c. It allows aeration of the external auditory canal.
    d. It decreases potential for acoustic feedback.

80. The auricle and concha of the ear increase high-frequency sound by collecting and resonating sound:
    a. Below 500 Hz
    b. 500 to 1000 Hz
    c. 1000 to 2000 Hz
    d. Above 2000 Hz

81. Which of the following hearing aid styles is least likely to be affected by excessive cerumen or perspiration?
    a. CIC
    b. RIC
    c. Full-shell
    d. Traditional BTE

82. An FM system consists of all the following *EXCEPT*:
    a. A microphone/transmitter
    b. An amplifier
    c. A receiver
    d. A probe

83. The hearing aid process generally begins with which of the following?
    a. Selection
    b. Verification
    c. Quality control
    d. Programming

84. Which of the following statements is true of target gain?
    a. It is based only on audiometric measures.
    b. It varies depending on the prescriptive measure selected.
    c. It is greater for patients who are using amplification for the first time.
    d. It is not dependent on patient age.

85. Which of the following statements is true of unilateral amplification when a patient has relatively symmetric hearing loss and is a bilateral candidate?
    a. It may improve long-term speech perception of the aided ear.
    b. It may improve long-term speech perception of the unaided ear.
    c. It may degrade long-term speech perception of the aided ear.
    d. It may degrade long-term speech perception of the unaided ear.

86. CROS or BiCROS systems are most appropriate for patients with which of the following?
    a. Symmetric hearing loss
    b. Significantly poorer hearing loss in one ear that will not benefit from amplification
    c. Symmetric word recognition scores
    d. Poor word recognition scores bilaterally

87. Earmold impressions are typically not contraindicated by which of the following?
    a. External otitis
    b. Inflammation
    c. Otomycosis
    d. Presence of a mastoid cavity

88. Electroacoustic analysis of a hearing aid measures all of the following *EXCEPT*:
    a. Frequency response
    b. Distortion
    c. Circuit noise
    d. Real ear resonance

89. Which of the following is verified by probe microphone measurements?
    a. Battery drain
    b. Distortion
    c. Circuit noise
    d. Real ear response

90. Objective verification of hearing aids includes which of the following?
    a. Loudness judgment ratings
    b. The Hearing Handicap Inventory for the Elderly
    c. Speech mapping
    d. Informal quality judgments from the patient

91. Subjective verification of hearing aid measures include all of the following *EXCEPT*:
    a. Assessment of real ear aided gain
    b. Loudness rating

c. The Client-Oriented Scale of Improvement

d. Speech-perception judgments

92. Which of the following is the ultimate priority of pediatric hearing aid fittings?
    a. Sound comfort
    b. Flexibility for continually changing listening needs, including manual controls
    c. Sound audibility
    d. Subjective measurements for verification due to limited patient feedback

93. Pediatric patients are generally fit with which of the following?
    a. Open-fit hearing aids
    b. BTE hearing aids
    c. ITE hearing aids
    d. CIC hearing aids

94. Compared with an adult ear, resonance characteristics of a pediatric ear:
    a. Generally result in a lower SPL delivered to the ear
    b. Are relatively stable over time
    c. Create the need for regular programming adjustments
    d. Can be disregarded until the child reaches 5 years of age

95. Which of the following statements is true of geriatric patients?
    a. They may have additional auditory processing changes that reduce their ability to understand speech.
    b. They maintain ability to hear spatially as they age.
    c. They are unlikely to benefit from amplification.
    d. They will likely need less digital processing in hearing aids due to decreased listening environment complexity.

96. Which of the following statements is true of patients with tinnitus?
    a. They generally do not benefit from amplification.
    b. They can use an ear-level masker to help alleviate tinnitus.
    c. They are a homogeneous population with obvious treatment options.
    d. They should pursue hearing aids only if their hearing loss is at least moderate in degree.

97. Which of the following is a common ALD used in school settings for children with hearing loss?
    a. AM system
    b. FM system
    c. Visual alerter
    d. Telephone amplifier

98. Which of the following statements is true of functional gain measurements?
    a. They compare aided and unaided performance.
    b. They can be performed only with speech stimuli.
    c. They require use of a probe microphone.
    d. They are not behavioral measurements.

99. Which of the following statements is true of hearing aid candidacy?
    a. It is the same for all patients.
    b. It is based solely on degree of hearing loss.
    c. It is based on communication challenges associated with hearing loss.
    d. It is unrelated to patient motivation.

100. Which of the following is the most critical aspect of hearing aid orientation?
    a. Hearing aid storage
    b. Battery use
    c. Maintenance
    d. Realistic expectations

CORE KNOWLEDGE

INDICATIONS FOR HEARING AID USE

- Hearing aid candidacy has expanded rapidly in recent years. Nearly all patients who seek hearing aids benefit from their use when properly fitted. Patient motivation is a significant indicator of prognosis for use.
- Patients over 50 years of age account for approximately 80% of hearing aid users in a sample population from Henry Ford Hospital. In general, the distribution of hearing aid users is negatively skewed (Figure 9-1).

- In populations of people with hearing loss, more people have mild hearing loss than severe or profound hearing loss. The majority of people who choose to use hearing aids have a loss that is at least moderate in degree (Figure 9-2).
- Degree of hearing loss is associated with hearing aid use but is not the only factor that determines candidacy. If a hearing impairment causes a problem with

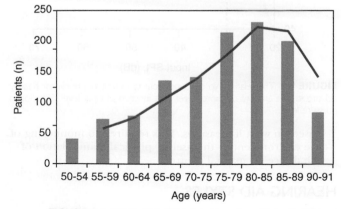

FIGURE 9-1 Distribution of hearing aid use by patient age.

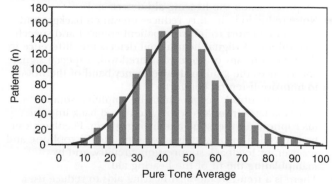

FIGURE 9-2 Distribution of hearing aid use by degree of hearing loss.

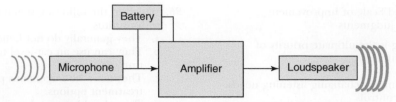

FIGURE 9-3 Schematic representation of the components of a hearing aid.

communication, the patient is typically a candidate for hearing aids. Similarly, a patient who does not notice communication difficulties related to the hearing loss may have limited success with amplification.

- Otologic factors such as anatomic abnormalities and recurrent external otitis as well as patient-specific factors such as cognitive limitations, dexterity, and perspiration will influence hearing aid candidacy and may in some cases preclude use of amplification altogether.

HEARING AID TECHNOLOGY

- Modern hearing aids can offer sophisticated digital processing for high-fidelity sound reproduction to enhance listening comfort with features such as adaptive directionality, feedback control, and noise reduction. These devices are readily programmable and provide substantial flexibility for precise fitting.
- A hearing aid consists of three basic components: a microphone, an amplifier, and a receiver. The amplifier adds gain to the level of the electric signal delivered to the hearing aid's transducer. The amplifier can differentially enhance higher or lower frequency and higher or lower intensity sounds. It also contains some type of limiting approach so that it does not deliver excessive energy to the ear (Figure 9-3).
- Hearing aid gain can be linear or nonlinear. In linear amplification, the same amount of amplification is applied to an input signal regardless of the intensity level of the input. Linear hearing aids are generally fit on ears with conductive hearing loss. In nonlinear amplification, gain is applied in a nonproportional manner, depending on the intensity of the input signal, to make low-intensity sounds audible, moderate sounds comfortable, and high-intensity sounds loud but not too loud. Nonlinear hearing aids are typically fit on ears with sensorineural hearing loss. Nonlinear amplification is accomplished through the use of compression and addresses the reduced dynamic range and abnormal loudness growth of patients with sensorineural hearing loss (Figures 9-4 and 9-5).
- Directionality improves the signal-to-noise ratio for speech perception by comparing signals from two or more separate microphones on a hearing aid. In many modern and mainstream instruments, this occurs automatically and adaptively when the hearing aid detects noise.
- Noise-reduction circuitry reduces unwanted background noise in an effort to improve patient comfort and speech recognition. A digital hearing aid detects the difference in the time constant of noise compared with a speech signal and reduces the gain in the frequency band of the noise to improve listening comfort.
- Acoustic feedback occurs when the amplified sound that emanates from a receiver is directed back into the microphone of the same amplifying system. Feedback can be controlled by physically separating the microphone and receiver, by feedback suppression circuitry, and by manipulating the fit of the hearing aid.
- There is a trend in modern hearing aids to reduce user control in favor of automatic adaptive control. The device samples the environment continuously and makes changes

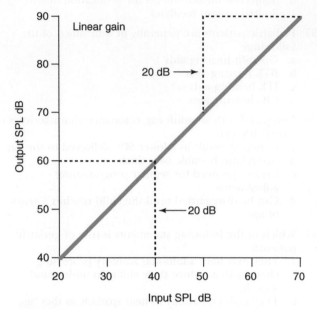

FIGURE 9-4 The relationship of sound input to output in a linear hearing aid circuit. Gain remains at a constant 20 dB regardless of input level. *SPL,* Sound pressure level.

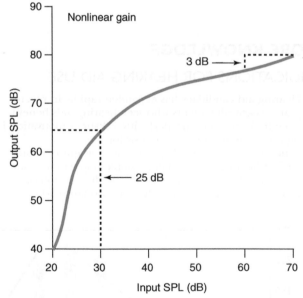

FIGURE 9-5 The relationship of sound input to output in a nonlinear hearing aid circuit. The amount of gain changes as a function of input level. *SPL,* Sound pressure level.

based on what it measures. This requires no monitoring of the environment by the user or physical manipulation of the device via manual controls.

HEARING AID STYLES

- BTE hearing aids consist of a microphone and an amplifier in a case that is worn behind the ear. The receiver may be located behind the ear or in the ear canal. The sound is delivered through a tube to a custom-fitted earmold or standard coupler.

- BTE hearing aids can be coupled in a manner referred to as open-fit or open-canal. The ear canal coupler is typically nonocclusive and does not completely fill the ear canal. It typically has thinner tubing than that found on traditional custom earmolds and often uses a standard rather than custom earmold. Open-canal fittings are especially useful for high-frequency hearing loss. Low-frequency sound is free to pass through the ear canal to permit natural hearing in the lower frequencies.
- If the receiver is in the ear canal and the microphone and amplifier are housed in the case behind the ear, the hearing aid is called a receiver-in-the-canal (RIC).
- An ITE hearing aid has all of the components contained in a custom-fitted case that fits into the outer ear or ear canal. A device that fills the outer ear concha is referred to as a full-shell hearing aid. A device that is smaller and fits into the ear canal is known as an in-the-canal (ITC) hearing aid. An even smaller device is known as a completely-in-the-canal (CIC) hearing aid and fits deeply in the canal.
- Many hearing aids offer external controls such as a volume control and/or a program button for manual user manipulation.
- Hearing aid style selection depends on many factors, including degree and configuration of hearing loss, acoustic feedback, occlusion, directional technology, ear canal structure, moisture, and patient dexterity and cognition.
- Assistive listening technologies may work with hearing aids or provide a solution to enhance the acoustic signal over background noise by the use of a remote microphone. This allows the signal to be received by the listener without the degrading effects of distance and reverberation.

SELECTION

- The process of hearing aid selection and fitting usually follows a course of selection, quality control, programming, verification, and adjustment.
- The starting point for determining the response of a hearing aid is to prescribe frequency gain characteristics based on audiometric measures. There are many prescriptive rules; some attempt to specify gain that will amplify average conversational speech to a comfortable level, some are simply based on the hearing thresholds at each frequency, and others incorporate type of hearing loss, whether one or both ears are being fitted, method of threshold determination, gender, hearing aid experience, loudness discomfort levels, or other factors into the prescription. The two most widely used procedures are the most recent versions of the National Acoustic Laboratories (NAL-NL2) and the Desired Sensation Level (DSLv5.0) methods.
- The process of hearing instrument selection first involves assessment of the patient's communication needs and other factors that may impact hearing aid use. This is followed by determination of the style and features that will be most appropriate. The fitting range of a hearing aid demonstrates the general response curve of the amplifier and is used to determine the ability of a particular hearing aid amplifier to provide necessary gain. This response curve can be manipulated with software controls to reduce or enhance specific frequency ranges to provide the necessary gain for a specific hearing sensitivity.
- Because of the inherent flexibility of the digital signal processing platform of modern hearing aids, a given

hearing aid can typically be programmed to fit a wide range of degree and configuration of hearing loss. In general, the factors that separate one hearing aid from another are related to features and processor algorithms rather than to the frequency gain response of the hearing aid.

- For most patients, it is best to fit both ears with hearing aids to take advantage of binaural hearing. The brain relies on differences in time and intensity of signals between the ears to localize the source of a sound in the environment. The use of two ears also improves the perception of sound quality and enhances hearing sensitivity and hearing in noise.
- If only one ear has hearing loss, and it can be effectively fitted with a hearing aid, then a monaural fitting is indicated. If the poorer ear cannot be effectively fitted, there are several methods of delivering a signal from the impaired side to the better hearing ear. This approach is generally referred to as contralateral routing of signals (CROS). In the typical model of CROS amplification, a microphone/transmitter is worn on the unaidable ear, and a receiver is worn on the normal ear where sound is delivered via a loudspeaker. When the hearing is also decreased in the better ear, the receiver device on the better ear can be integrated with or coupled to a traditional hearing aid. This allows the signal presented to the better ear to be amplified as needed. This is known as a bilateral CROS (BiCROS). The use of CROS or BiCROS devices does not allow patients to localize sound.

FITTING

- The fitting process begins with the making of impressions of the outer ear and external auditory meatus. The impressions are used by the manufacturer to create custom-fitted earmolds or ITE hearing aids.
- Earmold materials vary in softness and flexibility. Some materials are nonallergenic. Decisions regarding which material and style to use are based on issues relating to comfort and feedback. Decisions regarding bore size, tubing, and venting will impact the frequency gain of the hearing aid.
- Electroacoustic analyses of the hearing aids are made prior to programming to ensure that their output meets specified design parameters. This is done with the hearing aid placed in a test chamber of a hearing aid analyzer, in a 2-cc coupler, attached to a microphone. The amplified signal is sent to the analyzer, which is a sophisticated sound-level meter.
- Standard electroacoustic analysis of a hearing aid provides information about the hearing aid's gain, maximum output, and frequency response. It also provides a measure of circuit noise, distortion, and battery drain. Results of this analysis are compared with the hearing aid specifications provided by the manufacturer to ensure that the hearing aid is operating as expected.
- Programming of the hearing aids is accomplished via computer software that is proprietary for each manufacturer. Preliminary decisions are made about management of programming controls. Decisions are also made regarding the activation of manual controls, telecoil preferences, noise and feedback reduction responses, and level of sensitivity or responsiveness of adaptive technology. Furthermore, the gain response, maximum output, and prescriptive formula are evaluated to determine appropriateness of the fitting for each patient. These decisions are made based on the particular characteristics of the device and patient factors, including age and cognitive abilities, degree and configuration of hearing loss, patient experience with hearing aids, and communication needs.

- Following programming, the physical fit of the device is assessed. Appropriateness, comfort, and security of the fit are determined, as are the absence of feedback and appropriateness of the microphone location.
- As sound leaves the hearing aid, it is modified by the resonance characteristics of the ear canal. Therefore, the output of the hearing aid in the ear canal itself must be verified with real-ear testing. This testing assesses whether the targeted gains are achieved across the frequency range for a given input to the hearing aid.
- Probe-microphone measurements are made using a spectrum analyzer that delivers various calibrated signals to a loudspeaker located near the ears of a patient. A small thin tube is inserted into the ear canal close to the tympanic membrane. The other end of the tube is attached to a sensitive microphone that records sound from deep in the ear canal. This allows for measurement of the acoustic changes that occur due to the resonance of the patient's pinna and ear canal.
- In speech mapping, the signal presented through the loudspeaker is low-, average-, and high-intensity speech. The response of the hearing aid is measured near the patient's tympanic membrane, and adjustments are made to approximate targets for speech input. If the targets are correct and the output of the aid matches targets, then when the patient is wearing the hearing aids, low-intensity sounds should be audible, average sounds should be comfortable, and high-intensity sounds should be loud but tolerable.
- Following objective verification measures, the quality of the amplified sound is assessed with some form of subjective quality judgments and/or functional intelligibility procedures. Strategies include speech perception judgments, loudness judgment ratings, functional gain measurement, and speech recognition measures.
- Following the completion of hearing aid fitting and verification, the patient is oriented to the hearing aid and its use. Topics addressed typically include components and functioning of the hearing aids, battery use, and care and maintenance of the hearing aids. One of the most critical aspects of the hearing aid orientation is discussion of reasonable expectations of hearing aid use and strategies for adapting to different listening environments.
- At the end of the orientation and counseling session, patients are typically scheduled for a follow-up visit. At the follow-up appointment, benefit and satisfaction with the hearing aids are assessed, and any necessary adjustments are made. It is often at this follow-up that outcome measures are made to ensure that the patient's communication needs are being met and to help in planning of any additional rehabilitative services.

SPECIAL CONSIDERATIONS: INFANTS AND CHILDREN

- Hearing aid selection and fitting for infants and children is more challenging than for adults. There is a smaller volume of space between the end of the earmold and the tympanic membrane in children due to the smaller size of the ear canal, resulting in higher SPLs delivered to the ear than in adults. Children also have different resonance characteristics than adults, which means that certain frequencies are emphasized more than others. In addition, because children are growing over time, these physical factors also change over time and must be regularly accounted for in hearing aid adjustments.
- Because children are still in the process of learning speech and language, it is critical to provide consistent and

undistorted auditory input. They also have less control over their hearing aids, as most controls are disabled to protect against the child accidentally reducing the gain of the aid inappropriately.
- Children are always fitted with binaural hearing aids to maximize audibility unless contraindicated by medical factors or extreme hearing asymmetry. BTE hearing aids are used in most cases, because the auricle and ear canal grow in size, requiring that the custom portion of the hearing aid be frequently changed while the child is young. This is most appropriately accomplished by remaking the earmold of a BTE, rather than an entire custom hearing aid. Soft material is used for earmolds, and the earmolds are connected to pediatric earhooks for proper fitting.
- Functional measures are more frequently made for pediatric patients than for adult patients to verify the appropriateness of hearing aid output. Functional gain is the difference between the threshold with the hearing aid and without the hearing aid. Another useful functional measure is speech recognition with the hearing aids. Aided results can be compared with unaided results and with expectations for normal hearing ability under similar circumstances.

SPECIAL CONSIDERATIONS: AGING PATIENTS

- In some older patients, hearing sensitivity loss is compounded by changes in central auditory nervous system function. The consequence of such changes is typically reduction in speech recognition, even in quiet, reduced temporal processing of auditory information, and reduced ability to hear speech in background noise due to diminished ability to use two ears to hear spatially. Patients with significant changes in auditory nervous system function do not appear to benefit as much from hearing aid devices as their younger counterparts.
- In the older population, there may be greater difficulty with physical manipulation of the hearing aid and hearing aid batteries due to arthritis and other conditions. Special consideration may need to be given to hearing aid size and the use of rechargeable devices. Diminished vision may also be a problem.
- Patients with cognitive decline may have difficulty remembering how to effectively use and/or maintain their hearing aids and in general may have greater difficulty understanding speech, even when speech is made audible with hearing aids.

SPECIAL CONSIDERATIONS: TINNITUS

- Patients presenting with both hearing loss and tinnitus can often benefit simply through amplification targeted to remediate the hearing loss. Ear-level maskers can also be used alone or with hearing aid amplification in combination devices. In most cases, the audiologist can provide a multifaceted approach to tinnitus treatment.

SUMMARY

Although the details may change quickly, the following hearing aid rules-of-thumb have withstood the test of time:
- Two ears are better than one: the vast majority of patients will hear better with binaural amplification, will be more satisfied with sound quality and with hearing in noise, and will find better overall benefit. Two ears, two aids.
- Bigger is better: BTE hearing aids are considerably more durable than ITEs, are often less conspicuous, provide a

comfortable fit more easily, have fewer feedback issues, can have more features, and have better battery life.
- It is about communication, not the audiogram: if a patient is having difficulty communicating because of sensorineural hearing loss and is motivated for an amplification solution, one can be found.

- If you have not tried a hearing aid in 2 years, you have not tried a hearing aid. There is a technology arms race out there, and the result is higher quality devices, more flexible fitting opportunities, and better quality of life outcomes.

ANSWERS

TRUE OR FALSE QUESTIONS

1. F	14. T	27. T	40. T
2. T	15. F	28. T	41. F
3. T	16. T	29. T	42. F
4. F	17. T	30. T	43. F
5. T	18. T	31. F	44. T
6. T	19. T	32. F	45. T
7. T	20. F	33. F	46. T
8. T	21. T	34. F	47. T
9. F	22. F	35. F	48. T
10. T	23. F	36. T	49. F
11. F	24. T	37. F	50. T
12. F	25. F	38. T	
13. T	26. F	39. T	

SINGLE BEST ANSWER QUESTIONS

51. b	64. a	77. b	90. c
52. d	65. d	78. a	91. a
53. d	66. b	79. c	92. c
54. c	67. a	80. d	93. b
55. c	68. b	81. d	94. c
56. b	69. c	82. d	95. a
57. a	70. c	83. a	96. b
58. d	71. d	84. b	97. b
59. c	72. d	85. d	98. a
60. b	73. a	86. b	99. c
61. c	74. a	87. d	100. d
62. d	75. d	88. d	
63. c	76. b	89. d	

SUGGESTED READINGS

1. Bainbridge KE, Ramachandran V. Hearing aid use among older U.S. adults: the National Health and Nutrition Examination Survey, 2005-2006 and 2009-2010. *Ear Hear.* 2014;35(3):289-294.
2. Lewis DE, Eiten LR. Hearing instrument selection and fitting in children. In: Valente M, Hosford-Dunn H, Roeser RJ, eds. *Audiology: Treatment.* 2nd ed. New York: Thieme Medical Publishing; 2008:94-118.
3. Moore BCJ. Dead regions in the cochlea: conceptual foundations, diagnosis, and clinical applications. *Ear Hear.* 2004; 25:98-116.
4. Mueller HG, Ricketts TA, Bentler R. *Modern Hearing Aids: Pre-Fitting Testing and Selection Characteristics.* San Diego: Plural Publishing; 2014.
5. Palmer CV, Lindley GA, Mormer EA. Hearing aid selection and fitting in adults. In: Valente M, Hosford-Dunn H, Roeser RJ, eds. *Audiology: Treatment.* 2nd ed. New York: Thieme Medical Publishing; 2008:119-159.
6. Ramachandran V, Stach BA, Becker E. Reducing hearing aid cost does not influence device acquisition for milder hearing loss, but eliminating it does. *Hear J.* 2011;64(5): 10-18.
7. Silverman CA, Silman S. Apparent auditory deprivation from monaural amplification and recovery with binaural amplification: two case studies. *J Am Acad Audiol.* 1990; 1(4):175-180.
8. Stach BA. *Clinical Audiology: An Introduction.* Clifton Park, NY: Delmar Cengage Learning; 2010.
9. Sweetow RW, Bier J. Psychology of individuals with hearing impairment. In: Metz MJ, ed. *Sandlin's Textbook of Hearing Aid Amplification.* 3rd ed. San Diego: Plural Publishing; 2014:371-385.
10. Wilson C, Stephens D. Reasons for referral and attitudes toward hearing aids: do they affect outcome? *Clin Otolaryngol Allied Sci.* 2003;28:81-89.

10 Vestibular Function and Disease

S. Guan Khoo

TRUE OR FALSE QUESTIONS

T/F 1. Drop attacks with loss of consciousness, although rare, are due to vestibular disorders.

T/F 2. The macula of the vestibular system senses head rotation acceleration in all planes.

T/F 3. Caloric testing analyzes the function of all the semicircular canals.

T/F 4. Right beating nystagmus produced by cool water in the left ear during caloric testing is equivalent to that produced by warm water in the right ear.

T/F 5. There are three types of hair cells in the vestibular apparatus: types I, II, and kinocilia.

T/F 6. The crisis of Tumarkin occurs as a late stage manifestation of Meniere disease.

T/F 7. The cupula is the motion sense organ in the ampullae of the semicircular canals.

T/F 8. Nystagmus is considered second degree when the eye beats in the direction of the fast component and on straight gaze.

T/F 9. The slow phase of eye movement in paralytic vestibular pathology is away from the lesion.

T/F 10. Geotropic or ageotropic nystagmus is used to describe rotatory nystagmus in the Dix-Hallpike test.

T/F 11. Failure of ocular fixation suppression of nystagmus indicates a peripheral vestibular loss.

T/F 12. Caloric testing tests only low-frequency vestibular function.

T/F 13. When the head is rotated to the left, endolymph rotates to the left.

T/F 14. The slow phase of nystagmus is contralateral to the direction of endolymphatic flow.

T/F 15. Rotatory nystagmus elicited by the Dix-Hallpike test occurs immediately.

T/F 16. Dynamic posturography is a useful test of imbalance specifically due to pathological vestibular input.

T/F 17. In caloric testing, stimulation with cold water causes nystagmus to beat in a direction ipsilateral to the test ear.

T/F 18. Electronystagmography (ENG) measures the vestibuloocular reflex by measuring endolymphatic flow direction.

T/F 19. Vertigo is an uncommon symptom of vestibular schwannoma that arises from the vestibular portion of the eighth cranial nerve.

T/F 20. In the ENG assessment of nystagmus, ocular fixation occurs with the eyes closed.

T/F 21. Multisensory loss in the elderly is due primarily to vestibular hypofunction and commonly presents with vertigo.

T/F 22. The ability to suppress nystagmus by ocular fixation indicates a normal vestibular system.

T/F 23. T1-weighted magnetic resonance imaging (MRI) with gadolinium and T2-weighted MRI of the brain/internal auditory meatus (IAM) is the gold standard for diagnosing acoustic neuromas.

T/F 24. Trigeminal nerve signs are more common than facial nerve disorders with regard to acoustic neuromas.

T/F 25. Stapedial reflex decay is a constant feature and useful in the diagnosis of patients with acoustic neuromas.

T/F 26. Meniere disease is classically defined by fluctuating tinnitus, vertigo, hearing loss, and aural fullness, lasting seconds.

T/F 27. Much like the tonotropic arrangement of hair cell sensitivity to high- and low-frequency sounds in the cochlea, a similar arrangement is thought to exist for high- and low-frequency movement in the vestibule.

T/F 28. Vertical nystagmus associated with vertigo and bilateral internuclear ophthalmoplegia suggests multiple sclerosis as a diagnosis.

T/F 29. Oscillopsia occurs due to an uncompensated unilateral vestibular loss.

T/F 30. Nystagmus due to fractures of the vestibular apparatus in head injury is directed toward the side of the lesion.

T/F 31. Vestibular neuronitis is not associated with hearing loss.

T/F 32. Ototoxicity is a recognized cause of bilateral vestibular loss.

T/F 33. Lateral medullary syndrome is suspected in a patient with vertigo and Horner syndrome.

T/F 34. The use of diuretic therapy in Meniere disease is to decrease endolymphatic fluid through diuresis.

T/F 35. Low-dose aminoglycoside ototoxicity is associated with a mutation of the 12S mitochondrial rRNA gene.

T/F 36. The utricle is innervated by both the superior and inferior vestibular nerves.

T/F 37. Glycerol acts as a vestibular vasodilator in the glycerol test for Meniere disease.

T/F 38. Vertebrobasilar insufficiency causes vertigo and drop attacks with sudden loss of consciousness when looking upward.

T/F 39. Increasing aural fullness, tinnitus, and hearing loss relieved by a vertigo attack is a hallmark of Lermoyez syndrome.

T/F 40. Saccadic eye movements are mediated by the cerebellum.

T/F 41. Thirty percent of patients with recurrent vestibulopathy resolve their symptoms, with 60% evolving to Meniere disease and benign positional vertigo (BPV).

T/F 42. Gentamicin is more ototoxic than vestibulotoxic.

T/F 43. The inability to suppress the vestibuloocular reflex on horizontal head movement indicates a peripheral vestibular disorder.

T/F 44. Recurrent vestibulopathy is characterized by recurrent vertigo of unknown origin without the auditory signs and symptoms of Meniere disease.

T/F 45. Migraine is the most common central cause of chronic dizziness in adults.

T/F 46. Posture and movement coordination is mediated through the cerebellum and vestibular nuclei via afferent information from the vestibular system and visual system and proprioceptive feedback from the upper and lower limbs.

T/F 47. Endolymph is produced by the secretory cells of the stria vascularis and dark cells of the vestibular labyrinth.

T/F 48. Early detection of aminoglycoside vestibulotoxicity is crucial because good recovery of function can be expected.

T/F 49. Normal serum aminoglycoside level monitoring is adequate in preventing aminoglycoside vestibulotoxicity but not ototoxicity.

T/F 50. The Epley maneuver for BPV is effective in up to 75% of patients.

SINGLE BEST ANSWER QUESTIONS

51. Which of the following statements is true of vertigo?
    a. It is a hallucination of movement.
    b. It can be rotator.
    c. It can be described as swaying.
    d. All of the above are true.

52. The crisis of Tumarkin occurs in which of the following?
    a. Recurrent vestibulopathy
    b. Meniere disease
    c. BPV
    d. Vestibular schwannoma

53. Which of the following statements is true of nystagmus?
    a. It is directed toward the fast component of eye movement.
    b. It is third degree when it occurs on straight gaze and the direction of the fast component.

   c. Labyrinthine nystagmus can be suppressed by fixation.
   d. a and c

54. Which of the following statements is true of central nystagmus?
    a. It has slow and fast components.
    b. It is not suppressed by gaze fixation.
    c. Failure of vestibuloocular suppression is a peripheral vestibular sign.
    d. b and c

55. Which of the following statements is true?
    a. A change in a patient's position causing vertigo is due to BPV.
    b. A change in a patient's position resulting in light-headedness on upright positioning indicates a vestibular disorder.
    c. A change in a patient's position causing vertigo is nonspecific and cannot be attributed to positional vertigo alone.
    d. All of the above are true.

56. In Dix-Hallpike testing, which of the following statements is true?
    a. The rotatory nystagmus is best turned clockwise or anticlockwise based on the patient's point of view.
    b. The rotatory nystagmus is best turned clockwise or anticlockwise based on the examiner's point of view.
    c. Geotropic nystagmus is rotation of the patient's eyes away from the floor.
    d. Ageotropic nystagmus is rotation of the patent's eyes away from the floor.

57. Which of the following statements is true regarding nystagmus classical of BPV?
    a. It is not fatigable.
    b. It is ageotropic.
    c. It has a latent period.
    d. a and c

58. Which of the following statements is true regarding caloric testing?
    a. It is accomplished using water 7°C cooler and 7°C warmer than core body temperature.
    b. The patient is positioned 30 degrees from supine to allow the posterior semicircular canal to be in a vertical plane.
    c. With a patient's head 45 degrees from supine, ampullifugal endolymphatic flow in the lateral semicircular canal is established.
    d. a and b

59. Which of the following statements is true regarding a pathological result in caloric testing?
    a. It occurs when water at 44°C is irrigated in both ears at once.
    b. It relies on the difference between response from right and left inner ear hair cells.
    c. It occurs only when there is a difference in canal paresis of over 15%.
    d. It refers to pathology elicited by rapid head movement.

60. Which of the following statements is true regarding irritative vestibular pathology?
    a. It includes pathology caused by cholesteatoma.
    b. It causes nystagmus toward the diseased ear.
    c. It causes nystagmus away from the diseased ear.
    d. a and c

61. Which of the following statements is true regarding ENG?
    a. It is used in conjunction with caloric testing to measure vestibulospinal reflexes.

b. The electronic recording of nystagmus by ENG relates to the vestibuloocular reflex.

c. It measures the velocity of the fast phase of nystagmus.

d. b and c

62. Which of the following statements is true regarding the fistula test?

a. Medial tragal pressure causes nystagmus toward the pathologically affected ear.

b. Negative pressure causes nystagmus contralateral to the affected ear.

c. Both of the above are true.

d. None of the above is true.

63. Which of the following statements is true regarding dynamic posturography?

a. It can be useful in nonorganic vestibular loss.

b. It can identify defects in proprioceptive, ocular, and vestibular inputs separately.

c. It tests patients with eyes open and closed while standing on a soft platform only.

d. a and c

64. Which of the following statements is true regarding acoustic neuroma?

a. Vertigo is a prominent feature as the tumor arises off the vestibular nerve.

b. Loss of speech discrimination with regard to hearing loss is the principal manifestation.

c. It accounts for 50% of all lesions at the cerebellopontine angle.

d. b and c

65. Which of the following statements is true regarding Meniere disease?

a. Bilateral ears may be affected in up to 90% of cases in which disease has been present for 20 years or more.

b. Labyrinthectomy for Meniere disease has decreased in frequency due to the risk of bilateral involvement of the disease.

c. The presence of drop attacks increases the risk of bilateral ear involvement.

d. a and c

66. Which of the following statements is true regarding objective tests for Meniere disease?

a. Audiograms classically feature low-frequency sensorineural hearing loss.

b. ENG findings are constantly abnormal between each episodic attack.

c. Abnormal SP:AP ratios are shown on electrocochleography, which is the gold standard for diagnosis.

d. All of the above are true.

67. Which of the following statements is true regarding BPV?

a. Posterior semicircular canal occlusion is a recognized management option.

b. It is most commonly caused by canaliths within the ampullated end of the posterior semicircular canals.

c. It may be caused by occlusion of the anterior vestibular artery.

d. a and c

68. The following are recognized interventional management options for Meniere disease *EXCEPT:*

a. Labyrinthectomy

b. Glycerol application

c. Transtympanic dexamethasone injection

d. Silverstein MicroWick aminoglycoside application

69. Which of the following statements is true regarding oscillopsia?

a. It is the inability to maintain a stable horizon on walking.

b. It is a feature of Meniere disease.

c. It is due to otolithic dysfunction as opposed to semicircular canal pathology.

d. a and c

70. Which of the following statements is true regarding Meniere disease?

a. By definition, it cannot be diagnosed without the aural fullness component.

b. Remission occurs in 90% of patients if symptoms are of late onset.

c. Fluctuation in symptoms is thought to be secondary to rupture of the Reissner membrane of the inner ear.

d. a and b

71. Which of the following statements is true regarding posttraumatic vertigo?

a. It may cause Meniere syndrome as a result.

b. The most common cause of posttraumatic head injury vertigo is benign BPV.

c. It is more readily remedial to medical therapy.

d. a and b

72. Which of the following statements is true regarding a positive fistula test?

a. It is always indicative of a semicircular canal fistula.

b. It is due to stiffening of the stapes footplate.

c. It is diagnostic for superior semicircular canal dehiscence.

d. None of the above is true.

73. Which of the following statements is true regarding posttraumatic vertigo?

a. In conjunction with hearing loss it suggests a transverse temporal bone fracture rather than a longitudinal fracture.

b. It is common in patients in whom a middle ear hematoma is evident.

c. It is more common in temporal bone fractures longitudinal to the petrous apex.

d. None of the above is true.

74. Which of the following statements is true regarding vestibular rehabilitation?

a. It is not indicated when the patient is not symptomatic of his/her vertigo spell.

b. It will likely not benefit a patient with migraine-associated vertigo.

c. It is beneficial in patients with unilateral BPV or unilateral vestibular hypofunction.

d. b and c

75. Which of the following statements is true regarding vestibular neuronitis?

a. It is viral in origin; therefore, antivirals are a mainstay of primary treatment.

b. It causes debilitating vertigo that commonly lasts up to a week.

c. Spontaneous nystagmus is observed toward the side of the affected ear.

d. a and b

76. Which of the following statements is true regarding superior semicircular canal dehiscence?

a. It is associated with autophony in the affected side.

b. Measurement of ocular vestibular myogenic potential is the gold standard objective investigation for this condition.

c. It is related to temporal bone trauma in the majority of cases.
d. a and c

77. Which of the following statements regarding vestibular neuronitis is true?
   a. It classically affects one ear only.
   b. Episodes typically wax and wane, lasting minutes to hours.
   c. Complete resolution of symptoms is expected within 1 week.
   d. It occurs most commonly in the elderly.

78. Downbeating nystagmus occurs in which of the following?
   a. Arnold-Chiari malformation
   b. Psychotropic medication use
   c. Syringomyelia and syringobulbia
   d. All of the above

79. All of the following are communications between the inner ear and the temporal bone *EXCEPT:*
   a. Ductus reuniens
   b. Internal auditory canal
   c. Cochlear aqueduct
   d. Vestibular aqueduct

80. Which of the following statements is true regarding Wallenberg syndrome?
   a. It is suspected in a patient with vertigo, dysphagia, and vocal cord paralysis.
   b. It is secondary to disruption of the medial longitudinal fasciculus.
   c. It is also known as the lateral medullary syndrome.
   d. a and c

81. Which of the following statements is true regarding mal de debarquement syndrome?
   a. It is characterized by sway vertigo and imbalance due to endolymphatic hydrops similar to Meniere disease.
   b. Symptoms abate when the patient is in motion, such as in a car or train.
   c. It has an excellent prognosis with interventional vestibular rehabilitation.
   d. b and c

82. Which of the following statements is true regarding endolymph?
   a. It has high Na^+ and low K^+ content.
   b. It is resorbed in the endolymphatic sac.
   c. It is present in the scala tympani and scala media.
   d. None of the above is true.

83. Which of the following statements is true regarding nonorganic vertigo?
   a. It is intensified by head movement.
   b. It is associated with ataxia.
   c. Symptoms are accurately reproduced by hyperventilation.
   d. a and c

84. Which of the following statements is true regarding smooth pursuit assessment?
   a. It assesses the vestibulocerebellar tract.
   b. It is most likely to be affected by central nervous system pathology.
   c. It tests oculomotor function in addition to gaze stability and saccadic eye movement.
   d. b and c

85. Which of the following statements is true regarding compensation of a vestibular loss?
   a. It can be aided by vestibular rehabilitation therapy, which promotes central nervous system compensation.
   b. It is dependent on an intact vestibulocerebellum.

c. It involves desensitization of the balance system to movements that provoke vertigo.
d. All of the above are true.

86. Which of the following statements is true regarding the Halmagyi head thrust maneuver?
   a. It works on the premise that there is perfect compensatory conjugate eye movement to the contralateral side with respect to head movement.
   b. It assesses smooth pursuit function.
   c. It assesses refixation eye movements, termed *vergence movements.*
   d. b and c

87. Which of the following statements is true regarding the oscillopsia test?
   a. It is a test for unilateral vestibular loss.
   b. It is abnormal with a loss of two lines or more on reading a Snellen chart during repetitive head movement of 2 Hz.
   c. It is used to assess bilateral vestibular loss due to ototoxicity.
   d. It is a test of the vertical vestibuloocular reflex.

88. Which of the following statements is true regarding aminoglycoside therapy for intractable Meniere disease?
   a. Kanamycin and gentamicin are the most vestibulotoxic of the aminoglycoside group.
   b. Treatment protocols are divided into fixed-dose protocols and titration protocols.
   c. Efficacy is based on the accumulation of aminoglycoside within the hair cell.
   d. b and c

89. Which of the following statements is true regarding bilateral vestibular loss?
   a. It results in oscillopsia.
   b. It results in rotatory vertigo due to imbalance of afferent vestibular information.
   c. It results in loss of posture and coordination despite normal visual and proprioceptive feedback.
   d. a and b

90. Which of the following statements is true regarding Frenzel goggles?
   a. They allow the patient to focus on visual fixation.
   b. They remove the patient's ability to visually fixate.
   c. They are used primarily as a magnification tool to identify nystagmus.
   d. All of the above are true.

91. Which of the following statements is true regarding migraine-associated vertigo?
   a. Sumatriptan is not effective for vertigo spells.
   b. Prophylaxis includes antidepressants such as amitriptyline.
   c. Vertigo may occur as part of an aura, as part of the headache phase, or between headaches.
   d. All of the above are true.

92. Which of the following statements is true for betahistine use in Meniere disease?
   a. Betahistine is postulated to work via vasodilatory effects on blood supply to the inner ear.
   b. Betahistine is prescribed to decrease frequency and severity of vertiginous episodes.
   c. Betahistine is effective in arresting hearing loss.
   d. Betahistine is a H1-receptor agonist.

93. Which of the following statements is true regarding vestibular neuronitis?
   a. It is most commonly bilateral.
   b. It classically causes severe vertigo that lasts a week.

    c. Hearing loss is often a feature.

    d. a and c

94. Which of the following statements is true regarding mal de debarquement syndrome?

    a. Patients feel better getting off a moving vehicle.

    b. Objective caloric tests often show unilateral canal paresis.

    c. It can be treated effectively by vestibular rehabilitation.

    d. None of the above is true.

95. Which of the following statements is true regarding the doll's eye test?

    a. It is synonymous with the Halmagyi head thrust test.

    b. Catch-up saccades on turning the head swiftly to the left suggest right-sided vestibular hypofunction.

    c. It cannot be used in assessment of a comatose patient.

    d. a and c

96. The following objective tests of balance all serve to localize disease precisely to the central or peripheral vestibular system *EXCEPT*:

    a. Cervical vestibular myogenic potential

    b. Dynamic posturography

    c. ENG

    d. b and c

97. Which of the following statements is true regarding aminoglycoside ototoxicity?

    a. It is the most common cause of bilateral vestibular loss.

    b. Toxicity is associated with cumulative exposure to aminoglycosides.

    c. Hearing loss is a better indicator of toxicity than dizziness and imbalance.

    d. a and b

98. In attempting to diagnose the specific cause of peripheral vertigo, which answer is most useful to elicit from the patient?

    a. Aural fullness

    b. Duration of vertigo spell

    c. Sway or rotatory vertigo

    d. Associated tinnitus

99. Which of the following statements is true regarding Cogan syndrome?

    a. It is associated with interstitial keratitis and audiovestibular dysfunction.

    b. It typically causes unilateral audiovestibular symptoms.

    c. Anti–tumor necrosis factor therapy is first-line.

    d. It is a variant of Meniere disease.

100. Which of the following statements is true regarding central vestibular disorders?

    a. They are associated with a negative Romberg test.

    b. They are associated with fatigable nystagmus.

    c. They are associated with gaze-evoked nystagmus.

    d. a and b

CORE KNOWLEDGE

VESTIBULAR HISTORY

- Rotatory vertigo is often termed "true vertigo." However, a sway sensation is also characterized as a hallucination of movement and, therefore, vertigo (Figure 10-1).
- The duration of vertigo episodes is key to diagnosis.
- Drop attacks without loss of consciousness are associated with certain disorders such as Meniere disease and are termed crises of Tumarkin.
- Loss of consciousness is more indicative of a central disorder as opposed to a peripheral vestibular disorder.
- Vertigo associated with straining or heavy lifting, especially when associated with autophony, may be indicative of superior semicircular canal dehiscence.

NEUROOTOLOGICAL EXAMINATION (FIGURE 10-2)

- A positive fistula test suggests a labyrinthine fistula. Positive pressure stimulation of an affected ear causes nystagmus directed toward the ear, and negative pressure causes nystagmus away from the ear.
- First degree: nystagmus beats in the direction of gaze. Second degree: nystagmus on straight gaze and in the direction of the fast phase. Third degree: nystagmus in all three directions of gaze. The direction of nystagmus is indicated by the fast phase of nystagmus.
- The slow phase of nystagmus indicates direction of flow of endolymph.
- Paralytic pathology: causes nystagmus away from the side of the lesion (e.g., cholesteatoma, vestibular neuronitis). Irritative pathology: causes nystagmus toward the side of the disease (e.g., Meniere disease).

- The 4 Hs of the neurootological examination: headshake nystagmus, Halmagyi head thrust test (Figure 10-3), Dix-Hallpike test, and hyperventilation test.
- Headshake nystagmus may indicate high-frequency vestibular loss.
- Halmagyi head thrust: saccadic refixation when the head is turned quickly to the right indicates a right vestibular hypofunction; when the head is turned quickly to the left, it indicates a left vestibular hypofunction.
- Dix-Hallpike test (Figure 10-4): geotropic or ageotropic rotatory nystagmus with the head hanging to the left or right. Allow a latency period of up to 15 seconds before concluding whether the test is normal or abnormal. Use of Frenzel goggles during this test removes visual fixation and allows magnification of the eyes for assessment.
- Hyperventilation for 60 seconds: exact replication of dizziness symptoms would suggest a nonorganic psychogenic cause.
- Vestibuloocular suppression: peripheral nystagmus can be suppressed by visual fixation. Failure of vestibuloocular reflex suppression indicates a cerebellar disorder.
- Dynamic visual acuity test: the oscillopsia test. A positive test is indicative of bilateral vestibular hypofunction. The head is rotated to either side on a horizontal axis at 2 Hz and the patient asked to read the Snellen chart. A loss of four to five lines from the baseline norm for the patient when the head is not in motion is indicative of an abnormal test.

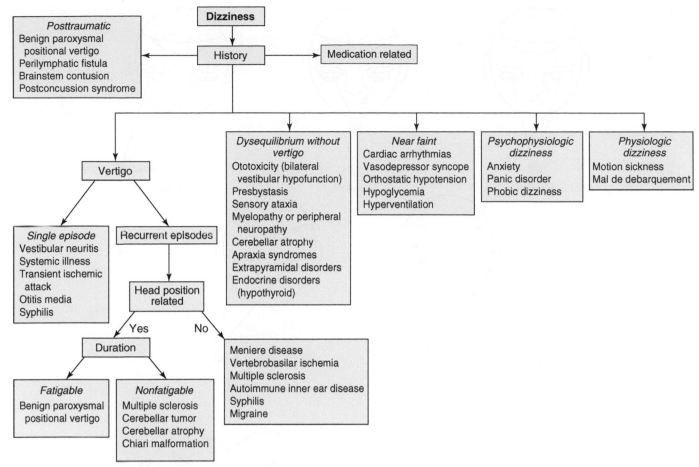

FIGURE 10-1 Algorithm for the differential diagnosis of dizziness based on information from the patient's history. (Modified from Baloh RW, Fife TD, Furman JM, Zee DS. The approach to the patient with dizziness. In: Mancall EL, ed: *Continuum: lifelong learning in neurology,* Cleveland, Advanstar Communication, 1996, pp 25-36.)

VESTIBULAR DISEASE

- *BPV* is the most common recognizable cause of true vertigo, occurring spontaneously or following significant head trauma. It is thought to be due to abnormal sensitivity of the semicircular canals, most commonly of the posterior canal, to free-floating canaliths. Canalithiasis causes paroxysms of this disorder, whereas cupulolithiasis, in which otoconia settle on the cupula, causes more long-lasting nystagmus. Recalcitrant BPV despite the Epley particle repositioning maneuver (Figure 10-5) may require vestibular rehabilitation for resolution, failing which surgical semicircular canal occlusion may be necessary.

- *Recurrent vestibulopathy* is the second most common diagnosis made of a vertiginous patient. Vertigo attacks are similar in nature to that experienced in Meniere disease, but without the cochlear symptoms of fluctuating hearing loss, tinnitus, and aural fullness. Some 60% to 70% of patients will resolve their vertigo symptoms; 15% will evolve to Meniere disease; and 10% will evolve to BPV.

- *Meniere disease* is a diagnosis of exclusion. Natural remission occurs in up to 60% of patients. Classification of Meniere disease has historically been according to the American Academy of Otolaryngology–Head and Neck Surgery guidelines of "possible, probable, definite, and certain" Meniere disease. Hearing loss is typically of the low frequencies. Up to 50% of patients may develop bilateral disease. Pathology is thought to be due to hypersecretion of endolymph by the stria vascularis, underabsorption of endolymph by the endolymphatic sac,

or a combination of both. Symptoms are caused by recurrent rupture and healing of the membranous labyrinth basement membranes. Low-salt diets and diuretics serve to attempt to reduce endolymph volume. Betahistine increases vasodilatory blood flow to the inner ear and reduces frequency and severity of vertiginous attacks. Recent reports suggest the use of Mycostatin suspension for treatment, ostensibly targeting fungal elements in the digestive tract that may play a role in antibody production directed toward the inner ear. The postulated autoimmune basis for Meniere disease has encouraged the use of transtympanic dexamethasone injection in recalcitrant cases with no reported risk of hearing loss. Transtympanic gentamicin use is effective, but there is controversy over which protocol to adopt: high-dose treatment with numerous injections over a number of weeks, or two injections over a 4-week period. Efficacy rates vary from 66% to 100% vertigo control with this technique. The risk of hearing loss with a high-dose regime can be as high as 30%. The previous gold standard labyrinthectomy for surgical management of Meniere disease has fallen by the wayside due to less invasive techniques available for good vertigo control and due to the high risk of development of bilateral Meniere disease.

- *Vestibular schwannomas/acoustic neuromas* arise from Schwann cells of the vestibular portion of the vestibulocochlear nerve. Most tumors cause few symptoms aside from unilateral sensorineural hearing loss. Up to 40% of patients report dizziness. Trigeminal nerve

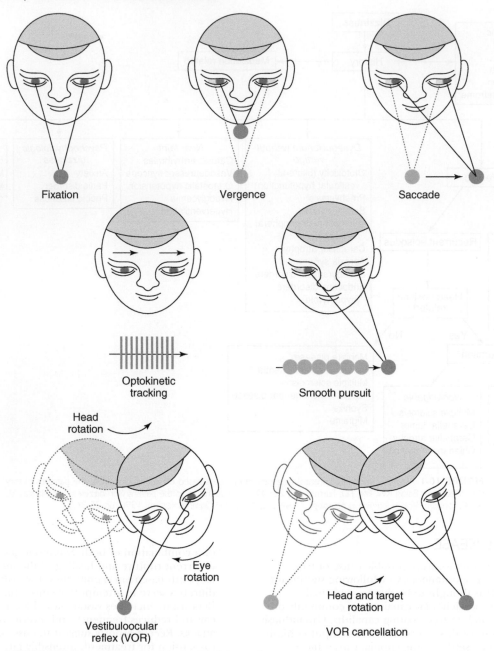

FIGURE 10-2 Schematic depiction of the functional classes of eye movements. Basic research in the neurophysiology of oculomotor control and clinical studies of eye movement disorders have been enhanced by the recognition of functionally distinct subsystems. Seven types of eye movements are shown.

symptoms are present in 8% of patients. Those that increase in size grow at a rate less than 2 mm/year in 92% of patients. Cerebellopontine angle tumors grow at a faster rate than those present within the internal acoustic meatus only. Up to 22% of these tumors regress in size. Even in tumors that do not grow, hearing continues to deteriorate. It is postulated that this may be due to long-term ischemia or protein shedding into the inner ear. Conservative management with MRI monitoring of these tumors has shown to be effective in avoiding surgery in 60% of patients over a 10-year period.

- *Vestibular neuronitis* is a postulated herpetic or zoster viral infection of the vestibular nerve. Labyrinthitis includes hearing loss as part of the disease spectrum. Vestibular neuronitis causes marked vertigo that can leave a patient bedridden for days to a week. Treatment is symptomatic

with antinausea medication. Vestibular sedatives should be discontinued after a week because they interfere with compensatory mechanisms. Long-term imbalance with head movement is not infrequent. Recurrence is rare (5%).

- *Mal de debarquement syndrome* causes a sway-type imbalance following a recent ship journey or flight. Patients classically are asymptomatic while on a moving vehicle. Symptoms recur when the patient alights from a moving vehicle. Visual-vestibular disturbance is not uncommon.

- *Bilateral vestibular loss* results in oscillopsia. This most commonly occurs after aminoglycoside vestibulotoxicity, with gentamicin most frequently the culprit. Toxicity occurs with cumulative exposure to the drug, and most cases occur after therapy of >5 days. Toxicity has historically been monitored via hearing loss, but by the

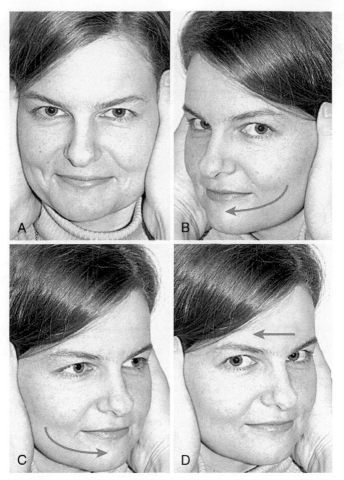

FIGURE 10-3 The head impulse sign in a patient with left unilateral horizontal canal hypofunction. Starting from a neutral position **(A),** a rapid head impulse to the right in the horizontal plane elicits compensatory eye movements to the left, and the patient's eyes remain stable on the examiner **(B).** With a similar movement to the left, a hypoactive labyrinth **(C)** results in a delayed catch-up saccade **(D)** to maintain gaze. The *arrow* in **D** shows the direction of the catch-up saccade. (From Hullar TE, Minor LB. The neurotologic examination. In: Jackler RK, Brackmann DE, eds. *Neurotology,* 2nd ed, St Louis, Mosby, 2004, pp 215-227.)

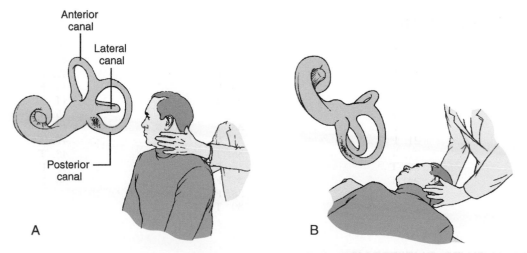

FIGURE 10-4 The Dix-Hallpike maneuver. Lowering the patient's head backward and to the side allows debris in the posterior canal **(A)** to fall to its lowest position, which activates the canal and causes eye movements and vertigo **(B).** (From Hullar TE, Minor LB: Vestibular physiology and disorders of the labyrinth. In Glasscock ME, Gulya AJ, eds. *Surgery of the ear,* ed 5, Toronto, 2003, BC Decker.)

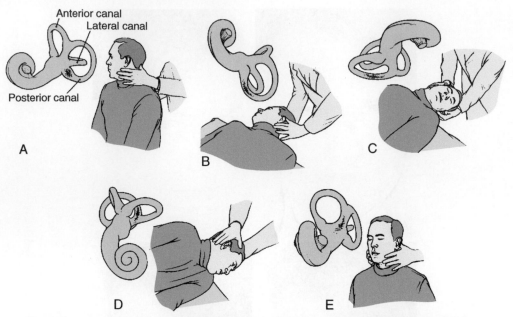

FIGURE 10-5 Canalith repositioning maneuver for treatment of benign paroxysmal positional vertigo (BPPV) affecting the posterior canal. **A,** A patient with right posterior canal BPPV. The patient's head is turned to the right at the beginning of the canalith repositioning maneuver. The location of the debris can be seen near the ampulla of the posterior canal; the diagram of the head in each panel shows the orientation from which the labyrinth is viewed. **B,** The patient is brought into the supine position with the head extended below the level of the gurney. The debris falls toward the common crus as the head is moved backward. **C,** The head is moved approximately 180 degrees to the left while keeping the neck extended with the head below the level of the gurney; debris enters the common crus as the head is turned toward the contralateral side. **D,** The patient's head is further rotated to the left by rolling onto the left side, until the patient's head faces down; debris begins to enter the vestibule. **E,** The patient is brought back to the upright position: debris collects in the vestibule. (From Hullar TE, Minor LB. Vestibular physiology and disorders of the labyrinth. In: Glasscock ME, Gulya AJ, eds. *Surgery of the ear,* 5th ed, Hamilton: 2003.)

time a hearing loss is evident, the vestibulotoxic effects have already occurred and may be irreversible. Hair cell apoptosis from excessive production of oxidative free radicals is the main mechanism of injury. Susceptibility to auditory loss is associated with mitochondrial DNA mutations, although this appears not to hold true for the vestibular apparatus. Toxicity may occur despite normal serum concentrations of the drug. Bilateral vestibular loss assessment can be clinically performed by dynamic visual acuity testing or the dynamic illegible "E" test.

ANSWERS

TRUE OR FALSE QUESTIONS

1. F	14. F	27. T	40. T
2. F	15. F	28. T	41. F
3. F	16. F	29. F	42. F
4. T	17. F	30. F	43. F
5. F	18. F	31. T	44. T
6. F	19. T	32. T	45. T
7. T	20. F	33. T	46. T
8. T	21. F	34. F	47. T
9. F	22. T	35. T	48. T
10. T	23. T	36. F	49. F
11. F	24. T	37. F	50. F
12. T	25. F	38. F	
13. T	26. F	39. T	

SINGLE BEST ANSWER QUESTIONS

51. d	56. d	61. b	66. a
52. b	57. c	62. a	67. d
53. d	58. a	63. a	68. b
54. c	59. b	64. b	69. c
55. c	60. b	65. b	70. c

71. d	79. a	87. c	95. a
72. d	80. d	88. d	96. b
73. a	81. b	89. a	97. c
74. d	82. b	90. b	98. b
75. b	83. c	91. d	99. a
76. a	84. d	92. c	100. c
77. a	85. d	93. b	
78. d	86. a	94. d	

SUGGESTED READINGS

1. Rutka J. Evaluation of vertigo. In: Blitzer A, ed. *Office-Based Surgery in Otolaryngology*. New York: Thieme Medical Publishers Inc; 1998:71-78.
2. Greenberg SL, Nedzelski JM. Medical and noninvasive therapy for Meniere's disease. *Otolaryngol Clin North Am.* 2010;43:1081-1090.
3. Bisdorff A, von Brevern M, Lempert T, Newman-Toker DE. Classification of vestibular symptoms: towards an international classification of vestibular disorders. *J Vestib Res.* 2009;19:1-13.
4. Ariano RE, Zelenitsky SA, Kasseum DA. Aminoglycoside-induced vestibular injury: maintaining a sense of balance. *Ann Pharmacother.* 2008;42(9):1282-1289.
5. Chen L, Wang WQ. Frequency perception and cell injury in the semicircular canal caused by gentamicin. *J Otolaryngol Head Neck Surg* 2011;40(6):446-452.
6. Szmulewicz DJ, Waterston JA, MacDougall HG, et al. Cerebellar ataxia, neuropathy, vestibular areflexia syndrome (CANVAS): a review of the clinical features and video-oculographic diagnosis. *Ann N Y Acad Sci.* 2011;1233: 139-147.
7. Rutka J. What would you do if you had a small vestibular schwannoma? An apocryphal tale. *Clin Otolaryngol.* 2008; 33(3):236-238.
8. Roy FD, Tomlinson RD. Characterization of the vestibulo-ocular reflex evoked by high-velocity movements. *Laryngoscope.* 2004;114(7):1190-1193.
9. Hajioff D, Raut VV, Walsh RM, et al. Conservative management of vestibular schwannomas: third review of a 10-year prospective study. *Clin Otolaryngol.* 2008;33(3):255-259.
10. Longridge NS, Mallinson AI. A discussion of the dynamic illegible "E" test: a new method of screening for aminoglycoside vestibulotoxicity. *Otolaryngol Head Neck Surg.* 1984; 92(6):671-677.

11 Neurotologic Skull Base Surgery

Paula Casserly

TRUE OR FALSE QUESTIONS

T/F 1. The principal blood supply to the temporalis muscle is the superficial temporal artery.

T/F 2. The middle meningeal artery passes through foramen spinosum.

T/F 3. No anatomical structures pass through foramen lacerum.

T/F 4. The frontal branches of the facial nerve are located superficial to the temporoparietal fascia.

T/F 5. The arcuate eminence corresponds consistently with the superior semicircular canal.

T/F 6. Vestibular schwannomas classically have a wide dural base on magnetic resonance imaging (MRI).

T/F 7. Epidermoid cysts can be distinguished from vestibular schwannoma on MRI following administration of gadolinium contrast.

T/F 8. Cholesterol granuloma typically demonstrates a hypointense signal on T1 MRI.

T/F 9. Erosion of the jugulocarotid spine on computed tomography (CT) scanning is characteristic of a glomus jugulare tumor.

T/F 10. The classical MRI appearance of lower cranial nerve neurinoma has been described as "salt and pepper."

T/F 11. Gallium citrate Ga-67 scan is highly specific for diagnosing necrotizing otitis externa (NOE).

T/F 12. In NOE CT scanning is useful for detecting early osteomyelitis.

T/F 13. Facial nerve palsy in an independent indicator for surgery in patients with NOE.

T/F 14. The majority of patients with trigeminal neuralgia have bilateral symptoms.

T/F 15. Paresthia in the distribution of the trigeminal nerve is commonly seen in trigeminal neuralgia.

T/F 16. Cerebrospinal fluid (CSF) has a composition almost identical to plasma.

T/F 17. CSF is produced by the choroid plexus.

T/F 18. CSF circulates from the subarachnoid space into the cerebral ventricles.

T/F 19. CSF is absorbed into the arachnoid villi.

T/F 20. CSF is produced at a rate of 150 mL/day.

T/F 21. Vestibular schwannomas constitute 40% of cerebellopontine angle (CPA) tumors.

T/F 22. Vestibular schwannomas arise from glial cells of the peripheral nervous system.

T/F 23. The facial nerve is located in the anterosuperior portion of the internal auditory meatus (IAM).

T/F 24. The facial nerve is separated from the cochlear nerve in the IAM by Bill bar.

T/F 25. Enhancement of the IAM seen on gadolinium-contrast MRI is pathognomonic of a vestibular schwannoma.

T/F 26. Preoperative carotid artery balloon test occlusion should be performed in Class A and B jugulotympanic glomus tumors as characterized by Fisch.

T/F 27. Following a translabyrinthine removal of a CPA tumor, the presence of a postauricular wound discharge, positive for β2-tranferrin, warrants immediate surgical intervention.

T/F 28. Preoperative embolization is generally indicated for a vestibular schwannoma tumor >4 cm.

T/F 29. Benign and malignant paragangliomas cannot be distinguished on histological examination.

T/F 30. Paragangliomas are associated with succinate dehydrogenase gene subunits and are inherited in an autosomal-dominant pattern.

T/F 31. During surgical approach to the IAM and CPA, division of the anterior inferior cerebellar artery (AICA) is often required to access the acoustic-facial bundle.

T/F 32. Chordomas are tumors derived from remnants of the notochord.

T/F 33. Chordomas are benign bone tumors that have a malignant potential.

T/F 34. Squamous cell carcinoma (SCC) accounts for 85% of malignant tumors of the temporal bone.

T/F 35. Nodal metastasis is always associated with a poor prognosis in SCC of the temporal bone.

T/F 36. Basal cell carcinomas involving the temporal bone generally arise from a cutaneous lesion.

T/F 37. Involvement of the temporal bone occurs in 80% of patients with head and neck rhabdomyosarcoma.

T/F 38. The embryonal subtype of rhabdomyosarcoma is considered to have the worst prognostic outcome.

T/F 39. Nodular basal cell carcinoma is the most common and most aggressive subtype found in the temporal bone.

T/F 40. The carotid artery lies anteromedial to the jugular foramen at the skull base.

T/F 41. Cranial nerve schwannomas are the most common tumors arising at the jugular foramen.

T/F 42. Paragangliomas arise from normal occurring neuroectocrine cells in vascular adventitia.

T/F 43. Endocrinologically active tumors occur in 20% of head and neck paragangliomas.

T/F 44. Ten percent of head and neck paragangliomas are bilateral.

T/F 45. Head and neck paragangliomas have malignant potential.

T/F 46. Glomus vagale tumors are the most common paraganglioma in the head and neck.

T/F 47. Neurofibromatosis type 2 (NF2) is inherited in an autosomal dominant pattern.

T/F 48. The manifestations of NF2 result from mutations in the *NF2* gene, located on the long arm of chromosome 22.

T/F 49. Longitudinal fractures comprise 80% of all temporal bone fractures.

T/F 50. Temporal bone fractures resulting in complete facial nerve palsy always require immediate surgical exploration.

SINGLE BEST ANSWER QUESTIONS

51. Which of the following structures passes through Dorello canal?
    a. Greater superficial petrosal nerve
    b. Subarcuate artery
    c. Vestibular aqueduct
    d. Abducent nerve
    e. AICA

52. Which of the following is the principal surgical landmark for middle cranial fossa procedures?
    a. Greater superficial petrosal nerve
    b. Arcuate eminence
    c. Foramen lacerum
    d. Foramen spinosum
    e. Gasserian ganglion

53. Which of the following foramina are found on the floor of the middle cranial fossa?
    i. Foramen spinosum
    ii. Foramen magnum
    iii. Superior orbital fissure
    iv. Foramen ovale
    v. Foramen rotundum
    a. i, iv, and v
    b. i, iii, iv, and v
    c. iv and v
    d. iii, iv, and v
    e. All of the above

54. Which of the following statements are true regarding clival chordomas?
    i. They are usually extradural.
    ii. They arise from embryonic remnants of the notochord.
    iii. They most commonly present with lower cranial nerve palsies.
    iv. They are sensitive to chemotherapy.
    v. They can occur anywhere on the axial skeleton.

    a. i and ii
    b. ii and iii
    c. ii, iv, and v
    d. i, ii, and v
    e. All of the above

55. Which of the following statements is *INCORRECT*?
    a. Meningiomas are the most common radiation-induced neoplasm of the central nervous system.
    b. Meningiomas have a malignant potential.
    c. Meningiomas rarely occur in children.
    d. Head trauma is an unequivocal risk factor for meningiomas.

56. Regarding meningiomas, which of the following statements is correct?
    a. Ninety percent of meningiomas occur in association with NF2.
    b. In asymptomatic patients <60 years, treatment options for a meningioma include a period of watchful waiting.
    c. All patients with meningiomas should have a full-body MRI.
    d. All patients with meningioma should have a 24-hour urine collection for vanillylmandelic acid, catecholamines, and metanephrines.

57. The retrosigmoid approach to the skull base:
    a. Is contraindicated in the presence of a contralateral hearing loss
    b. Has a lower postoperative risk of CSF fistula than a middle cranial fossa approach
    c. Is not suitable for cerebellopontine angle tumors extending to the fundus of the internal auditory meatus
    d. Avoids cerebellar retraction

58. Which of the following anatomical structures pass through the jugular foramen?
    i. Inferior petrosal sinus
    ii. Superior petrosal sinus
    iii. Meningeal branch of ascending pharyngeal artery
    iv. Cranial nerve (CN) IX
    v. CN XII
    a. i, iii, and iv
    b. i, ii, iii, and iv
    c. i and iv
    d. iii and iv
    e. All of the above

59. Regarding the infratemporal fossa, which of the following statements are true?
    i. It is bounded inferiorly by the digastric muscle.
    ii. It communicates with the orbit through the superior orbital fissure.
    iii. It contains the maxillary division of the trigeminal nerve (V_2).
    iv. It communicates with the middle cranial fossa through foramen spinosum.
    v. The lateral and medial pterygoid muscles lie within the infratemporal fossa.
    a. i, ii, iii, and iv
    b. i, ii, iii, and v
    c. ii, iii, and iv
    d. i, iv, and v
    e. All of the above

60. Regarding the contents of the IAM, which of the following statements is correct?
    a. The facial nerve is located anteroinferiorly in the IAM.
    b. The superior vestibular nerve is located posterosuperiorly in the internal auditory canal.

c. The cochlear nerve is located anterosuperiorly in the internal auditory canal.

d. The cochlear nerve is located posterosuperiorly in the internal auditory canal.

e. None of the above is correct.

61. Inadvertent opening of a dural sinus during surgery may lead to an air embolus. Signs of an air embolus include which of the following?

   a. Hypotension, tachycardia, and decreased end-tidal PCO_2

   b. Hypertension, tachycardia, and decreased end-tidal PCO_2

   c. Intravascular crepitation, hypertension, and decreased end-tidal PCO_2

   d. None of the above

62. Regarding the dural sinuses in skull base surgery, which of the following statements are correct?

   i. Small dural tears can usually be controlled with bipolar diathermy and/or oxidized cellulose gauze.

   ii. Inadvertent opening of the sigmoid sinus intraoperatively mandates identification and ligation of the internal jugular vein in the neck.

   iii. Air embolism is far more likely to be of clinical significance when the patient is operated on in the sitting position.

   iv. Rotating the operating table to a "reverse Tren-delenburg" position and application of digital pressure may help prevent a complication from an air embolus.

   a. i, ii, and iii

   b. i and iii

   c. ii and iii

   d. iii and iv

   e. All of the above

   f. None of the above

63. Regarding surgery of the CPA, which of the following statements is correct?

   a. Disruption of the AICA causes Wallenberg syndrome, characterized by vocal cord paralysis, ataxia, dysarthria, and ipsilateral Horner syndrome.

   b. Disruption of the posterior inferior cerebellar artery causes a lateral medullary infarction, characterized by vocal cord paralysis, ataxia, dysarthria, and contralateral Horner syndrome.

   c. The superior cerebellar artery gives a branch that travels in the IAM.

   d. The AICA is a branch of the internal carotid artery.

   e. Division of the petrosal vein (Dandy's vein) rarely has adverse neurological consequences.

64. Which answer best describes the MRI features of a vestibular schwannoma?

   a. Hyperintense on T1 imaging

   b. Decreased intensity with fat suppression

   c. Enhancement with gadolinium administration

   d. Isointense to CSF

65. Which of the following tumors is *LEAST* likely to involve the jugular foramen?

   a. Paraganglioma

   b. Schwannoma

   c. Meningioma

   d. Chondrosarcoma

   e. Craniopharyngioma

66. Which of the following is *NOT* histologically characteristic of a vestibular schwannoma?

   a. Antoni A cells

   b. Spindle-shaped nuclei

   c. Verocay body

   d. Antoni B cells

   e. Zellballen

67. Regarding the infratemporal fossa approach type A as described by Fisch, which of the following statements is correct?

   a. It is used for removal of tumors involving the petrous apex and clivus.

   b. It is contraindicated in tumors with intracranial extension.

   c. It provides access to the jugular foramen.

   d. Typically there is grade I House-Brackmann facial nerve function postoperatively.

68. Regarding malignant otitis externa (MOE), which of the following statemenonts are correct?

   i. The causative organism is always *Pseudomonas aeruginosa.*

   ii. The fissures of Santorini are implicated in spread of disease.

   iii. Cranial nerves IX, X, and XI are the most commonly affected cranial nerves.

   iv. Facial nerve involvement is an independent prognostic indicator.

   v. There is no difference in predisposition between type I and II diabetes.

   a. ii and v

   b. i and v

   c. ii, iv, and v

   d. ii and iv

   e. All of the above are correct.

69. Regarding MOE, which of the following statements are correct?

   i. Granulation tissue along the osteocartilaginous junction is pathognomonic for MOE.

   ii. A "picket fence" fever is a common sign in MOE.

   iii. Gallium citrate Ga-67 scanning is more useful than CT scanning in determining efficacy of therapy.

   iv. Facial nerve palsy is an indication for surgery.

   v. Ceftazidime is a third-generation cephalosporin that has demonstrated efficacy in the treatment of MOE.

   a. i, iii, and v

   b. iii, iv, and v

   c. i, ii, and iii

   d. i, iii, iv, and v

   e. ii, iii, iv, and v

70. Which of the following statements regarding temporal bone fractures involving the otic capsule is incorrect?

   a. They are generally associated with a sensorineural hearing loss (SNHL).

   b. They account for 10% to 20% of temporal bone fractures.

   c. Hemotympanum is the most common cause of hearing loss.

   d. They are more likely to result in facial nerve palsy than otic capsule–sparing fractures.

71. Regarding CSF fistula after temporal bone fracture, which of the following statements is *INCORRECT?*

   a. Diagnosis can be confirmed by evaluating the fluid for β2-transferrin.

   b. They can occur as a result of a dural tear after any type of temporal bone fracture.

   c. Initial management includes bed rest and placement of a lumbar drain.

d. CSF leak can be delayed after the initial trauma in 30% of cases.

72. Which of the following conditions most commonly causes pulsatile tinnitus?
    a. Glomus jugulare
    b. Glomus tympanicum
    c. Aberrant carotid artery
    d. Benign intracranial hypertension

73. The Pittsburgh classification system for staging of temporal bone SCC was modified in 2002. Patients with facial nerve paralysis were staged as a T4 tumor. According to that classification system, which of the following tumors are classified as stage III?
    i. T1, N2, M0
    ii. T1, N1, M0
    iii. T2, N1, M0
    iv. T3, N0, M0
    v. T4, N0, M0
    a. i, ii, ii, and iv
    b. iv
    c. ii and iv
    d. iv and v

74. In which of the following features of an acoustic neuroma would a middle cranial fossa approach be considered inappropriate?
    a. Only hearing ear
    b. Existing mastoid cavity
    c. 3-cm CPA tumor
    d. Age >60 years
    e. Unilateral peripheral vertigo

75. Anesthetic techniques to reduce brain edema during a middle cranial fossa approach include all EXCEPT:
    a. Elevated head position
    b. Mannitol
    c. Furosemide
    d. Hyperventilation to a PCO_2 of 25 to 30 mmHg
    e. Sevoflurane

76. Which of the following statements regarding neurofibromatosis is correct?
    a. Vestibular schwannomas are more commonly seen in neurofibromatosis type 1 (NF1).
    b. Bilateral vestibular schwannoma is diagnostic of NF1.
    c. All children of NF2 patients have a 50% chance of developing the disease.
    d. Hearing loss in NF2 can generally be rehabilitated with cochlear implantation.
    e. Twenty percent of cases of NF2 result from new mutations.

77. Which of the following are NOT features of NF2?
    a. Vestibular schwannomas
    b. Posterior subcapsular lenticular opacities
    c. Meningioma
    d. Lisch nodules
    e. Cataract

78. Regarding NF2, which of the following statements is INCORRECT?
    a. NF2 is inherited as an autosomal dominant condition.
    b. The manifestations of NF2 result from mutations of the NF2 gene and subsequent decreased function or production of gene product Merlin.
    c. Bilateral vestibular schwannomas are diagnostic of NF2.

d. Bevacizumab may improve hearing in some patients with unresectable vestibular schwannomas.
    e. The NF2 gene is located on the long arm of chromosome 17 at band 11.2.

79. Which of the following statements regarding lesions of the petrous apex is INCORRECT?
    a. Cholesterol granuloma is the most common petrous apex lesion.
    b. Cholesterol granuloma can usually be differentiated from cholesteatoma on CT scanning.
    c. Petrous apicitis associated with a CN IV palsy and facial pain is known as Gradenigo syndrome.
    d. Cholesterol granulomas demonstrate a hyperintense signal on T1 MRI.
    e. Clival chordomas may extend laterally to involve the petrous apex.

80. Which of the following statements regarding lesions of the CPA is correct?
    a. An enhancement of a dural tail after administration of gadolinium contrast is a characteristic MRI sign found in acoustic neuroma.
    b. Extension of a tumor into the internal auditory canal excludes the diagnosis of meningioma.
    c. Epidermoid cysts avidly enhance following administration of gadolinium contrast on MRI.
    d. Hitzelberger sign in acoustic neuroma is due to pressure on the sensory fibers carried in the nervus intermedius.

81. Regarding chondrosarcoma, which of the following statements is INCORRECT?
    a. Chondrosarcomas in the skull base are most commonly seen in the midline.
    b. Chondrosarcomas have radiologic features similar to chordomas.
    c. Chondrosarcomas are low-grade tumors that rarely require surgical intervention.
    d. On CT scanning, chondrosarcomas demonstrate matrix calcification and endosteal scalloping.

82. Regarding chondrosarcoma, which of the following statements is INCORRECT?
    a. Chondrosarcomas of the skull base may be associated with Maffucci syndrome.
    b. They account for 30% of intracranial neoplasms.
    c. They are most commonly located at the petrooccipital synchondrosis.
    d. Chondrosarcomas have a significantly better prognosis than chordomas.

83. A patient presents with a temporal bone SCC limited to the osseous external auditory canal. Which of the following is the most appropriate therapeutic intervention?
    a. Lateral temporal bone resection
    b. Sleeve resection
    c. Total temporal bone resection
    d. Radiation therapy
    e. Pinnectomy and sleeve resection

84. Regarding stereotactic radiotherapy for the treatment of vestibular schwannomas, which of the following statements is correct?
    a. Radiation doses of less than 40 Gy are not associated with facial neuropathies.
    b. It is generally considered as first-line treatment for acoustic neuromas >4 cm.
    c. After stereotactic radiation, hearing levels plateau 3 months posttreatment.

d. The cochlear dose is an independent predictor of hearing preservation.

e. It is contraindicated in patients <20 years.

85. Fluctuating deafness in a patient with temporal bone trauma is most likely due to which of the following?
    a. Hemotympanum
    b. Ossicular chain disruption
    c. Perilymph fistula
    d. Injury to internal acoustic meatus

86. In transverse fractures of temporal bone, the facial nerve is most commonly injured at which of the following?
    a. Mastoid segment
    b. Tympanic segment
    c. Labyrinthine segment
    d. Stylomastoid foramen
    e. IAM

87. Regarding the evaluation of a patient with a facial nerve injury, which of the following statements is *INCORRECT*?
    a. Conduction block only with no physical disruption of axonal discontinuity correlates with Sunderland's first-degree injury.
    b. Transection of the epineurium correlates with Sunderland's second-degree injury.
    c. Transection of the endoneurium correlates with Sunderland's third-degree injury.
    d. Synkinesis refers to the loss of discrete facial movements after facial nerve injury.
    e. Topodiagnostic testing has little correlation with the site of injury to the facial nerve.

88. Which of the following statements are correct?
    i. Griesinger sign refers to erythema and edema behind the mastoid process resulting from septic thrombi of the mastoid emissary veins in lateral sinus thrombosis.
    ii. Delta sign refers to the appearance of a lateral sinus thrombosis on contrast-enhanced radiographic imaging resulting from the nonenhancing clot surrounded by enhancing dural sinus wall.
    iii. The halo sign, a clinically detectable double ring resulting from CSF separating from blood when applied to filter paper, is diagnostic of a CSF fistula.

iv. Brown sign refers to blanching of the tympanic membrane when applying positive pressure and can be seen in glomus jugulare tumors.

v. Bezold sign refers to bruising behind the ear at the mastoid process and is seen in fractures of the petrous temporal bone.
    a. i, ii, iii, and iv
    b. i, ii, and iv
    c. ii, iii, and iv
    d. i, ii, and v
    e. All of the above

89. Which of the following is the most common cause of conductive deafness in a patient with a longitudinal fracture of the temporal bone?
    a. Hemotympanum
    b. Dislocation of malleus
    c. Tympanic membrane perforation
    d. Perilymph fistula
    e. Malleoincudal dislocation

90. An MRI of the brain and temporal bone demonstrates a lesion of the petrous apex, which is hyperintense on both T1 and T2 imaging and does not enhance with gadolinium. Which of the following is the most appropriate management?
    a. Wide en-bloc excision of petrous apex neoplasm
    b. Radiation therapy
    c. Excision of neoplasm followed by radiotherapy
    d. Surgical drainage of petrous apex granuloma

91. Which of the following is the most common complication in the treatment of vestibular schwannoma with the gamma knife?
    a. Delayed SNHL
    b. Immediate SNHL
    c. Immediate CN VII palsy
    d. Delayed CN VII palsy
    e. Malignant transformation

92. A 56-year-old woman presents to the outpatient clinic with an 8-month history of otalgia and otorrhea. Otoscopy reveals a large polyp filling the external auditory canal. Subsequent imaging is demonstrated in Figure 11-1. Which of the following statements represents the next single best step in managing this patient?

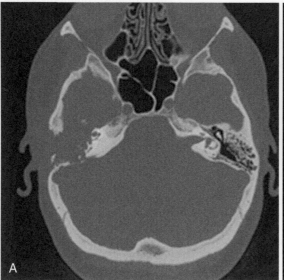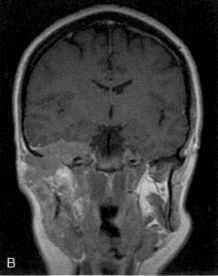

FIGURE 11-1 Imaging of patient with a large polyp in the external auditory canal.

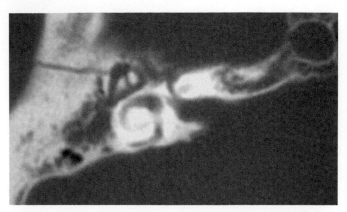

FIGURE 11-2 Axial high-resolution computed tomography (HRCT) of the temporal bone.

a. Balloon-test occlusion
b. Biopsy of the polyp
c. 24-hour urinary vanillylmandelic acid measurement
d. Referral to radiation oncology

93. Which of the following statements regarding vestibular schwannoma surgery is correct?
    a. The translabyrinthine approach cannot provide direct access to the CPA.
    b. The retrosigmoid approach involves a posterior craniotomy and thus avoids cerebellar retraction.
    c. The retrosigmoid approach to the CPA is not limited by tumor size.
    d. The middle cranial fossa approach is associated with a lower incidence of postoperative infection.

94. Which of the following statements regarding the management of temporal bone fracture complications is correct?
    a. The overall risk of damage to the otic capsule is about 80% in temporal bone fractures.
    b. Cable grafting of a transected facial nerve in patients with delayed complete facial nerve palsy will result in a House-Brackmann grade II facial nerve palsy in 80% of patients 18 months postoperatively.
    c. A patient with an otic capsule–involving fracture is likely to initially demonstrate third-degree nystagmus with the fast phase away from the fracture side.
    d. Facial nerve palsy is more likely to complicate temporal bone fractures in children· than in adults.

95. Figure 11-2 demonstrates an axial high-resolution CT (HRCT) of the temporal bone. What is the most likely presenting complaint?
    a. Pulsatile tinnitus
    b. Conductive hearing loss and facial nerve palsy
    c. SNHL and vertigo
    d. Foul-smelling otorrhea

96. Regarding MRI findings of paraganglioma, which of the following statements is correct?
    a. The "pepper" in "salt and pepper" appearance represents multiple areas of signal void of vessels.
    b. The "salt" in "salt and pepper" appearance represents multiple areas of signal void of vessels.
    c. The "salt and pepper" appearance is only appreciated on T2 imaging.
    d. The "empty delta" sign is pathognomonic of a carotid body tumor.

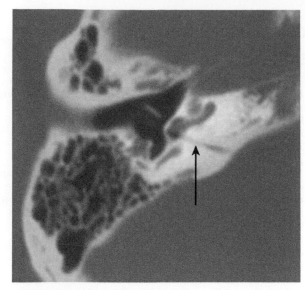

FIGURE 11-3 Axial high resolution computed tomographic scan.

97. Which of the statements regarding the arrowed structure on the axial HRCT scan shown in Figure 11-3 is correct?
    a. Its contents have an ionic composition similar to CSF.
    b. It most likely resulted from a blow to the temporoparietal region of the skull.
    c. When it is larger than normal, it is associated with Pendred syndrome in approximately one-third of cases.
    d. It cannot be appreciated on HRCT coronal plane images of the temporal bone.

98. Which of the following statements regarding fibrous dysplasia of the skull base is *INCORRECT*?
    a. Fibrous dysplasia is a developmental dysplastic disorder of bone in which the normal bone matrix is replaced by fibroblastic proliferation.
    b. Monostotic fibrous dysplasia may be associated with café-au-lait skin pigmentation in McCune-Albright syndrome.
    c. Craniofacial fibrous dysplasia typically presents before puberty and progresses throughout adolescence.
    d. Monostotic fibrous dysplasia is the most common form and accounts for 70% to 80% of cases.

99. Which of the following structures does *NOT* pass through the jugular foramen?
    a. CN IX
    b. Jacobson nerve
    c. Cervical sympathetic trunk
    d. Arnold nerve

100. A 48-year-old man sustained an immediate complete facial nerve palsy following a traumatic temporal bone fracture. He had an ipsilateral profound SNHL. Which of the following is the most appropriate surgical approach to decompress and explore the facial nerve?
    a. Transmastoid approach
    b. Retrosigmoid approach
    c. Middle cranial fossa approach
    d. Fisch A infratemporal fossa approach
    e. Translabyrinthine approach

CORE KNOWLEDGE

TEMPORAL BONE FRACTURES

- Temporal bone fractures are traditionally classified into longitudinal fractures and transverse fractures, depending on their orientation to the petrous apex. Some 80% to 90% of temporal bone fractures are thought to be longitudinal, running parallel to the petrous apex, and 10% to 20% transverse, running perpendicular to the petrous apex.
- Newer classifications are based on otic capsule sparing and otic capsule disrupting. An otic capsule–sparing fracture runs anterolateral to the otic capsule, is caused by a blow to the temporoparietal region, and accounts for 80% to 90% of temporal bone fractures. An otic capsule–disrupting fracture runs directly into the otic capsule, damaging the cochlea and semicircular canals, and is caused by a blow to the occipital region.
- Most temporal bone fractures are completely irregular following an oblique or mixed pattern. Therefore, rather than the type of fracture, the evaluation of function is the critical issue. However, these classification systems are useful to predict the pattern of injury.
- Longitudinal fractures typically spare the labyrinth, although intralabyrinthine extension is possible.
- Signs and symptoms of longitudinal fractures include bleeding into the ear canal from skin and tympanic membrane laceration, hemotympanum, external auditory canal (EAC) fractures, ossicular chain disruption, and conductive hearing loss. Twenty percent of longitudinal fractures injure the facial nerve and cause paralysis. The injury site is usually the horizontal segment of the nerve distal to the geniculate ganglion. CSF fistula is common but usually temporary.
- Transverse fractures more commonly involve the labyrinth, resulting in profound SNHL and vertigo. The intensity of the vertigo usually decreases over 4 to 6 weeks. Facial nerve injury occurs in 50% of transverse fractures. The injury site is most commonly at the labyrinthine segment of the facial nerve and geniculate ganglion.
- HRCT of the temporal bone should be acquired in all patients with a suspected complication of a temporal bone fracture.
- In the adult population, approximately 90% of temporal bone fractures are associated with concurrent intracranial injuries. Therefore, assessment of the complications associated with temporal bone fractures, in particular, examination of the facial nerve function, may not always be possible in the emergency setting.
- Patients with delayed-onset facial nerve paralysis almost always recover; delay in onset is the most important predictive factor for nerve recovery. Immediate incomplete paralysis implies a functional facial nerve and, in these subgroups, should be treated conservatively.
- Electrodiagnostic testing is usually unnecessary in patients with delayed-onset facial nerve palsy or immediate-onset incomplete palsy.
- The controversies regarding facial nerve paralysis involve the decision to operate, the timing of the operation, and the preferred surgical approach to the injured segment.
- Immediate complete paralysis is usually the result of a severed nerve and heralds a worse prognosis. That notwithstanding, spontaneous recovery rates have been reported as high as 60%.
- Patients with delayed facial palsy or incomplete palsy are managed conservatively with 10 to 14 days of systemic corticosteroids unless medically contraindicated.
- The decision to operate is made based on results of electrodiagnostic studies. The most common electrical tests are the maximum stimulation test, the nerve excitability test, electroneuronography, and electromyography.
- A complete palsy of immediate onset undergoes initial testing at 72 hours and at 3 weeks. If the nerve loses stimulability within 1 week or if >90% degeneration on electroneuronography occurs within 2 to 3 weeks, the threshold for surgical decompression should be considered.
- The surgical approach to facial nerve decompression will depend on the hearing status in the affected ear. A combination of middle cranial fossa and transmastoid surgery is adopted in patients with intact hearing, vwhereas a translabyrinthine approach is used in a nonhearing ear.
- Conductive hearing loss is frequently observed with longitudinal fractures and is caused by hemotympanum, tympanic membrane perforation, or partial or complete ossicular chain disruption. The incudostapedial joint is the most common site of ossicular chain disruption.
- CSF leaks tend to close spontaneously with conservative measures such as elevation of the head, bed rest, and stool softeners. Intermittent lumbar punctures or indwelling lumbar drains may help if the leak persists. However, surgical exploration may be indicated for CSF fistulas that last longer than 14 days.
- Vertigo is usually transient, and the possibility of posttraumatic benign positional paroxysmal vertigo or perilymph fistula should be considered for persistent vertigo.

TEMPORAL BONE SQUAMOUS CELL CARCINOMA

- SCC of the temporal bone is rare, accounting for <0.2% of all tumors of the head and neck.
- In the adult population, the most common type of primary temporal bone cancer is SCC, in contrast to the pediatric population, in which rhabdomyosarcoma is the most common malignancy.
- SCC of the temporal bone is an aggressive disease, and presentation is often at an advanced stage. The most common presenting symptoms are pain, discharge, and bleeding from the EAC.
- In the cartilaginous canal, the fissures of Santorini, foramen of Huschke, and bony-cartilaginous junctions are all implicated in spread of disease. In the middle ear or mastoid, tumors spread easily to the eustachian tube and nerves and vessels of the middle ear, providing a means of metastatic spread to the parotid, neck, and infratemporal fossa and through the base of skull to the middle and posterior cranial fossae. There is no universally accepted staging system for temporal bone SCC, although the staging system proposed by the University of Pittsburgh is most commonly applied.
- The Pittsburgh staging system is outlined in Tables 11-1, 11-2, and 11-3.
- Nodal involvement automatically confers an advance stage regardless of the initial T-stage and is a poor prognostic indicator.
- In general, all patients who are medically fit to undergo surgical treatment should do so. Palliative surgery should

Table 11-1 Tumor Size Staging According to the Pittsburgh Classification of External Auditory Canal (EAC) Squamous Cell Carcinoma

T1	Tumor limited to the EAC without bony erosion or evidence of soft tissue involvement
T2	Tumor with limited EAC bone erosion (not full thickness) with limited (<0.5 cm) soft tissue involvement
T3	Tumor eroding the osseous EAC (full thickness) with limited (<0.5 cm) soft tissue involvement or tumor involving the middle ear, mastoid, or both
T4	Tumor eroding the cochlea, petrous apex, medial wall of the middle ear, carotid canal, or jugular foramen or dura; or with extensive soft tissue involvement (>0.5 cm); patients presenting with facial nerve paralysis

Table 11-2 Lymph Node Staging for External Auditory Canal (EAC) Squamous Cell Carcinoma

N1	Single ipsilateral lymph node <3 cm
N2a	Single ipsilateral nodes >3 cm, <6 cm
N2b	Multiple ipsilateral nodes <6 cm
N2c	Bilateral or contralateral nodes <6 cm
N3	Nodes >6 cm

Table 11-3 Pittsburgh Staging for External Auditory Canal (EAC) Squamous Cell Carcinoma

Stage 0	Tis N0 M0
Stage I	T1 N0 M0
Stage II	T2 N0 M0
Stage III	T3 N0 M0, T1 N1 M0
Stage IV	T4 N0 M0, T2-4 N1 M0, any T N2 M0, any T N3 M0, any T any N M1

Hirsch BE. Staging System Revision. Arch Otolaryngol Head Neck Surg 2002; 128:93-94.

be considered in cases where curative resection is not thought possible.

- Workup for SCC of the temporal bone should include biopsy for histopathology, HRCT, MRI (with and without gadolinium contrast), and assessment of the internal carotid arteries and venous outflow. Balloon test occlusion may be required in cases where there is suspected tumor encroachment of the internal carotid arteries.
- Sleeve resection of a T1 tumor limited to the cartilaginous canal can be performed in rare circumstances, but it is generally accepted that a lateral temporal bone resection is the minimum operation for T1/T2 lesions. T3/T4 tumors require an extended temporal bone resection or subtotal temporal bone resection. There is a wide variety of procedures and nomenclature among surgeons, but most would concede that an adequate anterior margin for the temporal bone resection involves resection of the parotid gland, temporomandibular joint, and condyle. Supraomohyoid neck dissection provides staging information in the clinically node-negative neck. Modified radical neck dissection in the presence of positive lymph nodes does not confer a survival benefit. Involvement of the internal carotid arteries, dura, brain, and petrous apex portend a poor prognosis.

CEREBROSPINAL FLUID

- CSF occupies the subarachnoid space and the ventricular system around and inside the brain and spinal cord. It constitutes the content of the ventricles, cisterns, and sulci of the brain, as well as the central canal of the spinal cord.
- CSF is produced at a rate of 0.3 to 0.4 mL/min (500 mL/day) by the choroid plexus in the lateral, third, and fourth ventricles. This fluid is constantly reabsorbed, so that only 100 to 160 mL is present at any one time.
- CSF circulates within the ventricular system of the brain. The majority of CSF is produced from within the two lateral ventricles. From here, the CSF passes through the foramina of Monro to the third ventricle, then the cerebral aqueduct of Sylvius to the fourth ventricle. From the fourth ventricle, CSF passes through the foramen of Magendie on the midline, and two foramina of Luschka laterally, to enter the subarachnoid space. The CSF moves in a pulsatile manner throughout the CSF system with nearly zero net flow.
- Resorption takes place mostly in the arachnoid villi and granulations into the dural venous sinuses.
- An obstruction in CSF circulation, overproduction of CSF, or inadequate resorption results in hydrocephalus.
- Intraoperative techniques that can produce a reduction in intracranial pressure include patient positioning by elevating the head, administration of osmotic diuretics, avoidance of high doses of inhalation anesthetic agents that would increase intracranial pressure, hyperventilation to a PCO_2 of 25 to 30 mm Hg, and the placement of a lumbar subarachnoid drain.

VESTIBULAR SCHWANNOMA

- Vestibular schwannomas account for approximately 6% of intracranial tumors and approximately 80% to 90% of CPA tumors.
- Vestibular schwannomas can occur as sporadic tumors, which account for 95% of cases, or in association with NF2.
- Sporadic tumors tend to present later in life (50-60 years), whereas vestibular schwannomas in NF2 patients typically present at a younger age.
- Vestibular schwannomas arise from the Schwann cells of the superior and inferior vestibular nerves. The nerves are ensheathed in oligodendrocytes through the CPA. As the nerves enter the IAM the oligodendrocytes are replaced by Schwann cells in a region known as the zone of Obersteiner-Redlich.
- Histologically, schwannomas demonstrate Antoni A areas, composed of compact spindle cells, and Antoni B areas, composed of loose hypocellular areas. Most tumors have a mixture of both types.
- Three treatment strategies for vestibular schwannomas are available: continued observation with serial MRI, microsurgery, and stereotactic radiation.
- Continued observation is indicated in patients with small tumors or in whom there is a high probability of not needing any treatment for the rest of their predicted lifetime.
- The management of vestibular schwannomas >3 cm is microsurgical removal. The role of stereotactic radiotherapy is limited in tumors this size.
- The overall role of stereotactic radiotherapy in the treatment of vestibular schwannomas is expanding, and a fully balanced overview of the two treatment modalities should be considered at every step in the treatment algorithm.

- A variety of surgical approaches has been described for vestibular schwannoma surgery, but the most commonly used are the retrosigmoid, translabyrinthine, and middle cranial fossa approaches. Each has its advantages and disadvantages. Both the retrosigmoid and middle cranial fossa approaches require brain retraction, which is minimized using a translabyrinthine approach. The main disadvantage of the translabyrinthine approach is that hearing preservation is not possible. In selected patients, where hearing preservation is desired, a retrosigmoid or middle cranial fossa approach can be considered. The middle fossa approach allows complete exposure of the IAM but limited exposure of the CPA and is not appropriate for large tumors extending to the CPA. The retrosigmoid approach can be used for large and small tumors, and hearing preservation may be possible in tumors <2.5 cm that do not involve the lateral end of the IAM.
- Complications including hemorrhage, cerebral edema, cranial nerve deficits, CSF leak, meningitis, and arterial and venous hemorrhage can occur in any transcranial approach.
- There are three main cerebellar arteries: the posterior inferior cerebellar artery, the AICA, and the superior cerebellar artery. The AICA is a branch of the basilar artery and often loops into the vicinity of the IAM. The internal auditory artery, which traverses the IAM, most often originates from the AICA. Disruption of the AICA during surgery of the CPA and IAM results in the lateral pontine syndrome. Complete AICA syndrome results in extensive pontine infarction and is usually fatal. Less extensive infarction is characterized by ataxia, vertigo, ipsilateral facial nerve palsy, loss of facial sensation, and hearing loss. Loss of contralateral pain and temperature on the trunk and limbs is also seen.
- Occlusion of the posterior inferior cerebellar artery results in lateral medullary syndrome, or Wallenberg syndrome. It is characterized by sensory deficits affecting the contralateral trunk and extremities and ipsilateral sensory deficits affecting the face and cranial nerves. Specifically, there is a loss of pain and temperature sensation on the contralateral side of the body and ipsilateral side of the face. Clinical signs and symptoms include nausea and vomiting, dysphagia, dysarthria, ataxia, facial pain, vertigo, nystagmus, and ipsilateral Horner syndrome.
- The vein of Labbé bridges between the inferior surface of the temporal lobe and the transverse sinus. Interruption of this vein during dural incision or retraction of the temporal lobe may result in speech and memory impairment.
- CSF leak is the most common complication after vestibular schwannoma surgery, occurring in 5% to 15% of cases. It can present as leakage from the wound site or more commonly as otorhinorrhea.

MRI CHARACTERISTICS OF SKULL BASE LESIONS (Table 11-4)

Chordoma

- Chordomas are unusual, slow-growing neoplasms that originate from remnants of the primitive notochord.
- They are predominantly located in the sacrococcygeal region and in the region of the clivus in the skull base.
- Radiologically, cranial base chordomas usually appear as encapsulated tumors in the soft tissues with extensive bony destruction.
- Clival chordomas can extend to involve the petrous apex, sphenoid sinus, and CPA.

Table 11-4 **Comparative Radiological Features of Skull Base Lesions**			
Lesion	MRI T1	MRI T2	Gd
Chondrosarcoma	↓→	↑	Yes
Chordoma	↓→	↑	Yes
Schwannoma	↓→	↑→	Yes
Meningioma	↓	↑↓	Yes
Cholesterol granuloma	↑	↑	No
Cholesteatoma	↓	↑	No
Metastasis	↓	↑	Possible
Petrous apicitis	↓	↑	Rim enhancement
Paraganglioma	→	↑	Yes
Giant cell granuloma	↓→	↓→	Yes

Gd, Enhances with gadolinium; *MRI,* magnetic resonance imaging; ↑, hyperintense; ↓, hypointense; →, isointense.

- In most cases, complete surgical resection followed by radiation therapy offers the best chance of long-term control. Incomplete resection of the primary tumor makes controlling the disease more difficult and increases the odds of recurrence.

Chondrosarcoma

- Chondrosarcomas are thought to originate from primitive mesenchymal cells or from embryonal rest of the cartilaginous matrix of the cranium.
- They are relatively slow growing but locally aggressive. Metastatic disease is uncommon. Local resection is often the treatment of choice.
- Clinically they can be difficult to distinguish from chordomas, except that the majority of chondrosarcomas of the base of skull are located off the midline, most commonly along the petrooccipital synchondrosis. This contrasts with chordomas, which are usually midline.

Meningioma

- Meningiomas account for up to 20% of intracranial tumors and approximately 5% to 10% of CPA tumors. They are the second most common CPA tumor after vestibular schwannoma. They arise from the arachnoid "cap" cells of the arachnoid villi in the meninges. They are benign but locally aggressive tumors. Many meningiomas are asymptomatic and require no treatment other than periodic observation.
- Although the majority of meningiomas are benign, they may have malignant presentations. Classification of meningiomas is based on the World Health Organization classification system:
  Benign (Grade I) (90%): meningothelial, fibrous, transitional, psammomatous, angioblastic
  Atypical (Grade II) (7%): chordoid, clear cell, atypical with brain invasion
  Anaplastic/malignant (Grade III) (2%): papillary, rhabdoid, anaplastic

Cholesterol Granuloma

- Cholesterol granuloma can arise in any pneumatized space of the temporal bone but is most commonly seen at the petrous apex or middle ear.

- In contrast to middle ear cholesterol granulomas, petrous apex lesions can occur with no prior history of chronic suppurative otitis media.
- They present as expansile lesions of the petrous apex and are characteristically hyperintense on T1- and T2-weighted MRI. They do not enhance with gadolinium contrast, and these radiological features distinguish them from other petrous apex lesions.
- Total excision is usually unnecessary. Drainage can be achieved by a transmastoid or transcanal infracochlear approach to the petrous apex.

NEUROFIBROMATOSIS

- NF1 is inherited in an autosomal dominant pattern with the genetic defect located on chromosome 17q11.2. The gene product is neurofibromin, a tumor suppressor.
- Clinical diagnosis requires the presence of at least two of the following seven criteria to confirm the presence of NF1:
  1. Six or more café-au-lait spots or hyperpigmented macules 5 mm in diameter in prepubertal children and 15 mm postpubertal
  2. Axillary or inguinal freckles (more than two freckles)
  3. Two or more typical neurofibromas or one plexiform neurofibroma
  4. Optic nerve glioma
  5. Two or more iris hamartomas (Lisch nodules)
  6. Sphenoid dysplasia or typical long-bone abnormalities such as pseudarthrosis
  7. First-degree relative with NF1
- NF2 is inherited as an autosomal dominant condition. Half of affected individuals have NF2 as a result of a de novo gene mutation. The genetic defect is located on the long arm of chromosome 22. The *NF2* gene product is known as merlin, a tumor suppressor.
- Clinical diagnosis of NF2 requires that an individual present with at least one of the following clinical scenarios:
  1. Bilateral vestibular schwannomas
  2. A first-degree relative with NF2 *AND* unilateral vestibular schwannoma *OR* any two of the following: meningioma, schwannoma, glioma, neurofibroma, posterior subcapsular lenticular opacities
  3. Unilateral vestibular schwannoma *AND* any two of the following: meningioma, schwannoma, glioma, neurofibroma, posterior subcapsular lenticular opacities
  4. Multiple meningiomas *AND* unilateral vestibular schwannoma *OR* any two of the following: schwannoma, glioma, neurofibroma, cataract
- NF2 patients should be managed through a coordinated multidisciplinary approach involving teams from neurology, neurosurgery, neurotology, audiology, ophthalmology, dermatology, genetics, radiotherapy, and oncology.
- Treatment options for vestibular schwannomas in NF2 patients include observation with serial imaging, radiotherapy, and surgery. Hearing preservation is challenging, and all treatment options should be individualized to the patient, taking into account tumor growth patterns, cranial nerve function, and hearing status of both ears.
- Watchful waiting is reasonable in small vestibular schwannomas in an only hearing ear.
- Larger tumors may require surgical resection despite irreversible hearing loss, especially when there is evidence of brainstem compression, facial nerve palsy, or early hydrocephalus.

Table 11-5 The Fisch and Mattox Classification of Jugulotympanic Paragangliomas

Type A tumor	Tumor limited to the middle ear cleft (glomus tympanicum)
Type B tumor	Tumor limited to the tympanomastoid area with no infralabyrinthine compartment involvement
Type C tumor	Tumor involving the infralabyrinthine compartment of the temporal bone and extending into the petrous apex
Type C1 tumor	Tumor with limited involvement of the vertical portion of the carotid canal
Type C2 tumor	Tumor invading the vertical portion of the carotid canal
Type C3 tumor	Tumor invading the horizontal portion of the carotid canal
Type D1 tumor	Tumor with an intracranial extension <2 cm in diameter
Type D2 tumor	Tumor with an intracranial extension >2 cm in diameter

- Intracranial meningiomas may be quite slow growing; surgical resection should be considered only when symptomatic.
- Auditory brainstem implants allow electrical stimulation of the cochlear nucleus. They are used in patients with no serviceable hearing who are undergoing vestibular schwannoma removal. An auditory brainstem implant does not restore hearing but instead improves the patient's ability to appreciate environmental sounds and enhances communication.
- There is currently no cure for NF2. A trial of bevacizumab, an anti-vascular derived endothelial growth factor monoclonal antibody, has shown efficacy in some patients with NF2, with hearing improvement and reduction of tumor volume.

PARAGANGLIOMAS (TABLE 11-5)

- Paragangliomas are neuroendocrine tumors derived from the extraadrenal paraganglia of the autonomic nervous system. The sympathetic paraganglia are mostly located along the sympathetic nerve chains bordering the vertebrae and in the pelvis, while the parasympathetic ones are primarily located in the head and neck.
- Paragangliomas are rare vascular tumors, accounting for <1% of head and neck tumors. Approximately 3% of paragangliomas occur in the head and neck.
- The most common paraganglioma of the head and neck is the carotid body tumor, followed by the jugulotympanic and vagal paraganglioma. Paragangliomas have also been reported in the larynx, sinonasal chambers, and orbit.
- In contrast to the sympathetic tumors, only 2% to 5% of head and neck paragangliomas secrete catecholamines.
- Paragangliomas demonstrate early neural or blood vessel involvement and a propensity for skull base invasion and intracranial involvement.
- Histologically paragangliomas are characterized by Zellballen (densely packed nests of type I or chief cells) surrounded by spindled sustentacular cells (type II cells).
- It is estimated that 10% are multicentric and 5% to 10% are malignant. Multicentricity is more common in patients with familial paragangliomas.
- Familial paragangliomas account for 10% to 15% of cases. They are frequently multiple and bilateral and are

detected at an earlier age. The genes for familial paraganglioma have been identified as succinate dehydrogenase subunits C and B, inherited as autosomal dominant traits, and subunit D, transmitted in an autosomal dominant pattern with maternal imprinting.

- There are no histological or immunohistochemical criteria for diagnosing malignant paraganglioma, and the diagnosis can be made only when there is metastasis to nonneuroendocrine tissue.

- Temporal paragangliomas comprise tympanic (glomus tympanicum) and jugular (glomus jugulare) paragangliomas. They are thought to arise from the paraganglia located within adventitia of the jugular bulb and can be associated with either the auricular branch of the vagus nerve (Arnold nerve) or the tympanic branch of the glossopharyngeal nerve (Jacobson nerve).

- Jugulotympanic paragangliomas are benign, encapsulated, slow-growing, highly vascular, and locally invasive tumors. In the temporal bone they tend to expand along the pathway of least resistance, such as air cells, vascular lumen, skull base foramina, and eustachian tube.

- Pulsatile tinnitus and conductive deafness are the most common presenting symptoms in patients with jugulotympanic paragangliomas. A red mass behind an intact eardrum may also be seen. Blanching of the mass on pneumatic otoscopy is known as Brown sign. Lower cranial nerve palsy and facial nerve palsy indicate advanced disease.

- Radiographic evaluation includes CT and MRI. On HRCT, an irregular moth-eaten erosion of bone at the jugular foramen and erosion of the jugulocarotid spine can be seen. MRI defines soft tissue detail and intracranial, neural, and dural involvement. On MRI, all paragangliomas exhibit a high signal on T2-weighted imaging and a low signal on T1-weighted imaging. They demonstrate avid contrast enhancement. The classic "salt and pepper" appearance seen on MRI relates to the presence of hyperintense foci ("salt") interspersed with multiple areas of signal void ("pepper") due to high flow in vascular channels. This feature is reliably seen only in tumors >1 cm in size.

- Digital subtraction angiography is performed for jugular paragangliomas, and preoperative balloon embolization is performed to reduce intraoperative bleeding.

NECROTIZING OTITIS EXTERNA

- NOE or MOE is an infection of the EAC and temporal bone. The infection begins as an external otitis that can progress into an osteomyelitis of the skull base. Spread of the disease outside the EAC occurs through the fissures of Santorini and the osseocartilaginous junction, leading to involvement of the stylomastoid and jugular foramina and

eventually affecting cranial nerve function. It is generally seen in elderly patients with diabetes or in immunosuppressed patients. There is no difference in predisposition between diabetes types I and II.

- The hallmark of NOE is unrelenting pain disproportionate to the clinical findings. Granulation tissue along the floor of the EAC at the osseocartilaginous junction is virtually pathognomonic of NOE. Pyrexia and leukocytosis are uncommon.

- Levenson's criteria for diagnosis of MOE includes refractory otitis externa, severe nocturnal otalgia, purulent otorrhea, granulation tissue in the external canal, growth of *Pseudomonas aeruginosa* from the external canal, and the presence of diabetes or an immunocompromised state.

- The most common causative organism is *Pseudomonas aeruginosa*, although other organisms such as *Proteus mirabilis*, *Aspergillus fumigatus*, *Proteus* sp., *Klebsiella* sp., and *Staphylococci* have all been isolated.

- As the skull base is progressively involved, the adjacent exiting cranial nerves and their branches, especially the facial nerve and the vagus nerve, may be affected, resulting in facial paralysis and hoarseness, respectively.

- MRI and CT are complementary in evaluating patients with NOE. MRI has superior detection of bone marrow edema, which precedes the cortical bone erosion best seen on CT.

- Technetium-99 methylene diphosphonate bone scanning is based on binding to osteoblasts and depicts as little as a 10% increase in osteoblastic activity. It is of most use in the initial evaluation to confirm a clinical diagnosis; however, it is not useful in assessing response to therapy because results remain persistently positive long after clinical improvement due to continuous bone remodeling and reformation. The application of single-photon emission CT technology has improved the poor spatial resolution traditionally associated with this test.

- Gallium citrate Ga-67 scan is sensitive but not specific. Gallium binds to actively dividing cells, including inflammatory cells, tumor cells, and osteoblasts, and can be used to monitor response to treatment. Improvement of a positive test result correlates with therapeutic response.

- Complete resolution of NOE may take several months; antibiotics, aural toilet, and glucose control in diabetic patients are the cornerstones of treatment.

- The role of surgery in NOE is largely confined to tissue biopsy and abscess drainage.

- Removal of diseased bone and surgical resection is not recommended because of the spread of infection through vascular and fascial planes.

- Facial nerve palsy is not an independent indicator for surgical intervention, and facial nerve decompression is not indicated for patients with facial paralysis.

ANSWERS

TRUE OR FALSE QUESTIONS

1. F	10. F	19. T	28. F
2. T	11. F	20. F	29. T
3. F	12. F	21. F	30. T
4. T	13. F	22. T	31. F
5. F	14. F	23. T	32. T
6. F	15. F	24. F	33. F
7. T	16. F	25. F	34. T
8. F	17. T	26. F	35. T
9. T	18. F	27. F	36. T

37. F	41. F	45. T	49. T
38. F	42. T	46. F	50. F
39. F	43. F	47. T	
40. T	44. T	48. T	

SINGLE BEST ANSWER QUESTIONS

51. d	64. c	77. d	90. d
52. a	65. e	78. e	91. a
53. b	66. e	79. b	92. b
54. d	67. c	80. d	93. c
55. d	68. a	81. c	94. c
56. b	69. a	82. b	95. b
57. c	70. c	83. a	96. a
58. a	71. c	84. d	97. a
59. d	72. d	85. c	98. b
60. b	73. c	86. c	99. c
61. a	74. c	87. b	100. e
62. b	75. e	88. b	
63. e	76. c	89. a	

SUGGESTED READINGS

1. Bance M, Ramsden RT. Management of neurofibromatosis type 2. *Ear Nose Throat J.* 1999;78:91-94.
2. Bonneville F, Savatovsky J, Chiras J. Imaging of cerebellopontine angle lesions: an update. Part 2: intra-axial lesions, skull base lesions that may invade the CPA region, and non-enhancing extra-axial lesions. *Eur Radiol.* 2007;17: 2908-2920.
3. Conley GS, Hirsch BE. Stereotactic radiation of vestibular schwannoma: indications, limitations and outcomes. *Curr Opin Otolaryngol Head Neck Surg.* 2010;18:351-356.
4. Isaacson B. Cholesterol granuloma and other petrous apex lesions. *Otolaryngol Clin North Am.* 2015;Jan 30, [Epub ahead of print].
5. Green JD Jr, Brackmann DE, Nguyen CD, et al. Surgical management of previously untreated glomus jugulare tumors. *Laryngoscope.* 1994;104:917-921.
6. Nash JJ, Friedland DR, Boorsma KJ, Rhee JS. Management and outcomes of facial paralysis from intratemporal blunt trauma: a systematic review. *Laryngoscope.* 2010;120: 1397-1404.
7. Mendenhall WM, Amdur RJ, Vaysberg M, Mendehall CM, Werning JW. Head and neck paragangliomas. *Head Neck.* 2011;33:1530-1534.
8. Moffat DA, Wagstaff SA, Hardy DG. The outcome of radical surgery and postoperative radiotherapy for squamous carcinoma of the temporal bone. *Laryngoscope.* 2005;115: 341-347.
9. Moukarbel RV, Sabri AN. Current management in head and neck schwannomas. *Curr Opin Otolaryngol Head Neck Surg.* 2005;13:117-122.
10. Plotkin SR, Stemmer-Rachamimov AO, Barker FG 2nd, et al. Hearing improvement after bevacizumab in patients with neurofibromatosis type 2. *N Engl J Med.* 2009;361: 358-367.

12 Benign Neck Disease

Neville Patrick Shine

TRUE OR FALSE QUESTIONS

T/F 1. The majority of lateral neck masses presenting in the adult population are benign.

T/F 2. The majority of pediatric neck masses are congenital.

T/F 3. Lipoma is the second most common benign tumor of mesenchymal origin.

T/F 4. Branchial cleft cyst anomalies account for about 20% of congenital neck masses.

T/F 5. Most branchial cyst walls are thin and lined with stratified squamous epithelium.

T/F 6. Thyroglossal duct cysts represent a developmental anomaly of the third branchial arch.

T/F 7. Thyroglossal duct cysts most frequently present with an acute infection in the first decade.

T/F 8. Ultrasound evaluation easily delineates a thyroglossal duct cyst from a midline dermoid.

T/F 9. Recurrence of thyroglossal duct cyst after Sistrunk procedure is of the order of 5% to 10%.

T/F 10. Twenty percent of lymphangiomas arise in the cervicofacial region.

T/F 11. The majority of microcystic lymphangiomas spontaneously regress and are fully resolved by the age of 5 years.

T/F 12. Surgery for lymphangioma is generally recommended due to the risk of malignant degeneration.

T/F 13. Recurrence of lymphangioma after surgery is rare (<5%).

T/F 14. Schwannomas are benign tumors of Schwann cells; 25% to 40% of schwannomas occur in the head and neck.

T/F 15. Schwannomas are histologically characterized by a cellular pattern of alternating regions of compact spindle cells (Antoni A areas), loosely arranged hypocellular areas (Antoni B areas), and rows of nuclear palisading (Verocay bodies).

T/F 16. Schwannomas have a poorly defined or deficient capsule.

T/F 17. Neurofibromas are most frequently solitary lesions but may be multiple.

T/F 18. Neurofibromatosis type 1 (NF1) is inherited in an autosomal recessive manner.

T/F 19. Malignant degeneration is more frequent in neurofibromas associated with NF1.

T/F 20. Bronchogenic cysts are rare congenital anomalies of ventral foregut development.

T/F 21. Bronchogenic cysts in adults most frequently present in the neck.

T/F 22. Teratomas are tumors derived from two out of three germ cell layers.

T/F 23. The majority of teratomas occur in the cervicofacial region.

T/F 24. Teratomas of the head and neck can present antenatally with maternal polyhydramnios.

T/F 25. Malignancy is the most significant risk associated with cervical teratomas.

T/F 26. Plunging ranulas most frequently present as soft, painless, fluctuant swellings in the submandibular triangle.

T/F 27. Plunging ranulas egress the sublingual space to the neck via a dehiscence in the mylohyoid muscle.

T/F 28. Magnetic resonance imaging (MRI) is the most useful imaging modality for diagnosis of plunging ranulas.

T/F 29. Preservation of the ipsilateral sublingual salivary gland is an important component of the management of plunging ranulas.

T/F 30. Thymic cysts are rare abnormalities of the fourth pharyngeal pouch.

T/F 31. Cervical thymic cysts may present from the angle of the mandible to the lower midline neck.

T/F 32. Dermoid cysts are derived from all three germ cell layers (ectoderm, mesoderm, and endoderm).

T/F 33. Laryngoceles are abnormal dilations of the ventricular saccule.

T/F 34. Acquired laryngoceles have been reported in glass blowers and wind instrument musicians.

T/F 35. Most acquired laryngoceles are bilateral.

T/F 36. The head and neck account for the site of 30% of paragangliomas.

T/F 37. Of those paragangliomas occurring in the head and neck, carotid body tumors are the most common.

T/F 38. Paraganglioma syndrome (PGL1), caused by mutations of the D subunit of succinate dehydrogenase, is the commonest inherited genetic abnormality in families with paragangliomas.

T/F 39. Glomus jugulare paragangliomas are the most frequent bilateral tumor seen in hereditary paraganglioma syndromes.

T/F 40. The diagnosis of malignancy in paragangliomas can be made only with immunohistochemical analysis following total excision.

T/F 41. Kikuchi-Fujimoto disease is best treated by macrolide antibiotics.

T/F 42. Kikuchi-Fujimoto disease most often presents between the third and fourth decades.

T/F 43. Prevalence of Kimura disease is unaffected by gender.

T/F 44. Cat-scratch disease predominantly affects those younger than 20 years of age.

T/F 45. *Bartonella henselae* is the causative agent in cat-scratch disease.

T/F 46. Atypical mycobacterial infection most frequently affects the parotid and submandibular lymph node basins.

T/F 47. Prolonged combination therapy of macrolide antibiotics and rifampicin is the best treatment for atypical mycobacterial infection in immunocompetent patients.

T/F 48. Kawasaki disease affects children under 5 years of age in 80% of cases.

T/F 49. Kawasaki disease is the second most common cause of acquired heart disease in children in North America and Western Europe.

T/F 50. Massive lymphadenopathy is the main clinical manifestation of Rosai-Dorfman disease.

SINGLE BEST ANSWER QUESTIONS

51. Which of the following statements are correct regarding branchial cleft cysts?
    i. They most frequently present in childhood.
    ii. They most frequently arise from the second branchial cleft.
    iii. They contain a viscous, turbid, yellow-green liquid with cholesterin crystals in the sediment.
    iv. They occur with equal frequency in males and females.
    a. i, ii, and iii
    b. i and iii
    c. iii and iv
    d. All of the above

52. Which of the following statements is/are correct regarding third branchial arch cysts?
    i. They are rare.
    ii. They present in the lower neck, anterior to the sternocleidomastoid muscle.
    iii. They are located deep to fourth-arch derivatives including the superior laryngeal nerve and internal carotid artery.
    iv. They are located superficial to third-arch derivatives including the pharyngeal constrictors.
    a. i and iv
    b. i and ii
    c. i and iii
    d. i only
    e. All of the above

53. Which of the following statements are correct regarding anomalies of the branchial apparatus?
    i. They occur during embryogenesis between the second and seventh weeks of fetal life.
    ii. They may result in cyst, fistula, or sinus formation.
    iii. They most often present due to enlargement or infection.

iv. They account for almost 20% of congenital pediatric neck anomalies.
    a. i, ii, and iv
    b. ii, iii, and iv
    c. i and iii
    d. i and iv
    e. All of the above

54. The second branchial arch forms which of the following structures?
    i. Stylohyoid
    ii. Lesser cornu of hyoid
    iii. Stylopharyngeus
    iv. Anterior belly of digastric
    v. Maxillary artery
    a. iii, iv, and v
    b. ii and v
    c. i, ii, iii, and iv
    d. i and ii
    e. All of the above

55. The third branchial arch forms which of the following structures?
    i. Glossopharyngeal nerve
    ii. Stylohyoid muscle
    iii. Greater cornu of hyoid
    iv. Common carotid artery
    a. i, ii, and iii
    b. i, ii, and iv
    c. i and ii
    d. ii, iii, and iv
    e. i, iii, and iv

56. Which of the following statements is/are correct regarding plunging ranula?
    i. It is an extravasation salivary pseudocyst.
    ii. It most often presents as a swelling in the submental triangle.
    iii. It is more common in patients with a previous history of intraoral surgery.
    iv. It most often presents with an intraoral component.
    a. i only
    b. i and iv
    c. ii and iv
    d. i, iii, and iv

57. Which of the following statements is/are correct regarding plunging ranulas?
    i. Total excision via a transcervical approach is the standard of care.
    ii. Transoral excision of the sublingual gland with or without aspiration is appropriate in about 25% of cases.
    iii. Recurrence occurs in approximately 30% of cases.
    iv. Removal of the submandibular salivary gland is advisable at the time of ranula excision.
    a. i only
    b. i and ii
    c. i and iii
    d. ii and iv
    e. None of the above

58. Which of the following statements is/are correct regarding teratomas?
    i. The head and neck are the most common anatomical site of occurrence.
    ii. Malignancy is known to arise in 5% of congenital cervical teratomas.
    iii. The risk of malignancy increases with younger age of diagnosis.
    iv. They have a poor overall prognosis.

a. iv only
b. ii and iii
c. ii, iii, and iv
d. ii only
e. All of the above

59. Which of the following statements is/are correct regarding surgical intervention for teratomas?
i. It may be undertaken as an EXIT (ex utero intrapartum treatment)/OOPS (operation on placental support) procedure
ii. In cases of maternal polyhydramnios, surgical intervention should be deferred until at least 6 months of age.
iii. It has an associated mortality of <2%.
iv. In the absence of any airway compromise, surgical intervention should be deferred until the child weighs 15 kg.
   a. i and iv
   b. i, ii, and iv
   c. iii only
   d. i only
   e. All of the above

60. Teratomas may be diagnosed:
i. Secondary to maternal polyhydramnios
ii. On routine antenatal ultrasound
iii. During the second stage of labor
iv. In the neonatal period
v. In later childhood
   a. i, ii, iii, and iv
   b. i, iii, iv, and v
   c. i, ii, and iv
   d. All of the above

61. Which of the following statements are correct regarding chondromas of the neck?
i. They most frequently arise from the larynx.
ii. They may present as a lateral neck mass.
iii. They arise from immature hyaline cartilage.
iv. They have been reported arising from the hyoid.
   a. i and ii
   b. i, ii, and iii
   c. i and iv
   d. i, iii, and iv
   e. i, ii, and iv

62. Which of the following statements is/are correct regarding paragangliomas?
i. After the adrenal glands, the head and neck are the next most frequent site of occurrence.
ii. One percent to three percent of extraadrenal paragangliomas are secretory tumors.
iii. They are derived from paraganglionic cells of neural crest origin.
iv. In the head and neck they have a 20% rate of malignancy.
   a. i, ii, and iii
   b. i, iii, and iv
   c. ii only
   d. iii only
   e. ii and iii

63. Which of the following syndromes is/are associated with multiple paragangliomas and/or pheochromocytomas?
i. Multiple endocrine neoplasia 1
ii. Multiple endocrine neoplasia 2a
iii. Multiple endocrine neoplasia 2b
iv. von Hippel-Lindau disease
v. Carney's triad
   a. i, ii, iii, and iv
   b. iii, iv, and v

c. ii, iii, iv, and v
d. i only
e. All of the above

64. Which of the following statements is/are correct regarding hereditary paraganglioma syndromes?
i. Mutation of the B subunit of succinate dehydrogenase (SDH) is the most common abnormality.
ii. *SDHD* gene is found on chromosome 11.
iii. *SDHB* gene is found on chromosome 1.
iv. *SDHB* gene mutations confer a higher risk of secreting tumors and pheochromocytomas.
   a. i only
   b. ii only
   c. iii only
   d. iii and iv
   e. ii, iii, and iv

65. Which of the following statements are correct regarding carotid body tumors?
i. The carotid body is located in the adventitia of the posteromedial aspect of carotid bifurcation.
ii. The branchiomeric paraganglion group, from which the carotid body tumor grows, is derived from the third branchial cleft mesoderm.
iii. They are the most common bilateral paragangliomas in the head and neck.
iv. Bilateral carotid body tumors are best managed by single-stage bilateral surgery.
v. Carotid body tumors should always undergo preoperative embolization.
   a. ii, iii, iv, and v
   b. i, ii, iii, and iv
   c. i, iii, and v
   d. i, ii, and v
   e. i, ii, and iii

66. Genetic screening for hereditary paraganglioma *SDH* gene mutations should be considered in which of the following patients?
i. Patients <40 years of age
ii. Patients with a positive family history
iii. Patients with bilateral /multiple tumors
iv. Patients with tumors <2 cm
   a. All of the above
   b. i, ii, and iii
   c. ii, iii, and iv
   d. ii and iii

67. The classical features of carotid body tumors include which of the following?
i. The lyre sign
ii. Fontaine sign
iii. "salt and pepper" pattern on MRI
iv. Lower cranial nerve dysfunction
v. Horner syndrome
   a. i, ii, and iii
   b. i, iii, iv, and v
   c. i, iii, and v
   d. i and iii

68. Which of the following statements is/are correct regarding paragangliomas of the head and neck?
i. After carotid body tumors, glomus vagale is the next most common tumor.
ii. At altitude, there is a distinct male predominance in the gender distribution of carotid body tumors.
iii. Shamblin's classification may predict the necessity for carotid resection, with Shamblin type 1 conferring the highest risk.
iv. The dominant feeding vessel to carotid body tumors is the superior thyroid artery.

a. i, ii, and iii
b. i, ii, and iv
c. iv only
d. All of the above
e. None of the above

69. Which of the following statements is/are correct regarding schwannomas?
   i. Surgical excision is rarely associated with postoperative nerve dysfunction.
   ii. Demonstrates strong s100 immunohistochemical positivity.
   iii. Malignant transformation is reported in about 10%.
   iv. They are rarely multiple in the head and neck.
      a. ii, iii, and iv
      b. iii and iv
      c. ii only
      d. ii and iv
      e. All of the above

70. Which of the following statements are correct regarding cervical schwannomas?
   i. They tend to be slow growing.
   ii. They tend to be hypointense on T1-weighted MRI and hyperintense on T2-weighted MRI, depending on their cellularity.
   iii. There is marked enhancement of the solid component of the tumor following the administration of gadolinium.
   iv. A "salt and pepper" pattern may be seen in postgadolinium MRI.
      a. i, ii, and iii
      b. i and ii
      c. i and iv
      d. All of the above

71. Which of the following statements is/are correct regarding cervicofacial neurofibromas?
   i. They are most often seen in patients with neurofibromatosis type 2.
   ii. They are well-encapsulated tumors of peripheral nerve sheaths.
   iii. They are more frequently multiple than schwannomas.
   iv. When associated with neurofibromatosis, they have a higher risk of malignant degeneration.
   v. They should be routinely excised.
      a. i, iii, and iv
      b. iii and iv
      c. iii, iv, and v
      d. iii only
      e. ii only

72. Which of the following statements are correct regarding NF1?
   i. It has an incidence of 1 in 3000.
   ii. The *NF1* gene is located on chromosome 17.
   iii. Inheritance is by an autosomal dominant pattern.
   iv. It is associated with increased risk of malignant peripheral nerve sheath tumors.
      a. i, iii, and iv
      b. ii, iii, and iv
      c. i and iv
      d. All of the above

73. Which of the following statements are correct regarding bronchogenic cysts?
   i. A superficial presternal or suprasternal location is most common, while deep neck or laterally located bronchogenic cysts are comparatively rare.
   ii. Bronchogenic cysts of the cervical area are usually asymptomatic.

iii. In adults, the two most common locations of bronchogenic cyst are the mediastinum and the lung parenchyma.
iv. Most bronchogenic cysts are unilocular, filled with fluid, and not in communication with the airways.
   a. ii and iv
   b. i, ii, and iv
   c. i, ii, and iii
   d. iii and iv
   e. All of the above

74. Which of the following statements are correct regarding cervical bronchogenic cysts?
   i. Although congenital, they usually present in the third decade of life.
   ii. Surgery is the treatment of choice.
   iii. Malignant transformation has been reported.
   iv. They may become infected.
      a. ii, iii, and iv
      b. i, ii, and iv
      c. ii and iv
      d. All of the above

75. Which of the following statements are correct regarding cervical thymic cysts?
   i. They account for 1% of all cystic cervical masses.
   ii. They usually present in the first decade of life.
   iii. They are more common in males.
   iv. They are most often left sided.
   v. They can present anywhere in the neck from angle of mandible to suprasternal notch.
      a. i, ii, iii, and v
      b. i, ii, iv, and v
      c. i, iii, and iv
      d. i and v
      e. All of the above

76. Which of the following statements is/are correct regarding cervical thymic cysts?
   i. They have mediastinal extension in 50% of cases.
   ii. Distinction from third and fourth branchial arch cysts is made on MRI.
   iii. They are less common than branchial arch cyst anomalies.
   iv. They arise from the ventral foregut.
      a. i and iii
      b. ii and iv
      c. ii, iii, and iv
      d. i only
      e. None of the above

77. Which of the following statements is/are correct regarding the embryological development of the thyroid gland?
   i. It begins during the fifth week of gestation.
   ii. It begins at the foramen cecum, which lies rostral to the tuberculum impar.
   iii. Descent into the neck may go anterior, through, or ventral to the hyoid bone.
   iv. Obliteration of the migratory tract is normally complete by 18 weeks' gestation.
      a. i and iv
      b. ii and iii
      c. ii, iii, and iv
      d. i only
      e. i and iii

78. Which of the following statements is/are correct regarding thyroglossal duct cysts?
   i. They are the most common congenital neck anomaly.

ii. They may be present in up to 7% of the population.
iii. The majority present before the age of 10.
iv. They may present as lateral neck masses in adults.
   a. ii only
   b. iv only
   c. ii, iii, and iv
   d. i and ii
   e. All of the above

79. Which of the following statements are correct regarding thyroglossal duct cysts?
   i. They are most frequently infrahyoid.
   ii. They are suprahyoid in 25% of cases.
   iii. Radionuclide scans are required preoperatively.
   iv. They occur in cases in which thyroid cancer has been reported previously.
      a. i and ii
      b. i and iii
      c. i, ii, and iii
      d. i, ii, and iv

80. Which of the following statements is/are correct regarding surgical excision of thyroglossal duct cysts?
   i. It is associated with 15% recurrence rates if the central portion of the hyoid is excised as part of the procedure.
   ii. Simple cyst excision is associated with recurrence rates of 30%.
   iii. It is recommended predominantly for cosmetic reasons.
   iv. It should not be undertaken if the thyroglossal duct cyst represents the only functioning thyroid tissue.
      a. i only
      b. ii only
      c. iii and iv
      d. ii and iv
      e. None of the above

81. Which of the following statements is/are correct regarding lymphangiomas of the cervicofacial region?
   i. They most often present from the twelfth week of life onward.
   ii. They are best treated with propranolol.
   iii. Steroids may be of short-term benefit.
   iv. Sclerosants such as bleomycin and OK-432 are valid therapeutic options.
      a. i, ii, and iii
      b. ii, iii, and iv
      c. iv only
      d. None of the above

82. Which of the following statements are correct regarding cystic hygromas?
   i. They are the second most common congenital mass in the parotid region.
   ii. Oral cavity and tongue involvement may result in dysphagia and airway difficulties.
   iii. Within the neck, the anterior triangle is the most common site.
   iv. Rapid increase in size can occur secondary to spontaneous hemorrhage into the lesion.
      a. i, ii, and iv
      b. ii and iv
      c. i and ii
      d. All of the above

83. Which of the following statements are correct regarding laryngoceles?
   i. They arise from the saccule of the laryngeal ventricle.
   ii. They may present acutely with infection known as laryngopyoceles.

iii. They are frequently associated with laryngeal carcinoma.
iv. They demonstrate a male predominance.
v. They are unilateral in 90% of cases.
   a. ii, iii, and iv
   b. i, iv, and v
   c. i, ii, iv, and v
   d. i, iii, and v

84. Which of the following statements are correct regarding Kikuchi-Fujimoto disease?
   i. It is a self-limiting disease.
   ii. It most often occurs in the Japanese population.
   iii. It has a viral etiology.
   iv. It recurs in 30% of patients.
      a. ii, iii, and iv
      b. ii and iv
      c. i, iii, and iv
      d. i, ii, and iv

85. Which of the following statements are correct regarding Kikuchi-Fujimoto disease?
   i. It typically affects young adults.
   ii. It has a gradual onset.
   iii. Posterior cervical nodes are frequently involved (65% to 70% of the cases).
   iv. Lymph nodes tend to be mobile and firm.
   v. It occurs exclusively in Asian populations.
      a. i, ii, iii, and iv
      b. ii, iii, and iv
      c. ii, iv, and v
      d. All of the above

86. Which of the following statements is/are correct regarding adult rhabdomyoma?
   i. It is a rare benign tumor of smooth muscle differentiation.
   ii. It predominantly occurs in the head and neck.
   iii. It demonstrates a strong male predilection.
   iv. It generally presents in the over-40 age group.
   v. It may be multifocal in as many as 15% of patients.
      a. ii, iii, iv, and v
      b. i, iii, iv, and v
      c. i and v
      d. ii only
      e. All of the above

87. Which of the following statements is/are correct regarding Kimura disease?
   i. It presents as painless solitary or multiple subcutaneous nodules that are asymmetric, mostly in the head and neck region, with coexisting lymphadenopathy in 90% of the cases.
   ii. Typical areas for the nodules include preauricular, submandibular, and popliteal regions.
   iii. Renal involvement occurs in 30% of patients.
   iv. Hypereosinophilia and elevated serum immunoglobulin E are frequent findings.
      a. i only
      b. ii and iii
      c. iii and iv
      d. ii and iv
      e. All of the above

88. Which of the following statements are correct regarding Kimura disease?
   i. It is most common in Asian populations but has been reported in all populations.
   ii. A strong male predominance exists.
   iii. It most frequently presents in the third decade of life.

iv. Histopathology of excised specimens demonstrates a marked eosinophilic infiltrate and eosinophilic abscesses.
  a. i and iv
  b. i, ii, and iii
  c. i and iii
  d. All of the above

89. Which of the following statements is/are correct regarding cat-scratch disease?
  i. Presentation usually occurs 1 to 3 weeks after inoculation with tender lymphadenopathy.
  ii. Associated systemic symptoms are common.
  iii. Lymphadenopathy is usually the first to resolve.
  iv. Kittens have a greater capacity to transmit the disease than adult cats.
  a. ii, iii, and iv
  b. i, ii, and iii
  c. iii only
  d. iv only
  e. All of the above

90. Which of the following statements is/are correct regarding cat-scratch disease?
  i. *Bartonella quintana* is the causative agent.
  ii. It most often presents at 30 to 40 years of age.
  iii. It is more common in men.
  iv. It is a seasonal disease.
  v. It can occur in the absence of a history of feline contact.
  a. i, ii, iii, and iv
  b. iii, iv, and v
  c. i only
  d. All of the above

91. Which of the following statements are correct regarding cat-scratch disease?
  i. Positive serology is required for diagnosis.
  ii. Lymph node biopsy is required for diagnosis.
  iii. Antimicrobial therapy is indicated in most cases.
  iv. Azithromycin has been shown to reduce the risk of disseminated disease.
  a. i and iii
  b. ii and iv
  c. iii and iv
  d. None of the above

92. Which of the following statements is/are correct regarding atypical mycobacterial infection?
  i. *Mycobacterium avium* complex is the most common causative agent.
  ii. It most often presents in children <6 years of age.
  iii. It causes a shiny, violaceous discoloration of the skin overlying the affected lymph nodes.
  iv. Positive serology confirms the diagnosis.
  a. i, ii, and iv
  b. i, iii, and iv
  c. ii only
  d. iii only
  e. All of the above

93. Which of the following statements is/are correct regarding the treatment of atypical mycobacterial infections?
  i. It is generally supportive, because spontaneous resolution within 6 weeks is the norm.
  ii. Incision and drainage is the treatment of choice.
  iii. Prolonged antimicrobial therapy is preferred treatment in children.
  iv. Antibiotic therapy after surgical intervention may be indicated.

  a. iv only
  b. ii only
  c. iii and iv
  d. i and iv

94. Which of the following statements are correct regarding *Toxoplasma gondii* infection?
  i. It is associated with cervical adenitis in 90% of cases.
  ii. It is usually minimally symptomatic.
  iii. It is usually treated with azithromycin or pyrimethamine and sulfadiazine.
  iv. Seroprevalence in the United States is estimated between 11% and 22%.
  a. i, ii, and iv
  b. iii and iv
  c. ii and iv
  d. All of the above

95. Which of the following statements is/are correct regarding Kawasaki disease?
  i. Eighty percent of patients are 5 years of age or younger.
  ii. The male-to-female ratio is 1.5:1.
  iii. Cardiac sequelae occur in 5% of patients.
  iv. Early intervention with steroids reduces cardiac morbidity.
  v. Recurrence occurs in 20% of cases.
  a. i, ii, iii, and iv
  b. iii, iv, and v
  c. i, ii, and iii
  d. iii only

96. Which of the following are among the principal clinical findings utilized to diagnose Kawasaki disease?
  i. Cervical lymphadenopathy
  ii. Changes in lips and oral cavity
  iii. Polymorphous exanthema
  iv. Polyarthritis
  v. Changes in the extremities including erythema and desquamation
  a. i, ii, iii, and iv
  b. i, iii, iv, and v
  c. i, ii, iii, and v
  d. i and v

97. Which of the following statements are correct regarding Kawasaki disease?
  i. It is a systemic vasculitis with a predilection for the coronary arteries.
  ii. It may demonstrate seasonal incidence.
  iii. An inflammatory arteritis begins at day 6.
  iv. Aneurysm formation generally begins at day 12.
  a. i and iv
  b. i and ii
  c. iii and iv
  d. All of the above

98. Which of the following statements is/are correct regarding Rosai-Dorfman disease?
  i. It is also known as sinus histiocytosis with massive lymphadenopathy.
  ii. It most frequently involves the posterior triangle lymph nodes.
  iii. It most frequently affects those in the third and fourth decades of life.
  iv. It is usually treated with systemic corticosteroids.
  a. i, iii, and iv
  b. ii and iv
  c. i only
  d. iii only

99. Which of the following statements is/are correct regarding lipomas?
    i. They are hamartomatous proliferations of mature fat cells.
    ii. Twenty-five percent occur in the head and neck.
    iii. The anterior triangle of the neck is the most common site within the head and neck.
    iv. A peak incidence of lipoma formation is noted in fifth and sixth decades of life.
        a. ii and iii
        b. iv only
        c. i, ii, and iv
        d. All of the above

100. Which of the following syndromes are associated with lipoma formation?
    i. Gardner syndrome
    ii. Dercum disease
    iii. Madelung disease
    iv. von Recklinghausen disease
    v. Familial multiple lipomatosis
        a. i, iii, and v
        b. ii, iii, and iv
        c. i, ii, iii, and v
        d. i, ii, and iii

CORE KNOWLEDGE

BRANCHIAL CLEFT CYSTS

- Branchial anomalies are the result of altered development of the branchial apparatus during embryogenesis, between the second and sixth to seventh weeks of fetal life. The persistence of branchial remnants can lead to the development of cysts, sinuses, fistulas, or islands of cartilage.
- Anomalies of the second branchial cleft are the most frequent cause of neck masses of this type. They account for approximately 90% of all cases and are usually identified only in the second to fourth decades of life, when they become enlarged secondary to infection or rupture. They are seen with equal frequency in males and females.
- Third arch defects are rare and tend to occur in the lower neck anterior to the sternocleidomastoid muscle and deep to third-arch derivatives such as the glossopharyngeal nerve and internal carotid arteries but superficial to fourth-arch derivatives such as the superior laryngeal nerve and pharyngeal constrictors.
- They contain a viscous, turbid, yellow-green liquid with cholesterin crystals in the sediment. The walls are thin and coated with the stratified squamous nonkeratinized epithelium that covers the lymphoid tissue.

THYROGLOSSAL DUCT CYSTS

- On approximately the twenty-fourth day of gestation, the thyroid initially arises caudal to the tuberculum impar, which is also known as the median tongue bud, derived from the first pharyngeal arch. The foramen cecum begins rostral to the copula, also known as the hypobranchial eminence. This median embryologic swelling consists of mesoderm that arises from the second pharyngeal pouch (although the third and fourth pouches are also involved). The thyroid gland, therefore, originates from between the first and second pouches.
- Descent into the neck is complete by the seventh week of gestation, and the tract of migration obliterates by the eighth to tenth week.
- Failure of this obliteration can lead to a thyroglossal duct cyst (Figure 12-1), which may occur at any point along the tract.
- Thyroglossal duct cysts are reported to occur in 7% of the population, with 76% presenting under the age of 6.
- Most present as midline neck swellings, but a more lateral presentation can occur.
- Ultrasound is the investigation of choice to document the presence of a normal thyroid gland.
- Carcinoma is reported in 1% to 3% of cases.

LYMPHANGIOMAS

- Lymphangiomas are congenital lymphatic malformations due to failure of lymph spaces to connect to the rest of lymphatic system. They may also be classified on the basis of size of the cysts contained, as microcystic, macrocystic, and mixed lymphangiomas. Microcystic lymphangioma consists of cysts measuring <2 cm in size, whereas the size of cysts in case of macrocystic lymphangioma is >2 cm. These are also known as cystic hygromas. In about 80% of instances, the location of cystic hygromas is the cervicofacial region. More than 60% of cystic hygromas have onset at birth, and up to 90% become overt before the age of 2 years (Figure 12-2).
- Surgery is the mainstay of treatment, usually for cosmesis but occasionally for functional reasons. Surgery may be staged where necessary. Recurrence, even after apparent complete resection, can occur in up to a fifth of patients. Sclerosants including OK-432 and bleomycin have been successfully used in the management of cystic hygromas.

SCHWANNOMAS

- Schwannomas (Figure 12-3) are benign, slow-growing, well-encapsulated tumors that arise from Schwann cells of peripheral nerves. They are solid, but 4% demonstrate cystic degeneration, and thus schwannomas should be considered in the differential diagnosis of cystic neck lesions. They tend to be solitary but can be multiple on rare occasion.
- Twenty-five percent to 40% of schwannomas occur in the head and neck region, with the VIII cranial nerve the

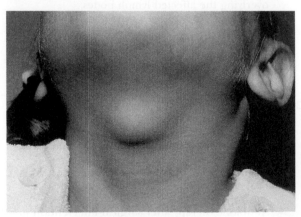

FIGURE 12-1 Thyroglossal duct cyst.

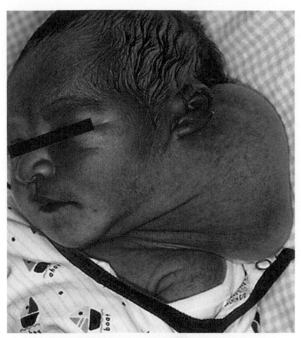

FIGURE 12-2 Left infrahyoid lymphangioma.

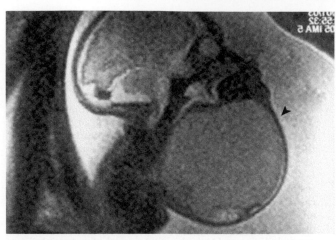

FIGURE 12-4 Sagittal fetal magnetic resonance imaging scan, showing cervical teratoma (arrowhead) from the floor of the mouth extending to the anterior chest wall. (From Shine NP, Sader C, Gollow I, Lannigan FJ. Congenital cervical teratomas: diagnostic, management and postoperative variability. *Auris Nasus Larynx* 2006;33:107-111.)

NEUROFIBROMAS

- Neurofibromas are unencapsulated, benign nerve sheath tumors of the peripheral nervous system. Most frequently they are multiple in association with NF1 but can occur in isolation.
- NF1 is an autosomal-dominant inherited condition with an incidence of 1 in 3000. The *NF1* gene has been identified on chromosome 17.
- In patients with NF1 there is an increased risk of malignant peripheral nerve sheath tumors.

LIPOMAS

- Lipomas are hamartomatous proliferations of mature fat cells. They are the most common benign tumor of mesenchymal origin. Twenty-five percent of lipomas occur in the head and neck, with the posterior triangle the most common site. A peak incidence of lipoma formation is noted in fifth and sixth decades of life.
- The following syndromes are associated with lipoma formation: Gardner syndrome, Dercum disease, Madelung disease, and familial multiple lipomatosis.

BRONCHOGENIC CYSTS

- Bronchogenic cysts are congenital malformations of ventral foregut development.
- A superficial presternal or suprasternal location is most common, whereas deep neck or laterally located bronchogenic cysts are comparatively rare. Bronchogenic cysts of the cervical area are usually asymptomatic. In adults, the two most common locations of bronchogenic cyst are the mediastinum and lung parenchyma. Most bronchogenic cysts are unilocular, filled with fluid, and not in communication with the airways.

TERATOMAS

- Teratomas (Figure 12-4) are congenital germ cell tumors. The sacrococcygeal region is the most common site, but they also occur in the gonads, retroperitoneum, liver, and brain. Within the head and neck, there is a predilection for the cervical region, but teratomas in the nasopharynx, orbit, palate, and tonsil have been reported.

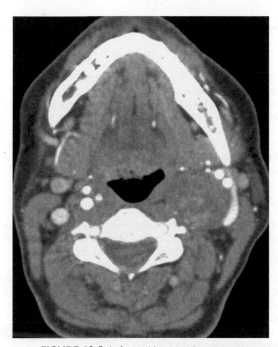

FIGURE 12-3 Left carotid space schwannoma.

most commonly affected nerve, followed by the vagus, cervical sympathetic plexus, and the brachial plexus.

- Histopathological analysis demonstrates the classical cellular pattern of alternating regions of compact spindle cells (Antoni A), loosely arranged hypocellular areas (Antoni B), and rows of nuclear palisading (Verocay bodies). Schwannomas demonstrate strong s100 immunohistochemical positivity.
- Surgery is associated with a high rate of nerve dysfunction.
- Although very rare, sarcomatous transformation has been reported.

- Less than 5% of congenital cervical teratomas are malignant, with the risk of malignancy increasing with increasing age at diagnosis.
- Diagnosis may be made antenatally on routine ultrasound. In about 20% of cases, and more frequently in larger tumors, maternal polyhydramnios occurs, secondary to impaired fetal swallowing.
- The major risk posed by large cervical teratomas is that of neonatal airway obstruction. If at the time of delivery there is no respiratory compromise, the mortality from these tumors is around 3%, increasing substantially (up to 43%) if there is respiratory embarrassment. Most neonates (70%) with large cervical teratomas have some degree of respiratory compromise, which is severe in 50% of these cases. There is a direct relationship between tumor size and the presence of airway compression symptoms. A distressed neonate requires intervention to secure an imperiled airway. Once this vital period of potential airway difficulty is successfully negotiated, the prognosis is good following excision of these tumors.
- Securing the airway has been successfully achieved using EXIT/OOPS procedures.
- Definitive management of these tumors is surgical excision. This should be performed expeditiously to remove the threat of respiratory impairment and prevent less common sequelae related to the teratoma, including sepsis, ulceration, coagulopathy, and hemodynamic disturbance; additionally the removal of the tumor eliminates the risk of malignant degeneration. It should be noted that surgery is not without risk; an operative mortality of 15% has been reported.

PLUNGING RANULA

- Plunging ranula is an extravasation pseudocyst. Extravasation of saliva from the duct of the sublingual gland elicits localized pseudocyst formation. Egress into the neck is mostly through small dehiscences in the mylohyoid muscle. Most ranulas present with a soft, painless, submandibular triangle swelling with an associated intraoral ranula. Cases may arise, however, without an intraoral component. Plunging ranulas occur more frequently where there is a history of surgery of the floor of the mouth. MRI is the best imaging modality, highlighting the relationship of the pseudocyst and the sublingual gland.
- Surgery is curative. Excision of the sublingual gland is the crucial part of the procedure, and this may be undertaken with pseudocyst excision or aspiration.

THYMIC CYSTS

- Thymic cysts are unusual epithelial-lined lesions that may occur anywhere along the course of descent of the thymus. The thymus is a third pharyngeal pouch derivative that appears at 6 weeks' gestation, with descent inferior to the clavicles at 9 weeks' gestation. The course of descent is from the mandibular ramus to the midline neck.
- The usual presentation is during the first decade, more frequently in males and left sided. About 50% will have mediastinal extension. Surgery is both diagnostic and therapeutic.

LARYNGOCELES

- Laryngoceles are abnormal dilations of the laryngeal saccule. They may be internal, confined within the larynx, or combined with external extension through the thyrohyoid membrane. Laryngoceles can be congenital or

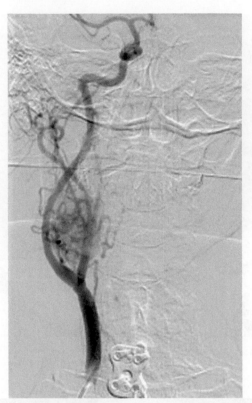

FIGURE 12-5 Digital subtraction angiogram demonstrating right carotid body tumor.

acquired, with the latter more common in wind instrument musicians and glass blowers.
- Most laryngoceles are unilateral (two-thirds) and most frequently present in males during the fifth or sixth decade of life.
- Presentation may occasionally occur with infection, a laryngopyocele, or rarely in association with laryngeal carcinoma.

PARAGANGLIOMAS

- Paragangliomas are the most common benign vascular tumor of the head and neck. They arise from extraadrenal paraganglionic cells from the neural crest.
- Ninety percent of all paragangliomas arise from the adrenal glands and are known as pheochromocytomas. Of the remaining 10%, 85% are intraabdominal, 12% intrathoracic, and 3% occur in the head and neck.
- Of those in the head and neck, carotid body tumors (Figure 12-5) are the most common, followed by jugulotympanic and vagal paragangliomas.
- The carotid body is located in the adventitia of the posteromedial aspect of carotid bifurcation. The branchiomeric paraganglion group, from which the carotid body arises, is derived from the third branchial cleft mesoderm.
- Sensory innervation is from the nerve of Hering, a branch of the glossopharyngeal nerve that originates 1.5 cm distal to the jugular foramen.
- The carotid body has a chemoreceptor role in modulation of respiratory and cardiovascular function via the autonomic nervous system in response to alteration in arterial pH, PCO_2, and PO_2.
- Most carotid body tumors are sporadic (85%) but may be familial (10%) or hyperplastic in response to chronic hypoxia, for example, living at altitude.

- Multiple paragangliomas, including pheochromocytomas, are seen in familial syndromes such as MEN 2a/2b, NF1, von Hippel-Lindau disease, and Carney triad.
- Isolated hereditary *PGL* gene mutations may also occur; the most frequently identified mutations occur in genes that code for SDHD/B/C on chromosomes 11/1/1, respectively.
- Germline mutations in SDHD/B/C are termed hereditary PGL syndromes 1/4/3, respectively.
- Those with hereditary PGL syndrome have an earlier presentation of tumors, a higher incidence of multiple and/or bilateral tumors, and malignancy.
- PGL1, caused by mutations of the D subunit of succinate dehydrogenase, is the most common inherited genetic abnormality in families with paragangliomas.
- Eighty-six percent of people with gene mutation will develop a tumor by 50 years of age.
- *SDHB* gene mutations are less common but confer a higher risk of pheochromocytomas and extraadrenal catecholamine-secreting tumors.
- Clinical presentation of these tumors in the neck is that of a slow-growing, painless, laterally mobile, pulsatile mass. Less mobility is demonstrable in the craniocaudal direction known as Fontaine sign.
- With enlargement, lower cranial nerve deficits may appear and cause symptoms.
- Overall, 1% to 3% of extraadrenal paragangliomas are secreting tumors.
- Screening for secreting tumors is required for multiple tumors and in those who have symptoms and/or a familial history.
- Multiplicity occurs in 10% of patients, with bilateral carotid body tumor most common. In familial paragangliomas, multiplicity occurs in 30% to 50%.
- Malignancy is reported in 6% of tumors. The diagnosis of malignancy should be made by evidence of spread to regional lymph nodes or distant sites.
- Treatment options include surgery, external beam radiotherapy, or observation, depending on the individual patient.
- In bilaterally operated carotid body tumors, baroreflex failure syndrome characterized by unopposed sympathetic outflow resulting in labile blood pressure and tachycardia can occur. Compensation occurs over time but may be variable and unpredictable. Bilateral carotid body tumors should undergo staged surgeries to minimize the risk of baroreflex failure syndrome.

KIKUCHI-FUJIMOTO DISEASE

- Kikuchi-Fujimoto disease is a rare, self-limiting disorder of lymph nodes typically affecting cervical lymph nodes and characterized by a histiocytic necrotizing lymphadenitis.
- It occurs mostly in Japanese patients and those between 20 and 30 years of age.
- The cause is unknown.
- The clinical presentation is lymphadenopathy, fever, rash, and headache. Treatment is supportive.
- Recurrence is rare, occurring in 3% of cases.

KIMURA DISEASE

- Kimura disease is a chronic inflammatory condition presenting as multiple painless, solitary, subcutaneous nodules localized mostly in the region of the head and neck with coexisting lymphadenopathy and peripheral eosinophilia.
- This uncommon condition is found almost exclusively in Asian individuals in the second to fourth decades of life, mostly in males (70% to 80%).

- The etiology is unknown.
- Kimura disease may affect kidneys in up to 60% of patients.
- Hypereosinophilia and elevated serum immunoglobulin E are found in Kimura disease.

CAT-SCRATCH DISEASE

- Cat-scratch disease is an infectious disease caused by *Bartonella henselae,* a small, aerobic, fastidious, Gram-negative bacillus. A history of feline contact is found in 90% of cases but is not necessary for diagnosis. There is a male predominance, and most cases occur in those <20 years of age. It displays seasonal variations in North America, Europe, and Japan.
- The classical clinical picture is of local lymphadenopathy with or without rash and malaise.
- It is generally a self-limiting disease in immunocompetent patients and requires no active treatment.

TOXOPLASMOSIS

- Toxoplasmosis is a parasitic infection caused by *Toxoplasma gondii.* In the immunocompetent host, this protozoan primary infection tends to be with few or no symptoms and self-limiting. Of those who do experience symptoms, lymphadenopathy is the most frequent, occurring in 90% of patients. Most patients require no treatment, but in the immunocompromised group, pyrimethamine and sulfadiazine combined or azithromycin are suitable therapeutic agents.

ATYPICAL MYCOBACTERIA

- Atypical mycobacteria are a variety of acid-fast saprophytes that do not cause tuberculosis but may cause infectious disease in human hosts. Of those infections that occur in immunocompetent populations, most occur between the ages of 2 and 5 years and are rare after the age of 12 years. *Mycobacterium avium-intracellulare* is the most common pathogen identified.
- Typical presentation is with a firm, painless, discrete cervical mass that fails to respond to conventional antibiotics. Progression is characterized by enlargement, fluctuance, and development of a characteristic violaceous hue. Subsequent spontaneous discharge and fistula formation result. There is a predilection for lymph nodes in the upper-neck echelons or major salivary glands.
- Spontaneous regression in immunocompetent individuals is the norm but may take years to occur and may do so with unsightly scarring.
- Surgery to excise the affected nodes is the recommended first-line treatment to expedite resolution and minimize scar formation. Given the sites of predilection, surgery frequently entails risk to the branches of the facial nerve.
- Antibiotics have also been used in the management of atypical mycobacteria both alone as an alternative to surgery and as a postoperative adjunct. The optimal drug of choice, dose, and duration of treatment remain unclear, but drugs that have been used include clarithromycin, azithromycin, ethambutol, and rifampicin, usually in combination form.

KAWASAKI DISEASE

- Kawasaki disease, or mucocutaneous lymph node syndrome, is a systemic vasculitis of unknown etiology with a predilection for the coronary arteries. The majority of patients (80%) are <5 years of age, and it is the most

common cause of acquired heart disease in children in Japanese, North American, and European populations.
- Accurate diagnosis and early intervention reduces the risk of coronary artery aneurysm from 20% to 5%, but a specific diagnostic test does not exist.
- A male predominance exists, and it can occur in siblings.
- Diagnosis is made on the presence of at least four of the five principal features associated with a fever persisting for at least 5 days:
  - Changes in extremities: acute: erythema and edema of hands and feet; convalescent: membranous desquamation of fingertips
  - Polymorphous exanthema
  - Bilateral, painless bulbar conjunctival injection without exudate
  - Changes in lips and oral cavity: erythema and cracking of lips, strawberry tongue, diffuse injection of oral and pharyngeal mucosae
  - Cervical lymphadenopathy (≥1.5 cm in diameter), usually unilateral
  - Other clinical, radiological, and hematological factors can be considered.

- Aspirin and immunoglobulin are the mainstay of initial treatment.
- Cardiac surveillance and interventions as appropriate may be required.

ROSAI-DORFMAN DISEASE

- Rosai-Dorfman disease, also known as sinus histiocytosis with massive lymphadenopathy, is a non–Langerhans cell histiocytosis.
- Children, adolescents, and young adults are more frequently affected by this disorder, but it may also occur in older adults.
- Lymphadenopathy is the main clinical manifestation. Lymph node enlargement occurs more frequently in cervical and submandibular regions, but enlarged lymph nodes in mediastinal and retroperitoneal regions have also been described. Extranodal involvement has been reported, most frequently in the skin.
- The clinical course of Rosai-Dorfman disease is unpredictable, regardless of treatment. The evolution of the disease is slow and it may regress spontaneously.

ANSWERS

TRUE OR FALSE QUESTIONS

1. F	14. T	27. T	40. F
2. T	15. T	28. T	41. F
3. F	16. F	29. F	42. T
4. T	17. T	30. F	43. F
5. T	18. F	31. T	44. T
6. F	19. T	32. F	45. T
7. F	20. T	33. T	46. T
8. F	21. F	34. T	47. F
9. T	22. F	35. F	48. T
10. F	23. F	36. F	49. F
11. F	24. T	37. T	50. T
12. F	25. F	38. T	
13. F	26. T	39. F	

SINGLE BEST ANSWER QUESTIONS

51. c	64. e	77. e	90. b
52. b	65. e	78. e	91. d
53. e	66. b	79. d	92. a
54. d	67. a	80. e	93. a
55. e	68. e	81. c	94. b
56. d	69. d	82. d	95. c
57. e	70. d	83. c	96. c
58. d	71. b	84. d	97. d
59. d	72. d	85. a	98. c
60. d	73. e	86. a	99. c
61. e	74. a	87. d	100. c
62. e	75. e	88. d	
63. c	76. a	89. e	

SUGGESTED READINGS

1. Prosser JD, Myer CM 3rd. Branchial cleft anomalies and thymic cysts. *Otolaryngol Clin North Am.* 2015;48(1):1-14.
2. De Tristan J, Zenk J, Kunzel J, Psychogios G, Iro H. Thyroglossal duct cysts: 20 years' experience (1992-2011). *Eur Arch Otorhinolaryngol.* 2014;[Epub ahead of print].
3. Welander J, Söderkvist P, Gimm O. Genetics and clinical characteristics of hereditary pheochromocytomas and paragangliomas. *Endocr Relat Cancer.* 2011;18(6):R253-R276.
4. Makino N, Nakamura Y, Yashiro M, et al. Descriptive epidemiology of Kawasaki disease in Japan, 2011-2012: from the results of the 22nd nationwide survey. *J Epidemiol.* 2015;25(3):239-245.
5. Zimmermann P, Tebruegge M, Curtis N, Ritz N. The management of non-tuberculous cervicofacial lymphadenitis in children: a systematic review and meta-analysis. *J Infect.* 2015;71(1):9-18.

6. Samant S, Morton RP, Ahmad Z. Surgery for plunging ranula: the lesson not yet learned? *Eur Arch Otorhinolaryngol.* 2011;268(10):1513-1518.

7. Martinez Devesa P, Ghufoor K, Lloyd S, Howard D. Endoscopic CO_2 laser management of laryngocele. *Laryngoscope.* 2002;112(8 Pt 1):1426-1430.

8. Perkins JA, Manning SC, Tempero RM, et al. Lymphatic malformations: review of current treatment. *Otolaryngol Head Neck Surg.* 2010;142(6):795-803.

9. Kadlub N, Touma J, Leboulanger N, et al. Head and neck teratoma: from diagnosis to treatment. *J Craniomaxillofac Surg.* 2014c;42(8):1598-1603.

10. Dalia S, Sagatys E, Sokol L, Kubal T. Rosai-Dorfman disease: tumor biology, clinical features, pathology, and treatment. *Cancer Control.* 2014;21(4):322-327.

13 Tonsils and Adenoids

J. Scott McMurray

TRUE OR FALSE QUESTIONS

T/F 1. Lymphoma is the most common neoplasm of palatine tonsil.

T/F 2. The blood supply to the tonsillar fossa includes branches from the internal carotid artery.

T/F 3. The most common method of wound closure following transoral tumor extirpation of tonsillar carcinoma is to allow the wound bed to heal by secondary intention.

T/F 4. Human papillomavirus is increasingly associated with tonsillar carcinoma as the sole risk factor in patients.

T/F 5. Adenotonsillectomy is the first line of therapy for obstructive sleep apnea (OSA) in otherwise healthy children.

T/F 6. Adenotonsillectomy is the first line of therapy for OSA in complex patients with adenotonsillar hypertrophy.

T/F 7. The cure rate of OSA after adenotonsillectomy varies among studies but in general is about 60%.

T/F 8. Bleeding is the most common complication after tonsillectomy.

T/F 9. Codeine has been shown to be the best analgesia after tonsillectomy in children.

T/F 10. Adenoidectomy is recommended in children with persistent eustachian tube dysfunction, requiring multiple sets of tympanostomy tubes.

T/F 11. Biofilms were found on a significant number of adenoid specimens after adenoidectomy for chronic rhinosinusitis.

T/F 12. Adenoidectomy alone improved symptoms of chronic rhinosinusitis in only 15% of children who had the operation.

T/F 13. Group A beta-hemolytic *Streptococcus* infection of the tonsils is no longer the leading cause of bacterial tonsillitis.

T/F 14. Tonsillectomy has been shown to be initially successful in treating periodic fever with aphthous stomatitis, pharyngitis, and adenitis (PFAPA).

T/F 15. Although pediatric nasopharyngeal carcinoma (NPC) is rare, accounting for <1% of pediatric malignancies, NPC accounts for 20% to 50% of pediatric tumors of the nasopharynx.

T/F 16. The most common type of nasopharyngeal carcinoma seen in children is World Health Organization (WHO) type III, undifferentiated carcinoma (lymphoepithelial).

T/F 17. When combined, adenoidectomy and tonsillectomy effectively remove all of the lymphoid tissue of the nasopharynx, oropharynx, and hypopharynx.

T/F 18. Bacterial pharyngitis and tonsillitis are significantly more common than viral infections in adults compared with children.

T/F 19. Groups A beta-hemolytic *Streptococcus* pyogenes (GABHS) is the most common cause of bacterial tonsillitis in adults.

T/F 20. Because of incision and drainage risk of injury to the great vessels, surgical management of a peritonsillar abscess requires a transcervical approach.

T/F 21. Retropharyngeal abscess secondary to adenoidal infections can commonly be drained transorally.

T/F 22. Adenotonsillectomy is often curative of adult OSA.

T/F 23. Similar to adenoidectomy in children, adult adenoidectomy often decreases the nasal symptoms of chronic rhinosinusitis.

T/F 24. Complete removal of a type II branchial anomaly often requires tonsillectomy.

T/F 25. Nasopharyngeal carcinoma with neck metastasis most commonly presents in level I lymph nodes.

T/F 26. The epithelial lining of the tonsillar fossa and palatine tonsil is derived from the second pharyngeal pouch.

T/F 27. Because of their common embryonic origin, fistulas associated with third branchial anomalies originate in the tonsillar fossa.

T/F 28. The adenoid is also known as the pharyngeal tonsil.

T/F 29. Rheumatic fever is a common complication of streptococcal tonsillitis.

T/F 30. Antibiotics have been shown to alter the natural course of acute glomerulonephritis secondary to streptococcal tonsillitis.

T/F 31. Lymphoma in Waldeyer ring is more typically Hodgkin lymphoma in the pediatric patient.

T/F 32. Atlantoaxial subluxation is caused by laxity of the ligaments secondary to inflammation after adenoidectomy.

T/F 33. The tonsils and adenoids as a common part of Waldeyer ring share the same histologic epithelial covering: nonkeratinized stratified squamous epithelium.

T/F 34. The majority of the blood supply to the tonsillar fossa comes from branches of the facial artery.

T/F 35. Tonsillectomy is indicated in children with four infections over a year.

T/F 36. Adenoidal tissue is abundant at birth.

T/F 37. Maximal growth of the adenoid is seen between ages 3 to 5.

T/F 38. Antibiotics are helpful in the initial treatment of rheumatic fever.

T/F 39. Asymmetric tonsillar size is an indication for tonsillectomy.

T/F 40. Because they are both a part of Waldeyer ring, the risk of postoperative velopharyngeal insufficiency (VPI) is the same for tonsillectomy and adenoidectomy.

T/F 41. The muscular sling medial to the tonsillar fossa is the palatopharyngeus.

T/F 42. The muscular sling lateral to the tonsillar fossa is the palatopharyngeus.

T/F 43. Preservation of the palatoglossus muscular sling is most important to prevent velopharyngeal incompetence after tonsillectomy.

T/F 44. Tonsilliths, or stones in the tonsillar crypts, are formed in a manner similar to that of uric acid stones in the kidney.

T/F 45. Patients with human papilloma virus type 16 (HPV 16)–positive tonsil carcinoma have a better overall prognosis than patients whose tonsil cancer specimens are HPV-negative.

T/F 46. Velocardiofacial syndrome may be associated with medial displacement of the internal carotid artery at the nasopharynx, making adenoidectomy and VPI surgery potentially life threatening.

T/F 47. Tornwaldt cyst is an uncommon midline nasopharyngeal cyst that arises from the pharyngeal bursa or pouch of Luschka in the posterior nasopharynx.

T/F 48. The development of Tornwaldt cyst has been linked to scarring from previous adenoidectomy.

T/F 49. Children under the age of 2 years have a fivefold reduction in the risk of adenoidal regrowth after adenoidectomy because of the small size of their adenoidal beds.

T/F 50. Tonsillectomy was associated with more severe paralytic bulbar polio.

SINGLE BEST ANSWER QUESTIONS

51. Which of the following is the most common neoplasm of the tonsil?
    a. Lymphoma
    b. Metastatic carcinoma
    c. Squamous cell carcinoma
    d. Salivary neoplasm

52. Which of the following is the most common complication after pediatric tonsillectomy?
    a. VPI
    b. Oropharyngeal stenosis

c. Bleeding
d. Dehydration

53. Blood supply to the palatine tonsil is derived from branches of which of the following arteries?
    a. Internal carotid
    b. External carotid
    c. Common carotid
    d. Both internal and external carotid

54. The pathology specimen in a patient with squamous cell carcinoma of the tonsillar fossa without a history of smoking or drinking often is positive for which of the following?
    a. HPV
    b. Epstein-Barr virus (EBV)
    c. Cytomegalovirus (CMV)
    d. Herpes simplex virus (HSV)

55. Pediatric nasopharyngeal carcinoma has a more favorable prognosis than adult nasopharyngeal carcinoma and is more closely associated with which of the following?
    a. HPV
    b. EBV
    c. CMV
    d. HSV

56. Tonsillitis associated with a gray membrane covering the surface of the tonsil but that may be removed without bleeding is often associated with which of the following?
    a. HPV
    b. EBV
    c. CMV
    d. HSV

57. Which of the following is the leading cause of bacterial tonsillitis after 2002?
    a. Methicillin-resistant *Staphylococcus aureus* (MRSA)
    b. Intermediate-resistant *Streptococcus pneumoniae* (IRSP)
    c. GABHS
    d. Vancomycin-resistant enterococcus

58. Which of the following is the most common cause of tonsillitis?
    a. Viral infection
    b. Bacterial infection
    c. Environmental allergens
    d. Gastropharyngeal reflux

59. When comparing the WHO classification for nasopharyngeal carcinoma in children versus adults, children most commonly have more of which of the following?
    a. Type 1: squamous cell carcinoma
    b. Type 2: nonkeratinizing carcinoma
    c. Type 3: undifferentiated carcinoma
    d. No difference in WHO classification between adults and children

60. Which of the following does *NOT* adversely affect prognosis in pediatric nasopharyngeal carcinoma?
    a. Metastatic disease in the cervical lymph nodes
    b. Skull base involvement
    c. Extent of the primary tumor
    d. Cranial nerve involvement

61. Type II branchial fistulas that open into the pharynx most commonly can be found at which of the following locations?
    a. The junction of hard and soft palates
    b. Tonsillar fossa
    c. Pyriform sinus
    d. Cricopharyngeus muscle

62. Type III branchial fistulas that open into the pharynx most commonly can be found at which of the following locations?
    a. The junction of the hard and soft palates
    b. Tonsillar fossa
    c. Pyriform sinus
    d. Cricopharyngeus muscle

63. The rare complication of atlantoaxial subluxation seen after adenotonsillectomy is known as which of the following?
    a. Grisel syndrome
    b. Gaucher disease
    c. Gilbert syndrome
    d. Gilles de la Tourette syndrome

64. DiGeorge syndrome (22q11.2 deletion syndrome) has which of the following typical heritance profiles?
    a. Sex linked
    b. Autosomal recessive
    c. Autosomal dominant
    d. Spontaneous deletion

65. The abnormal velopharyngeal closure pattern associated with VPI in children with 22q11.2 deletions is often described as which of the following?
    a. Poor anteroposterior closure
    b. Poor lateral closure
    c. Poor circumferential closure (black hole)
    d. Poor Passavant ridge formation

66. Tonsillar concretions or tonsilloliths commonly form in which percentage of the population?
    a. 5%-10%
    b. 25%-40%
    c. 60%-75%
    d. Nearly 100%

67. Tonsillar concretions or tonsilloliths are typically composed of which of the following?
    a. Uric acid salts
    b. Sodium bismuthate salts
    c. Potassium hydroxide salts
    d. Calcium carbonate apatite salts

68. The immune cells responsible for antigen presentation from the surface of the tonsils are known as:
    a. M cells
    b. B cells
    c. T cells
    d. Natural killer cells

69. The tonsils have been shown to produce which of the following lymphocytes in a manner similar to but different from either thymus or bone marrow?
    a. M cells
    b. B cells
    c. T cells
    d. Macrophages

70. HPV-associated oropharyngeal carcinoma is most commonly caused by which HPV strain?
    a. 6
    b. 11
    c. 16
    d. 69

71. Which of the following is the most common complication after adenotonsillectomy in both adults and children?
    a. VPI
    b. Same day hemorrhage
    c. Hemorrhage at around 1 week
    d. Dehydration

72. Which of the following is the most common life-threatening complication after adenotonsillectomy in both adults and children?
    a. VPI
    b. Same day hemorrhage
    c. Hemorrhage at around 1 week
    d. Dehydration

73. Who first described the use of the snare to remove tonsils?
    a. Hippocrates of Kos (400 BCE)
    b. Galen (25-50 CE)
    c. Ambrose Pare (1600s)
    d. Joseph Lister (1860s)

74. Who first described the practice of partial tonsillotomy or incomplete tonsillar removal to decrease the risk of bleeding?
    a. Aetius (490 CE)
    b. Ambrose Pare (1600s)
    c. Joseph Lister (1860s)
    d. Peter Koltai (2000s)

75. The removal of adenoidal tissue to improve eustachian tube function is thought to be effective due to which of the following?
    a. Clearing the eustachian tube nasopharyngeal orifice of obstruction
    b. Decreasing the bacterial load of the nasopharynx
    c. Tightening the muscular attachments to the eustachian tube
    d. Changing the epithelial lining type of the nasopharynx after adenoidectomy

76. Patients requiring revision adenoidectomy were most likely to be from which age group at time of primary adenoidectomy?
    a. <2 years
    b. 2-4 years
    c. 15-20 years
    d. >67 years

77. Which of the following is the classic presentation after adenoidectomy for Grisel syndrome?
    a. Fever and neck pain
    b. Dehydration
    c. VPI
    d. "Cock robin" deformity

78. Rotatory atlantoaxial subluxation following adenoidectomy can generally be treated with which of the following?
    a. Open reduction and screw pedicle fixation
    b. Closed reduction and halo fixation
    c. Closed reduction with cervical collar
    d. Soft cervical collar and conservative treatment

79. VPI immediately after adenoidectomy:
    a. Often spontaneously resolves within 12 weeks
    b. Often requires voice therapy to resolve
    c. Often requires a pharyngeal flap to resolve
    d. Often requires a palatal sphincteroplasty to resolve

80. Patients with Down syndrome who have had normal flexion and extension neck radiographs in the past should preoperatively have which of the following?
    a. New radiographs before every head and neck surgery
    b. New radiographs once a year
    c. New radiographs once every 5 years
    d. No new radiographs without new neurological findings

81. Regarding pediatric autoimmune neuropsychiatric disorder associated with streptococcal infections (PANDAS), when is tonsillectomy indicated?
    a. Always, as it is curative.
    b. Never, as it does no help.
    c. It is indicated if there is an increased incidence of streptococcal tonsillitis.
    d. It is indicated if there is a failure of antibiotic therapy.

82. Patients with sickle cell disease should be transfused to a hemoglobin S concentration of less than which percentage to prevent perioperative complications?
    a. 5%
    b. 25%
    c. 40%
    d. 75%

83. Patients with PFAPA best benefit from which of the following?
    a. Adenoidectomy
    b. Tonsillectomy
    c. Adenotonsillectomy
    d. No benefit from surgical treatment

84. When looking at the risk of HPV-related oropharyngeal cancer, white nonsmoking males have which of the following risks compared with females?
    a. 1 to 4, with a female predominance
    b. 1 to 1 (males equal to females)
    c. 4 to 1, with a male predominance
    d. Related not to gender but to economic class

85. Which of the following is the fastest growing segment of the oral and oropharyngeal cancer population?
    a. Healthy nonsmokers in the 25-50 age range
    b. Healthy nonsmokers in the 50-75 age range
    c. Healthy smokers in the 25-50 age range
    d. Healthy smokers in the 50-75 age range

86. In the oral/oropharyngeal environment, HPV 16 manifests itself primarily in which of the following locations?
    a. Tonsillar crypts
    b. Adenoidal tissue
    c. Pyriform sinus
    d. Uvula

87. Every day in the United States, about 12,000 people ages 15 to 24 are infected with HPV. The vast majority of them will:
    a. Become chronically infected and continually shed virus
    b. Develop oropharyngeal carcinoma
    c. Clear the virus without any sequelae
    d. Develop palatal papilloma

88. Which of the following is correct regarding antibiotics after tonsillectomy or adenotonsillectomy?
    a. They should routinely be given as a single preoperative dose within 30 minutes of incision.
    b. They should not be routinely given.
    c. They should be given postoperatively to decrease pain and halitosis.
    d. They should be given to recurrent tonsillitis patients only.

89. Which of the following is correct regarding codeine after tonsillectomy?
    a. It is the most effective narcotic for pain control.
    b. It has polymorphism for metabolism and therefore may lead to overdose.
    c. It decreases the time to first oral intake compared with acetaminophen alone.
    d. It is safer than ibuprofen because of its therapeutic index.

90. Intraoperative dexamethasone is given during tonsillectomy at a dose of 0.5 mg/kg for which of the following reasons?
    a. It decreases postoperative nausea and vomiting.
    b. It decreases immediate hemorrhage.
    c. It decreases delayed hemorrhage.
    d. It decreases postoperative pain.

91. Waldeyer ring, the name of the tonsil, adenoid, and lingual tonsil ring of lymphoid tissue, was named after which of the following anatomists?
    a. Galen
    b. Anton Johannes Waldeyer
    c. Waldeyer Sigurdsson
    d. Heinrich Wilhelm Gottfried von Waldeyer-Hartz

92. When comparing tonsillectomy specimens for recurrent tonsillitis versus tonsillar hypertrophy, the incidence of EBV detection in pediatric patients is:
    a. The same in both specimen groups
    b. Higher in the hypertrophy group than the recurrent infection group
    c. Higher in the recurrent infection group than the hypertrophy group
    d. Absent in both groups

93. Which of the following tonsils are commonly referred to as "the tonsils"?
    a. Lingual
    b. Palatine
    c. Cerebellar
    d. Pharyngeal

94. Which of the following types of immunological activity best describes Waldeyer ring?
    a. Secretory
    b. Filter
    c. Cell mediated
    d. Humoral

95. PFAPA typically afflicts patients in which of the following age groups?
    a. 1-2 years
    b. 2-5 years
    c. 9-15 years
    d. >25 years

96. Which of the following ethnic groups most commonly suffers from nasopharyngeal carcinomas?
    a. North American Caucasians
    b. Inuit of Alaska and Canada
    c. Southeast Chinese
    d. North Africans

97. In an African American teenaged female with unilateral otitis media with effusion and an ipsilateral 2-cm firm posterior triangle lymph node, which of the following must be ruled out?
    a. Eustachian tube dysfunction from adenoidal hypertrophy
    b. Nasopharyngeal carcinoma
    c. Recurrent rhinosinusitis causing inflammatory eustachian tube dysfunction
    d. OSA from adenotonsillar hypertrophy

98. When performing adenoidectomy in a patient with 22q11.2 deletion, which of the following is the most important variant to consider?

a. Aberrant internal carotid
b. Poor velopharyngeal function and the possibility of VPI postoperatively
c. Atlantoaxial ligament laxity
d. Potential airway compromise secondary to retrognathia

99. Congenital hypoplasia of the adenoids contributing to the incidence of VPI is seen in four-fifths of which genetic syndrome?
a. Down syndrome
b. Turner syndrome

c. Fragile X syndrome
d. Velocardiofacial syndrome

100. The posterior pillar of the tonsillar pillar is the most important tonsillar structure for velopharyngeal competence and is made of which of the following muscles?
a. Tonsillopharyngeus
b. Palatoglossus
c. Pharyngoglossus
d. Palatopharyngeus

CORE KNOWLEDGE

TONSILS

- Before performing tonsillectomy, clinicians should refer children with sleep-disordered breathing for polysomnography if they exhibit the following: obesity, Down syndrome, craniofacial anomalies, neuromuscular disorders, sickle cell disease, or mucopolysaccharidoses.
- Clinicians should advocate for polysomnography prior to tonsillectomy for sleep-disordered breathing in children without any comorbidities and for whom the need for surgery is uncertain or when there is discordance between tonsillar size on physical examination and the reported severity of the sleep-disordered breathing.
- Clinicians should communicate the results of the polysomnography to the anesthesiologist prior to induction for tonsillectomy.
- Clinicians should admit children with OSA documented in results of polysomnography for inpatient overnight monitoring after tonsillectomy if the patient is <3 years of age or has severe OSA (apnea-hypopnea index of 10 or more obstructive events/hour, oxygen saturation nadir less than 80%, or both).
- In children for whom polysomnography is indicated to assess sleep-disordered breathing prior to tonsillectomy, clinicians should obtain laboratory-based polysomnography, when available.
- Peritonsillar abscess often requires operative intervention under general anesthesia in children.
- PFAPA is often self-limiting after a prolonged course. Tonsillectomy has been shown to be effective in resolving symptoms, but the risk to benefit ratio needs to be explored with the family.
- The incidence of immediate posttonsillectomy bleeding is not statistically different in patients with the bleeding disorders of von Willebrand disease or hemophilia. There is a significant increase in delayed bleeding in patients with bleeding disorders.
- In tumor-free tonsillectomy specimens, oncogenic and nononcogenic HPVs were present at a relatively high frequency in children and adults.
- The evidence suggests that a single intravenous dose of dexamethasone is an effective, safe, and inexpensive treatment for reducing morbidity from pediatric tonsillectomy.
- Due to common embryonic origin, second branchial cleft anomalies can originate in the tonsillar fossa.

ADENOIDS

- Adenoiditis is an important contributing factor to pediatric chronic rhinosinusitis, especially in younger children.

- The ability of adenoids to serve as a bacterial reservoir for pediatric chronic rhinosinusitis is independent of adenoid size.
- Adenoidectomy is an effective first-line surgical procedure for children up to 12 years of age with chronic rhinosinusitis.
- Adenoidectomy can have a beneficial effect in patients with pediatric chronic rhinosinusitis that is independent of endoscopic sinus surgery.
- Tonsillectomy (without adenoidectomy) is an ineffective treatment for pediatric chronic rhinosinusitis.
- Endoscopic sinus surgery is an effective procedure for treating pediatric chronic rhinosinusitis that is best performed after failure of medical therapy and/or adenoidectomy.
- Young age at first adenoidectomy and evidence of gastroesophageal reflux disease was associated with a higher

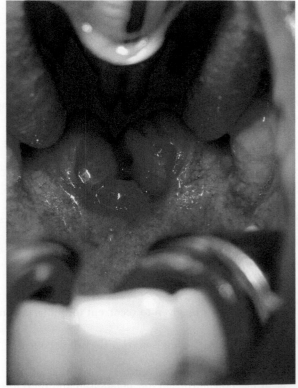

FIGURE 13-1 Tonsillar hypertrophy seen with obstructive sleep apnea.

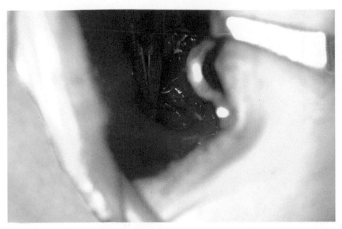

FIGURE 13-2 Lacrimal duct probe to the right of the forceps entering the tonsillar fossa from a type 2 branchial anomaly.

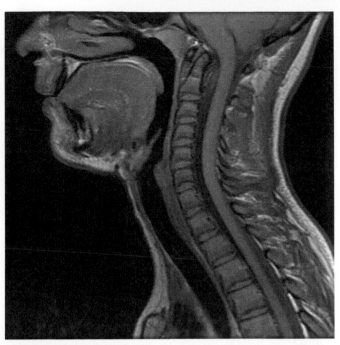

FIGURE 13-4 Sagittal magnetic resonance image demonstrating the nasopharynx and a small adenoid pad.

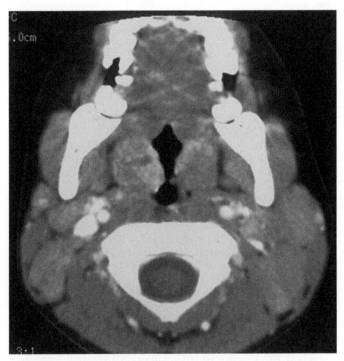

FIGURE 13-3 Computed tomography scan demonstrating tonsillar enlargement.

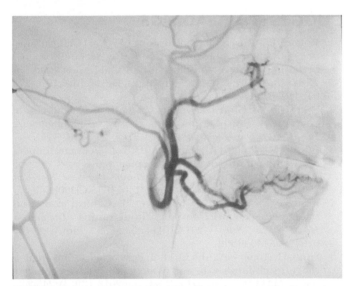

FIGURE 13-5 Angiogram in a patient with recurrent tonsillar hemorrhage demonstrating a pseudoaneurysm on the ascending pharyngeal artery.

incidence of adenoidal regrowth requiring revision adenoidectomy.
- Primary bleeding is 0.5% after both adenoidectomy and tonsillectomy.
- Delayed bleeding after adenoidectomy is extremely rare.
- In children, the risk of a serious primary hemorrhage following an adenotonsillectomy is double that of either procedure when performed alone.

- Adenoidectomy should be considered in children with persistent and recurrent otitis media with effusion requiring more than a single set of pressure equalization tubes.
- Figures 13-1 to 13-5 demonstrate tonsillar hypertrophy, lacrimal duct probe, computed tomography (CT) scan, sagittal magnetic resonance imaging (MRI), and angiogram.

ANSWERS

TRUE OR FALSE QUESTIONS

1. F	5. T	9. F	13. F
2. F	6. T	10. T	14. T
3. T	7. T	11. T	15. T
4. T	8. F	12. F	16. T

17. F	26. T	35. F	44. F
18. F	27. F	36. F	45. T
19. T	28. T	37. T	46. T
20. F	29. F	38. T	47. T
21. T	30. F	39. T	48. T
22. F	31. F	40. F	49. F
23. F	32. T	41. T	50. T
24. T	33. F	42. F	
25. F	34. T	43. F	

SINGLE BEST ANSWER QUESTIONS

51. c	64. c	77. d	90. a
52. d	65. c	78. d	91. d
53. b	66. a	79. a	92. a
54. a	67. d	80. d	93. d
55. b	68. a	81. c	94. a
56. b	69. c	82. c	95. b
57. c	70. c	83. b	96. c
58. a	71. d	84. c	97. b
59. c	72. c	85. a	98. a
60. a	73. b	86. a	99. d
61. b	74. a	87. c	100. d
62. c	75. b	88. b	
63. a	76. a	89. b	

SUGGESTED READINGS

1. Roland PS, Rosenfeld RM, Brooks LJ, et al. Clinical practice guideline: polysomnography for sleep-disordered breathing prior to tonsillectomy in children. *Otolaryngol Head Neck Surg.* 2011;145(1 suppl):S1-S15. doi:10.1177/0194599811409837.

2. Schraff S, McGinn JD, Derkay CS. Peritonsillar abscess in children: a 10-year review of diagnosis and management. *Int J Pediatr Otorhinolaryngol.* 2001;57(3):213-218.

3. Burton MJ, Pollard AJ, Ramsden JD. Tonsillectomy for periodic fever, aphthous stomatitis, pharyngitis and cervical adenitis syndrome (PFAPA). *Cochrane Database Syst Rev.* 2010;(9):CD008669, doi:10.1002/14651858.CD008669.

4. Brietzke SE, Shin JJ, Choi S, et al. Clinical consensus statement: pediatric chronic rhinosinusitis. *Otolaryngol Head Neck Surg.* 2014;151(4):542-553. doi:10.1177/0194599814549302.

5. Sun GH, Auger KA, Aliu O, et al. Posttonsillectomy hemorrhage in children with von Willebrand disease or hemophilia. *JAMA Otolaryngol Head Neck Surg.* 2013;139(3):245-249. doi:10.1001/jamaoto.2013.1821.

6. Dearking AC, Lahr BD, Kuchena A, Orvidas LJ. Factors associated with revision adenoidectomy. *Otolaryngol Head Neck Surg.* 2012;146(6):984-990. doi:10.1177/0194599811435971.

7. Tomkinson A, Harrison W, Owens D, Fishpool S, Temple M. Postoperative hemorrhage following adenoidectomy. *Laryngoscope.* 2012;122(6):1246-1253. doi:10.1002/lary.23279.

8. Duray A, Descamps G, Bettonville M, et al. High prevalence of high-risk human papillomavirus in palatine tonsils from healthy children and adults. *Otolaryngol Head Neck Surg.* 2011;145(2):230-235. doi:10.1177/0194599811402944.

9. Steward DL, Grisel J, Meinzen-Derr J. Steroids for improving recovery following tonsillectomy in children. *Cochrane Database Syst Rev.* 2011;(8):CD003997, doi:10.1002/14651858.CD003997.pub2.

10. Fishman G, Zemel M, DeRowe A, et al. Fiber-optic sleep endoscopy in children with persistent obstructive sleep apnea: inter-observer correlation and comparison with awake endoscopy. *Int J Pediatr Otorhinolaryngol.* 2013;77(5):752-755. doi:10.1016/j.ijporl.2013.02.002.

Pediatric Airway | 14

Anna H. Messner | Mai Thy Truong

TRUE OR FALSE QUESTIONS

T/F 1. The stridor of laryngomalacia is always biphasic.

T/F 2. The diagnosis of laryngomalacia can be made by listening to the stridor.

T/F 3. Gastroesophageal reflux disease (GERD) is common in patients with laryngomalacia.

T/F 4. The incidence of laryngomalacia is higher in African American infants compared with Caucasian infants.

T/F 5. Laryngeal penetration and aspiration are common in the child with severe laryngomalacia.

T/F 6. A supraglottoplasty performed for laryngomalacia is typically performed as an outpatient procedure.

T/F 7. Laryngomalacia occurs only in infants.

T/F 8. A supraglottoplasty is less likely to be successful in a neurologically impaired child.

T/F 9. The median time to spontaneous resolution of stridor due to laryngomalacia in infants who do not undergo surgery is 24 months.

T/F 10. The most likely etiology of laryngomalacia is neuromuscular hypotonia.

T/F 11. Supraglottoplasty and aryepiglottoplasty are the same procedure.

T/F 12. The term "stertor" is derived from the Latin word *stertere*, which means "to snore."

T/F 13. If an infant is diagnosed with a left vocal fold paralysis (VFP) after cardiac surgery, the patient most likely had a patent ductus arteriosus ligation or repair of an interrupted aortic arch.

T/F 14. Iatrogenic VFP can result after tracheoesophageal fistula repair.

T/F 15. Diagnosis of VFP is best made in the operating room with the patient under general anesthesia spontaneously ventilating.

T/F 16. If an infant is diagnosed with a unilateral VFP, the parents should be counseled that a gastrostomy tube will be needed.

T/F 17. A tracheotomy is usually required in the child with bilateral VFP.

T/F 18. An ex utero intrapartum treatment procedure should be performed for a patient with congenital high airway obstruction syndrome (CHAOS).

T/F 19. The term "stertor" is used to describe noisy breathing from the vibration of tissues above the larynx.

T/F 20. Subglottic infantile hemangiomas (IHs) are more common in males than females.

T/F 21. A beta-adrenergic blocking agent can be used to treat IHs.

T/F 22. Most commonly, an infant diagnosed with a subglottic cyst was born between 24 and 31 weeks' gestation.

T/F 23. Intubation in the newborn period is the primary precipitating factor in the development of a subglottic cyst.

T/F 24. A bifid epiglottis is defined as a cleft of the tip of the epiglottis.

T/F 25. Polydactyly has been reported in approximately 75% of patients with a bifid epiglottis.

T/F 26. Pallister-Hall syndrome is also called "congenital hypothalamic hamartoblastoma syndrome."

T/F 27. A laryngotracheoesophageal cleft (LTEC) leads to abnormal communication between the trachea and esophagus.

T/F 28. A laryngeal cleft is best diagnosed on flexible laryngoscopy in the awake patient.

T/F 29. Type I laryngeal clefts almost always need to be surgically repaired.

T/F 30. The prognosis of a patient with an LTEC that extends to the carina is poor.

T/F 31. The laryngeal saccule is a pouch of mucous membrane that rises superiorly between the false vocal fold, the base of the epiglottis, and the inner surface of the thyroid cartilage.

T/F 32. External laryngoceles pass through the cricothyroid membrane.

T/F 33. Laryngoceles typically contain air.

T/F 34. Saccular cysts typically contain air.

T/F 35. Surgical treatment of laryngoceles and saccular cysts is typically endoscopic marsupialization.

T/F 36. Laryngeal agenesis is a common cause of CHAOS.

T/F 37. All infants with congenital stridor should undergo a direct laryngoscopy and bronchoscopy in the operating room.

T/F 38. GERD can cause stridor.

T/F 39. Airway obstruction due to laryngeal papillomas typically occurs within the first 3 months of life.

T/F 40. Bilateral choanal atresia cannot typically be diagnosed prenatally.

T/F 41. The "EXIT" in EXIT procedure stands for "extrication in time."

T/F 42. Type 3 glottic webs typically have associated subglottic stenosis.

T/F 43. Infants with a type 4 glottic web typically require a tracheotomy.

T/F 44. A vallecular cyst can cause sudden death in an infant.

T/F 45. Thyroid follicles are often found in a vallecular cyst on pathologic examination.

T/F 46. All newborns with a suspected vallecular cyst should undergo computed tomography (CT) or magnetic resonance imaging (MRI) of the airway.

T/F 47. The initial surgical intervention for a vallecular cyst should be aspiration of the cyst only.

T/F 48. Exercise-induced laryngomalacia results when enough inspiratory force occurs during exercise to draw the aryepiglottic folds into the larynx and partially obstruct the glottis.

T/F 49. If an infant has only quiet stridor, the airway is stable.

T/F 50. A diagnosis of laryngomalacia should be given to all infants with stridor until proven otherwise.

SINGLE BEST ANSWER QUESTIONS

51. Which of the following is the most common complication after a supraglottoplasty?
    a. Unilateral VFP
    b. Bilateral VFP
    c. Subglottic stenosis
    d. Supraglottic stenosis
    e. Posterior glottic stenosis

52. Which of the following improves after supraglottoplasty?
    a. Growth curve percentile
    b. Sleep mechanics
    c. Incidence of aspiration
    d. Frequency of stridor
    e. All of the above

53. Which of the following anatomic abnormalities lead(s) to laryngomalacia?
    a. Short aryepiglottic folds
    b. Posterior collapse of the epiglottis
    c. Anterior prolapse of the mucosa overlying the arytenoid cartilages
    d. a and c only
    e. a, b, and c

54. Children with congenital anterior laryngeal webs should undergo genetic testing for abnormalities of which of the following chromosomes?
    a. 22
    b. 21
    c. 7
    d. 13
    e. 1

55. A 3-month-old infant diagnosed with recurrent croup most likely has which of the following airway abnormalities?
    a. Laryngomalacia
    b. Tracheomalacia
    c. Subglottic hemangioma
    d. Vallecular cyst
    e. Paradoxical vocal fold motion

56. The stridor from VFP is typically which of the following?
    a. High-pitched, inspiratory, or biphasic
    b. High-pitched, inspiratory only
    c. Low-pitched, inspiratory, or biphasic
    d. Low-pitched, inspiratory only
    e. Low-pitched, inspiratory, biphasic, or expiratory

57. Which of the following cardiac procedures is most commonly associated with an iatrogenic VFP?
    a. Ventricular septal defect repair
    b. Tetralogy of Fallot repair
    c. Patent ductus arteriosus ligation
    d. Repair of an interrupted aortic arch
    e. Atrial septal defect repair

58. Evaluation of the infant with idiopathic bilateral VFP should include which of the following?
    a. Ultrasound of the head
    b. MRI of the brain
    c. CT of the brain
    d. Positron emission tomography scan
    e. Modified barium swallow study

59. What percentage of idiopathic unilateral VFP diagnosed in infants will resolve spontaneously?
    a. 5%
    b. 20%
    c. 50%
    d. 70%
    e. 100%

60. Which of the following is true of an infant with paradoxical vocal fold motion?
    a. The stridor is loudest when the baby is sleeping.
    b. Diagnosis should be made on direct laryngoscopy performed in the operating room.
    c. The stridor is present on both inspiration and expiration.
    d. The stridor will be constantly present.
    e. The stridor typically resolves within the first few months of life.

61. Which of the following symptoms is typically seen in an infant with a type 3 glottic web?
    a. No symptoms
    b. Mild hoarseness
    c. Hoarse, weak cry, stridor with exertion
    d. Severe hoarseness, moderate airway obstruction
    e. Aphonia, severe airway obstruction

62. Which of the following diagnoses would be most likely to cause CHAOS?
    a. Bilateral VFP
    b. Congenital subglottic stenosis
    c. Laryngeal atresia
    d. Supraglottic stenosis
    e. Subglottic hemangioma

63. Congenital subglottic stenosis is defined as a cricoid diameter of less than:
    a. 1.5 mm
    b. 2.5 mm
    c. 3.5 mm
    d. 4.5 mm
    e. 5.5 mm

64. Which of the following is the correct description of the elliptical cricoid found in infants with congenital subglottic stenosis?
    a. The transverse and anteroposterior diameters are equal.
    b. The transverse diameter is significantly smaller than the anteroposterior diameter.

c. The anteroposterior diameter is significantly smaller than the transverse diameter.
d. The superior-inferior length of the posterior portion of the cricoid ring measures ≤10 mm.
e. The superior-inferior length of the posterior portion of the cricoid ring measures ≥10 mm.

65. Which of the following is *NOT* a feature of PHACE syndrome?
a. Sternal defect
b. Hemangioma
c. Cardiac anomalies
d. Arterial anomalies
e. Ear anomalies

66. An infant with a thyroglossal duct cyst at the foramen cecum will have which of the following signs/symptoms?
a. Midline neck mass, stridor, feeding difficulties
b. Midline neck mass, muffled voice, cyanotic episodes
c. Stridor, feeding difficulties, muffled voice
d. Stridor, failure to thrive, hoarseness
e. Failure to thrive, cyanotic episodes, hoarseness

67. Congenital anomalies that occur in association with a bifid epiglottis include all of the following *EXCEPT:*
a. Cleft lip
b. Cleft palate
c. Bifid uvula
d. Micrognathia
e. Microglossia

68. Which of the following features characterize the congenital hypothalamic hamartoblastoma syndrome?
a. Bifid uvula, cleft lip, laryngotracheal cleft, micrognathia
b. Cleft palate, congenital hamartomas, cretinism, macroglossia
c. Bifid uvula, cleft tongue, congenital hamartomas, micrognathia
d. Bifid epiglottis, polydactyly, pituitary dysfunction, imperforate anus, laryngotracheal cleft
e. Bifid epiglottis, cleft palate, polydactyly, macroglossia

69. All infants with a congenitally bifid epiglottis should undergo which of the following tests?
a. MRI of the brain
b. Endocrine evaluation
c. Genetics consultation
d. a and c
e. a, b, and c

70. Following LTEC repair, which of the following is a negative prognostic indicator for the success of the repair?
a. Preoperative aspiration
b. Chromosomal anomalies
c. History of a tracheoesophageal fistula
d. Congenital heart disease
e. Hypospadias

71. An LTEC that extends into the cervical trachea would be classified as which of the following?
a. Benjamin-Inglis type I, Myer-Cotton LI
b. Benjamin-Inglis type II, Myer-Cotton LII
c. Benjamin-Inglis type II, Myer-Cotton LIII
d. Benjamin-Inglis type III, Myer-Cotton LTEI
e. Benjamin-Inglis type IV, Myer-Cotton LTEII

72. Laryngeal and LTECs can be associated with all of the following syndromes *EXCEPT:*
a. Velocardiofacial syndrome
b. Opitz-Frias syndrome
c. Townes-Brock syndrome

d. Chromosome 1q43 deletion
e. Trisomy 21

73. Which of the following is/are possible symptoms/signs of a type I laryngeal cleft?
a. Chronic cough
b. Chronic aspiration
c. Consolidation/reticular opacities in the lung on chest radiography
d. b and c
e. a, b, and c

74. Typical conservative management for patients with a type I laryngeal cleft includes which of the following?
a. Placement of a gastrostomy tube and nothing by mouth
b. Thickening of liquids
c. Nissen fundoplication
d. Positioning the infant at a 30-degree angle for feeding
e. b and d

75. Which of the following laryngeal clefts can be surgically treated endoscopically?
a. Type I
b. Type II
c. Type III
d. Type IV
e. Types I and II

76. An infant with a long LTEC may experience airway obstruction due to which of the following mechanisms?
a. Prolapse of interarytenoid mucosa into the airway
b. Aspiration of stomach contents
c. Severe tracheomalacia
d. Severe tracheal stenosis
e. Severe bronchomalacia

77. Which of the following surgical approaches to a type III or type IV laryngeal cleft is most commonly used?
a. Lateral thoracotomy
b. Lateral pharyngotomy
c. Anterior laryngofissure
d. Median sternotomy
e. c and d

78. Laryngoceles may be described as which of the following?
a. Internal
b. External
c. Combined internal and external
d. a and b
e. a, b, and c

79. Which of the following is typically true of laryngoceles?
a. Upper airway obstruction is intermittent.
b. Vocal quality is normal.
c. They rarely need to be treated.
d. a and b
e. b and c

80. Which of the following airway diagnoses is/are typically a consequence of neonatal intubation?
a. Laryngeal cysts
b. Posterior glottis stenosis
c. Subglottic cysts
d. a and c
e. b and c

81. Features of CHAOS on fetal MRI include which of the following?
a. Polyhydramnios, enlarged heart, normal lungs, fluid-filled lower airways

b. Oligohydramnios, enlarged heart, enlarged lungs, nonvisible lower airways

c. Enlarged lungs, compressed heart, nonvisible lower airways

d. Enlarged lungs, inverted diaphragm, massive ascites, dilated fluid-filled lower airways

e. Oligohydramnios, normal diaphragm, compressed heart, normal lungs

82. A fetus diagnosed with CHAOS will require which of the following?
    a. Immediate intubation at birth
    b. Prone positioning immediately following birth
    c. Immediate tracheotomy at birth
    d. Nasopharyngeal airway at birth
    e. b and d

83. Parents of a fetus diagnosed with CHAOS should be counseled that:
    a. Significant congenital anomalies often accompany the airway obstruction.
    b. Patients with laryngotracheal agenesis will eventually be able to have their airway replaced.
    c. They will need to decide whether to proceed with tracheotomy within 24 hours of the birth.
    d. There is no hope for survival and the pregnancy should be terminated.
    e. A vaginal delivery is the preferred method of delivery.

84. Infantile airway hemangiomas are most commonly associated with cutaneous hemangiomas in which of the following locations?
    a. Scalp distribution
    b. Back
    c. Extremities
    d. Area of beard distribution
    e. Chest and abdomen

85. Which of the following is/are potential side effects of long-term steroid use in children?
    a. Cushing syndrome
    b. Diabetes
    c. Growth retardation
    d. Hypertension
    e. All of the above

86. Which of the following is the initial preferred treatment for an infant with an airway hemangioma?
    a. Oral steroids
    b. Intravenous steroids
    c. Endoscopic laser therapy
    d. Oral propranolol
    e. Inhaled racemic epinephrine

87. Following supraglottoplasty in an infant with severe laryngomalacia and failure to thrive, which of the following is/are expected?
    a. Improvement in sleep mechanics
    b. Improvement in growth curve percentile
    c. Decreased incidence of aspiration
    d. b and c
    e. a, b, and c

88. The presenting symptoms of an infant with a unilateral VFP typically include which of the following?
    a. Weak cry only
    b. Weak cry and feeding difficulties only
    c. Weak cry, feeding difficulties, and aspiration only
    d. Weak cry, feeding difficulties, aspiration, and intermittent stridor
    e. Any of the above

89. Which of the following would cause a characteristic "washing machine" type of stridor?
    a. Laryngomalacia, tracheomalacia, foreign body aspiration
    b. Tracheomalacia, tracheal stenosis, vascular ring
    c. Vascular ring, bilateral VFP, vallecular cyst
    d. Bilateral VFP, LTEC, subglottic cysts
    e. Subglottic cysts, bilateral VFP, saccular cyst

90. Which of the following can lead to aphonia?
    a. Laryngeal web
    b. Paradoxical vocal fold motion
    c. Saccular cyst
    d. Choanal atresia
    e. Subglottic hemangioma

91. Which of the following cause stertor (as opposed to stridor)?
    a. VFP
    b. Nasolacrimal duct cyst
    c. Posterior glottis stenosis
    d. Subglottic stenosis
    e. Tracheomalacia

92. GERD is commonly associated with which of the following airway diagnoses?
    a. Bilateral choanal atresia
    b. Robin sequence
    c. Laryngomalacia
    d. Tracheomalacia
    e. Unilateral VFP

93. Which of the following airway diagnoses is typically diagnosed within the first 48 hours of life?
    a. Bilateral choanal atresia
    b. Laryngomalacia
    c. Laryngeal papillomatosis
    d. Subglottic hemangioma
    e. Unilateral VFP

94. Which of the following airway diagnoses is typically associated with increased stridor while crying?
    a. Bilateral choanal atresia
    b. Nasolacrimal duct cyst
    c. Laryngomalacia
    d. Bilateral VFP
    e. Macroglossia

95. Which of the following airway diagnoses is typically associated with a change in vocal quality (i.e., hoarseness)?
    a. Bilateral choanal atresia
    b. Laryngomalacia
    c. Unilateral VFP
    d. Bilateral VFP
    e. Subglottic stenosis

96. Which of the following airway diagnoses is typically treated medically (as opposed to surgically)?
    a. Bilateral choanal atresia
    b. Congenital subglottic stenosis
    c. Subglottic cysts
    d. Subglottic hemangioma
    e. Tracheal stenosis

97. Which of the following airway diagnoses will typically improve spontaneously with age?
    a. Laryngeal web
    b. Bilateral VFP
    c. Tracheal compression due to a vascular ring
    d. Tracheomalacia
    e. Tracheal stenosis

98. Which of the following airway diagnoses typically warrants surgery within the first week of life?

a. Bilateral choanal atresia
b. Laryngomalacia
c. Unilateral VFP
d. Subglottic cysts
e. Subglottic hemangioma

99. Which of the following airway diagnoses is more common in infants born prematurely?
   a. Laryngomalacia
   b. Bilateral VFP
   c. Subglottic cysts

d. Bifid epiglottis
e. Tracheomalacia

100. The evaluation of the pediatric airway begins with the assessment of which of the following?
   a. Noisy breathing
   b. Ability to feed
   c. Ability to gain weight
   d. Presence of suprasternal and subcostal retractions
   e. All of the above

CORE KNOWLEDGE

LARYNGOMALACIA

- Laryngomalacia is the most common cause of stridor in infants. The stridor is typically inspiratory, worsens with feeding, and is associated with GERD. The median time to spontaneous resolution of stridor is 7 to 9 months of age.
- The stridor of laryngomalacia results from the collapse of the supraglottic larynx, which creates a narrow airway and turbulent airflow. It appears to be related to neuromuscular hypotonia.
- Severe laryngomalacia can result in GERD, laryngeal penetration and aspiration, failure to thrive, apnea, pectus excavatum, and cyanosis.
- Supraglottoplasty (aryepiglottoplasty) is the standard treatment for severe laryngomalacia.
- Laryngomalacia can occur in older children and be a cause of obstructive sleep apnea, particularly in neurologically impaired children.

VOCAL FOLD DYSFUNCTION

- The stridor of VFP is inspiratory or biphasic, with a high-pitched musical quality.
- Unilateral VFP typically presents with a weak cry or stridor, aspiration, dysphagia, or feeding difficulties. Infants with bilateral VFP often have severe airway obstruction (Figure 14-1) that requires a tracheotomy.
- Approximately 70% of noniatrogenic unilateral VFP will resolve spontaneously, most within the first 6 months of life. The vocal folds spontaneously become mobile in up to 65% of patients with noniatrogenic bilateral VFP, usually within 24 to 36 months.

- Iatrogenic left VFP is a known complication of thoracic surgery, particularly patent ductus arteriosus ligation or repair of an interrupted aortic arch. Tracheoesophageal fistula repair, thyroidectomy, and transcervical resection of branchial anomalies can also cause iatrogenic VFP.
- Surgical options to improve the airway of a patient with bilateral VFP include lateral cordotomy, arytenoidectomy, arytenoidopexy, posterior laryngeal graft, and lateralization of the paralyzed vocal fold.
- Paradoxic vocal fold motion in a neonate typically resolves spontaneously within the first few months of life.

LARYNGEAL WEB/ATRESIA

- Anterior congenital laryngeal webs typically cause aphonia or stridor. Occasionally a minor web will present as hoarseness in an older child.
- The Cohen classification of glottic webs is as follows:
  Type 1: <35% obstruction (mild hoarseness)
  Type 2: 35% to 50% obstruction (hoarse, weak cry, stridor with exertion)
  Type 3: 50% to 75% obstruction (severe hoarseness, moderate airway obstruction)
  Type 4: 75% to 90% obstruction (aphonia, severe airway obstruction)
- The most severe form of a laryngeal web is total atresia of the larynx. Laryngeal atresia (Figure 14-2) is associated

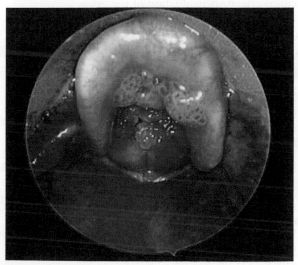

FIGURE 14-1 Laryngeal papillomas.

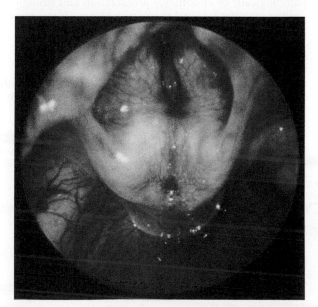

FIGURE 14-2 Laryngeal atresia. (From Benjamin B. The pediatric airway, In *Slide Lecture Series, American Academy of Otolaryngology–Head and Neck Surgery,* 1992.)

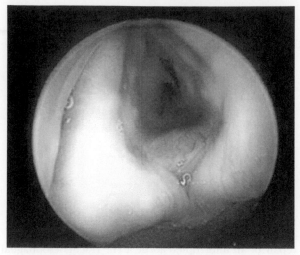

FIGURE 14-3 Subglottic hemangioma.

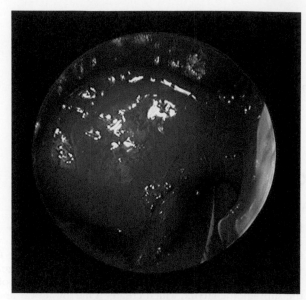

FIGURE 14-4 Vallecular cyst.

with CHAOS. CHAOS on fetal MRI is characterized by enlarged echogenic lungs, inverted diaphragm, massive ascites, and dilated fluid-filled lower airways. Delivery by ex utero intrapartum treatment procedure is necessary to secure the airway by immediate tracheotomy while the neonate remains on placental support.

- Anterior laryngeal webs may be associated with deletions of chromosome 22q11.2 (velocardiofacial syndrome, DiGeorge syndrome, Shprintzen syndrome).

SUBGLOTTIC DISEASE

- Subglottic stenosis is defined as a cricoid diameter of <3.5 mm in a newborn.
- An elliptical cricoid is often present in congenital subglottic stenosis with a transverse diameter that is significantly smaller than the anteroposterior diameter.
- Subglottic infantile hemangiomas (IH) are characterized pathologically by endothelial proliferation and strongly positive staining for erythrocyte-type glucose transporter protein isoform 1.
- Symptoms of a subglottic IH include biphasic stridor, barking cough, and temporary improvement with oral steroids. Often the symptoms will resemble those of nonresolving croup. IHs grow rapidly in the first 6 months of life, stabilize for approximately a year, and then slowly involute.
- First-line treatment for IH is oral propranolol.
- Subglottic cysts may mimic the symptoms of subglottic hemangiomas (Figure 14-3). Intubation trauma is believed to be the source of these cysts. Typically the infants were born prematurely at 24 to 31 weeks.

CYSTS

- Ductal cysts can occur at any site within the larynx and originate from obstruction of the submucosal glands.
- Vallecular cysts (Figure 14-4) occur in the midline and can become large and cause lethal airway obstruction in the neonate. They are often of thyroglossal duct origin. The pathologic diagnosis may be thyroglossal duct cyst or vallecular cyst, depending on the presence or absence of thyroid follicles, respectively.

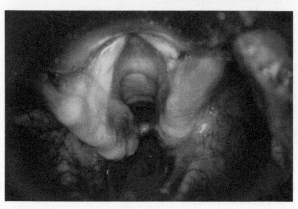

FIGURE 14-5 Laryngotracheal cleft: Benjamin-Inglis type III. (From Benjamin B. The pediatric airway, In *Slide Lecture Series, American Academy of Otolaryngology–Head and Neck Surgery*, 1992.)

- Saccular cysts and laryngoceles are unusual causes of respiratory obstruction in children. Treatment entails endoscopic marsupialization of the cyst.

LARYNGEAL OR LARYNGOTRACHEOESOPHAGEAL CLEFT

- A laryngeal cleft is caused by failure of fusion of the posterior cricoid lamina, which leads to abnormal communication between the posterior portion of the larynx and esophagus. An LTEC results from extension of a laryngeal cleft to involve the tracheoesophageal septum.
- Multiple classification schemes exist for laryngeal cleft and LTEC. The most commonly used are the Benjamin-Inglis (Figure 14-5) and Myer-Cotton staging systems.
- A laryngeal cleft should be considered in any newborn with feeding problems and recurrent aspiration. Definitive diagnosis is made at the time of direct laryngoscopy. A laryngeal cleft can be missed if only flexible laryngoscopy or flexible bronchoscopy is performed.
- The deeper the cleft, the more severe the symptoms of aspiration and pneumonia. Airway obstruction can occur

as a result of the prolapse of interarytenoid mucosa into the airway. The prognosis is poor for an infant with a type 4 LTEC.
- Medical management is often adequate for type 1 laryngeal cleft because aspiration resolves as the patient grows older.

BIFID EPIGLOTTIS

- A bifid epiglottis is a rare anomaly defined as a cleft of the epiglottis that encompasses at least two-thirds of its length. It is commonly associated with other anomalies, especially midline defects.

ANSWERS

TRUE OR FALSE QUESTIONS

1.	F	14.	T	27.	T	40.	T
2.	F	15.	F	28.	F	41.	F
3.	T	16.	F	29.	F	42.	T
4.	T	17.	T	30.	T	43.	T
5.	T	18.	T	31.	T	44.	T
6.	F	19.	T	32.	T	45.	T
7.	F	20.	F	33.	T	46.	F
8.	T	21.	T	34.	F	47.	F
9.	F	22.	T	35.	T	48.	T
10.	T	23.	T	36.	T	49.	F
11.	T	24.	F	37.	F	50.	F
12.	T	25.	T	38.	T		
13.	T	26.	T	39.	F		

SINGLE BEST ANSWER QUESTIONS

51.	d	64.	b	77.	e	90.	a
52.	e	65.	e	78.	e	91.	b
53.	e	66.	c	79.	a	92.	c
54.	a	67.	a	80.	e	93.	a
55.	c	68.	d	81.	d	94.	d
56.	a	69.	e	82.	c	95.	c
57.	c	70.	c	83.	a	96.	d
58.	b	71.	d	84.	d	97.	d
59.	d	72.	a	85.	e	98.	a
60.	e	73.	e	86.	d	99.	c
61.	d	74.	b	87.	e	100.	e
62.	c	75.	e	88.	e		
63.	c	76.	a	89.	b		

SUGGESTED READINGS

1. Thompson DM. Abnormal sensorimotor integrative function of the larynx in congenital laryngomalacia: a new theory of etiology. *Laryngoscope.* 2007;117(suppl 114 6 Pt2):1-33.
2. Lim J, Hellier W, Harcourt J, Leighton S, Albert D. Subglottic cysts: the great Ormond Street experience. *Int J Pediatr Otorhinolaryngol.* 2003;67(5):461-465.
3. Balakrishnan K, Cheng E, de Alarcon A, et al. Outcomes and resource utilization of endoscopic mass-closure technique for laryngeal clefts. *Otolaryngol Head Neck Surg.* 2015;153(1):119-123.
4. Ojha S, Ashland JE, Hersh C, et al. Type 1 laryngeal cleft: a multidimensional management algorithm. *JAMA Otolaryngol Head Neck Surg.* 2014;140(1):34-40.
5. Chen EY, Lim J, Boss EF, et al. Transoral approach for direct and complete excision of vallecular cysts in children. *Int J Pediatr Otorhinolaryngol.* 2011;75(9):1147-1151.
6. Nicollas R, Triglia JM. The anterior laryngeal webs. *Otolaryngol Clin North Am.* 2008;41(5):877-888.
7. Setlur J, Hartnick CJ. Management of unilateral true vocal cord paralysis in children. *Curr Opin Otolaryngol Head Neck Surg.* 2012;20(6):497-501.
8. Lesnik M, Thierry B, Blanchard M, et al. Idiopathic bilateral vocal cord paralysis in infants: case series and literature review. *Laryngoscope.* 2014;125(7):1724-1728.
9. Miyamoto RC, Cotton RT, Rope AF, et al. Association of anterior glottic webs with velocardiofacial syndrome (chromosome 22q11.2 deletion). *Otolaryngol Head Neck Surg.* 2004;130(4):415-417.
10. Durr ML, Meyer AK, Huoh KC, Frieden IJ, Rosbe KW. Airway hemangiomas in PHACE syndrome. *Laryngoscope.* 2012;122(10):2323-2329.

15 Laryngeal Pathology and Trauma

Guri Sandhu | Karan Kapoor

TRUE OR FALSE QUESTIONS

T/F 1. When performing flexible nasal endoscopy, asking the patient to sniff can assist in assessing vocal cord abduction.

T/F 2. The external branch of the superior laryngeal nerve innervates the cricothyroid muscle.

T/F 3. The hyoid articulates with the corniculate cartilage of the larynx.

T/F 4. The recurrent laryngeal nerve has no sensory fibers.

T/F 5. The narrowest point of the pediatric and adult airway is the glottis.

T/F 6. The vocal fold structure in a neonate has a single layer of lamina propria.

T/F 7. The macula flavae connect the vocalis muscle to the thyroid cartilage and arytenoid cartilage.

T/F 8. The lymphatic drainage of the supraglottic larynx is bilateral.

T/F 9. The recurrent laryngeal nerve innervates all intrinsic muscles of the larynx.

T/F 10. In a patient with impending airway obstruction from laryngeal trauma, early endotracheal intubation may be necessary. A tracheostomy should be considered where safe.

T/F 11. The American Joint Committee on Cancer stages a cancer that is limited to both vocal cords as T2.

T/F 12. When performing a laryngectomy it is advisable to resect the medial head of sternocleidomastoid.

T/F 13. Post intubation trauma is seen most commonly on the medial surface of the posterior commissure due to pressure necrosis.

T/F 14. Laryngeal papillomatosis secondary to the human papillomavirus virus is considered a sexually transmitted disease due to its orogenital transmission pathway.

T/F 15. Stroboscopy works on the principle of synchronizing the light pulses to the same frequency as the vocal fold vibration and matching the same speed in order to allow visualization of the vocal cord waveform.

T/F 16. With regard to perceptual voice assessment, the GRBAS (grade, roughness, breathiness, asthenia, strain) scale has good interrated reliability.

T/F 17. The commonest site for vocal cord nodules is the midpoint of the membranous vocal fold.

T/F 18. Any impaired mobility of the vocal fold upstages laryngeal squamous cell carcinoma to T3 or above as per American Joint Committee on Cancer criteria.

T/F 19. Patients with ballistic trauma to the neck should have mandatory C-spine immobilization and clearance prior to management of the penetrating injury.

T/F 20. In patients with a neck stabbing, the laceration can be explored in the emergency department with a gloved finger to assess depth of penetration.

T/F 21. In less than 1% of cases does angiography alter the management of asymptomatic patients with penetrating neck trauma.

T/F 22. Laryngopharyngeal reflux is a risk factor for dysplasia in the larynx.

T/F 23. *Jitter* is defined as the cycle to cycle variation in the fundamental frequency of the voice.

T/F 24. The cough reflex is diminished during sleep.

T/F 25. The pediatric larynx is proportionately larger than the adult larynx when compared to their respective tracho-bronchial tree.

T/F 26. In electroglottography, the conductance of the electrical conductance across the neck decreases as the vocal folds touch each other in phonation, which results in a change in the trace.

T/F 27. The clinical management of low grade laryngeal chondrosarcoma is akin to a chondroma.

T/F 28. Exacerbations of laryngotracheal granulomatosis with polyangiitis (Wegener granulomatosis) should be treated with systemic steroids and cyclophosphamide.

T/F 29. Injection thyroplasty aims to medialize the vocal fold by augmenting the vocal ligament and hence improving glottis apposition.

T/F 30. Idiopathic subglottic stenosis is seen almost exclusively in women.

T/F 31. Recurrent laryngeal nerve palsy is idiopathic in 10% of cases.

T/F 32. When approaching the vocal cords externally, they run perpendicular to the upper border of the thyroid cartilage.

T/F 33. The principle of endoscopic subglottis stenosis management is to circumferentially excise the stenotic segment down to cartilage, allowing fresh healthy mucosa to regrow.

T/F 34. Acute laryngotracheobronchitis is best treated with a third-generation cephalosporin and antipyretic agents.

T/F 35. Laryngomalacia has no sex preponderance.

T/F 36. Patients with laryngeal carcinoma most commonly present with symptoms of stridor.

T/F 37. A cricothyroid approximation procedure has a negative effect on vocal range.

T/F 38. The Myer-Cotton grading system was developed for pediatric tracheal stenosis.

T/F 39. A laryngeal cleft is more common in boys than girls in a ratio of 5:3.

T/F 40. In the pediatric larynx the arytenoid vocal process takes up ½ the length of the vocal cord.

T/F 41. A full-term neonate should be intubated with a size 3.0 mm pediatric endotracheal tube. If a smaller tube is required, subglottis stenosis should be considered.

T/F 42. Idiopathic subglottic stenosis does not affect or infiltrate the cartilaginous framework of the airway.

T/F 43. Mucous membrane pemphigoid of the larynx should primarily be treated with radical surgery to ablate diseased areas followed by immunosuppression.

T/F 44. The most common bacteria to colonize airway stents and tracheostomies are *Staphylococcus aureus* and *Pseudomonas aeruginosa*.

T/F 45. A stridulous patient with respiratory distress at presentation following significant laryngeal trauma should immediately proceed to have a tracheotomy under local anesthesia.

T/F 46. Reduction of an anterior dislocation of the cricoarytenoid joint can be achieved using a straight bladed anesthetic laryngoscope to lift the arytenoid anterosuperiorly.

T/F 47. Cricotracheal resection should never be used in the management of idiopathic subglottic stenosis.

T/F 48. The neonatal larynx lies at the level of C3 vertebra and descends during the first three years of life to its adult position at the level of C6 vertebra.

T/F 49. The position of the neonatal larynx is the reason it is more likely to sustain direct trauma.

T/F 50. Abductor spasmodic dysphonia is more common than adductor spasmodic dysphonia.

SINGLE BEST ANSWER QUESTIONS

51. Which of the following is the fundamental frequency range of the normal female voice?
   a. 50 to 150 Hz
   b. 100 to 200 Hz
   c. 150 to 250 Hz
   d. 200 to 300 Hz

52. The superior limit of the glottis defined as the arcuate line is anatomically:
   a. The free edge of the false cord
   b. The superior limit of the aryepiglottic fold
   c. The apex of the laryngeal ventricle
   d. 1 cm above the free edge of the true cord

53. Which of the following muscles is not involved in adduction of the vocal cords?
   a. Thyroarytenoid
   b. Transverse and oblique arytenoid muscles
   c. Posterior cricoarytenoid
   d. Vocalis and cricothyroid muscles

54. Edema within the airway changes the resistance to flow because of Poiseuille's law, which states that:
   a. Resistance $= 1/r^8$
   b. Resistance $= 1/r^4$
   c. Resistance $\propto 1/r^8$
   d. Resistance $\propto 1/r^4$

55. Which of the following is the most common complaint of those presenting with laryngeal trauma?
   a. Hoarseness
   b. Dysphagia
   c. Pain
   d. Surgical emphysema

56. In patients with known laryngeal trauma, a concomitant cervical spine injury is found in:
   a. 0.1% of cases
   b. 1% of cases
   c. 5% of cases
   d. 10% of cases

57. Iatrogenic laryngeal trauma from long-term intubation is seen in what percentage of patients?
   a. 25%
   b. 55%
   c. 75%
   d. 95%

58. The cricoarytenoid joint is a
   a. Synovial joint
   b. Syndesmotic joint
   c. Synarthrotic joint
   d. Synchondrotic joint

59. The wavelength of the carbon dioxide (CO_2) laser is
   a. 514 nanometers
   b. 1064 nanometers
   c. 10.6 micrometers
   d. 20.1 nanometers

60. Which of the following is the ideal position for microlaryngoscopy?
   a. Neck flexed, head flexed
   b. Neck flexed, head extended
   c. Neck extended, head extended
   d. Neck extended, head flexed

61. With which of the following is Reinke edema *NOT* associated?
   a. Smoking
   b. Elevated progesterone levels
   c. Hypothyroidism
   d. Elevated estradiol levels

62. When considering penetrating neck injuries, which of the following is *NOT* contained in Zone 1?
   a. Subclavian artery
   b. Thyroid
   c. Thyroid cartilage
   d. Esophagus

63. Which of the following is treated principally by voice therapy?
   a. Vocal fold nodules
   b. Hemorrhagic vocal cord polyp
   c. Reinke edema
   d. Vocal cord granulomas

64. A type I Isshiki thyroplasty indicates which of the following?
    a. Lateralize the cord.
    b. Shorten the cord.
    c. Medialize the cord.
    d. Lengthen the cord.

65. All of the following affect maximum phonatory time *EXCEPT*:
    a. Vowel choice
    b. Forced expiratory volume in 1 second
    c. Vital capacity
    d. Repetition

66. Hemorrhagic vocal cord polyps more commonly present:
    a. In women
    b. As bilateral
    c. On anticoagulants
    d. In professional singers

67. Which of the following would raise the fundamental frequency?
    a. Type IV Isshiki thyroplasty
    b. Reinke edema
    c. Spasmodic dysphonia
    d. T2 laryngeal squamous cell carcinoma

68. A workup for patients with suspected relapsing polychondritis should routinely undergo all the following *EXCEPT*:
    a. Antineutrophil cytoplasmic antibody testing
    b. VDRL testing
    c. HIV testing
    d. Hepatitis screening

69. In the Schaefer-Fuhrman classification of laryngeal trauma, exposed cartilage would be graded as which of the following?
    a. Group 1
    b. Group 2
    c. Group 3
    d. Group 4
    e. Group 5

70. When considering tracheal resection for a stenotic segment, which of the following is the advised maximum length of resection in an adult, without other surgical maneuvers?
    a. 2 cm
    b. 4 cm
    c. 6 cm
    d. 8 cm

71. Which of the following statements is true regarding vocal fold nodules?
    a. They are related to smoking.
    b. Early surgical intervention is advised.
    c. They can be premalignant.
    d. They are always bilateral.

72. Dysphonia is defined as decreasing ability to vocalize because of which of the following?
    a. An abnormality in articulating
    b. A laryngeal disorder
    c. Cerebral dysfunction
    d. A neuromuscular disorder

73. Which of the following statements is true regarding the larynx?
    a. The corniculate cartilages articulate with the summit of the arytenoid cartilage.
    b. Mucous glands are present throughout the glottis and subglottis.

c. The recurrent laryngeal nerve is motor to the cricothyroid muscle.
d. The lateral cricoarytenoid muscle abducts the vocal cord.

74. The acronym LASER stands for which of the following?
    a. Light Array with Simultaneous Emission of Radiation
    b. Longwave Amplification of Stimulated Enhanced Radiation
    c. Light Amplification by Stimulated Emission of Radiation
    d. Lightwaves Aligned by Serial Emission of Radiation

75. Which of the following statements is true regarding laryngoceles?
    a. They are always bilateral.
    b. They can be a presentation of laryngeal cancer.
    c. They never extend outside the larynx.
    d. They exit the larynx though the cricothyroid membrane.

76. Which of the following statements is true regarding the recurrent laryngeal nerve?
    a. It is purely motor in its fibers.
    b. It is tethered by the ligamentum arteriosum in the left thorax.
    c. It is tightly attached to the inferior thyroid artery as it enters the larynx.
    d. It is involved in innervating the cardiac plexus.

77. Which of the following statements is true regarding acute epiglottitis?
    a. It is most commonly a viral infection.
    b. It is commonly caused by *Streptococcus pneumoniae*.
    c. Lateral plain radiographs may show the "steeple sign."
    d. It should be treated with a third-generation cephalosporin empirically.

78. Vocal fold mucosal vibration is unaffected by which of the following?
    a. Edema
    b. A sulcus
    c. Nodules
    d. Radiotherapy

79. With regard to elective tracheostomy, which of the following is true?
    a. The Björk flap is placed superiorly.
    b. The first tracheal ring may be excised.
    c. The first elective tube change must take place after a week.
    d. The largest tube should be used to reduce cuff pressure within the trachea.

80. When performing a surgical myotomy, which of the following muscles is divided?
    a. Inferior constrictor
    b. Cricopharyngeus
    c. Radial fibers of muscularis propria
    d. All of the above

81. From which of the following do the vocal cords develop?
    a. Third branchial arch
    b. Fourth pharyngeal pouch
    c. Primordial foregut
    d. Midgut

82. With regard to the Cotton-Myer grading system, grade II would represent as an airway stenosis of which of the following?
    a. 31% to 50%
    b. 41% to 60%
    c. 51% to 70%
    d. 61% to 80%

83. Which of the following is true of a type III laryngeal cleft?
   a. It is an interarytenoid defect that extends inferiorly no further than the level of the true vocal folds.
   b. It is a defect that partially involves the cricoid lamina with extension of the cleft below the level of the true vocal folds.
   c. It is a total cricoid cleft that extends completely through the cricoid cartilage with or without extension into the cervical trachea.
   d. It is a defect extending into the posterior wall of the thoracic trachea extending as far as the carina.

84. From which of the following is the cricoid cartilage derived?
   a. Third pharyngeal pouch
   b. Fourth pharyngeal pouch
   c. Fifth branchial arch
   d. Sixth branchial arch

85. Which of the following is the most common symptom of a laryngeal cleft?
   a. Choking on thin fluids
   b. Stridor
   c. Recurrent pneumonia
   d. Cough

86. If required, a full-term neonate should undergo endotracheal intubation with a pediatric tube of which of the following sizes?
   a. 3.0 mm
   b. 3.5 mm
   c. 4.0 mm
   d. 4.5 mm

87. The following statements are true of pertussis (whooping cough) *EXCEPT*:
   a. It is a notifiable infection.
   b. The most common cause is *Bordetella*.
   c. It is most severe in children, particularly infants.
   d. The first-line treatment is tetracycline-based antibiotics.

88. Which of the following are proven risk factors for adult-acquired subglottic stenosis?
   a. Female sex
   b. Human papillomavirus infection
   c. Peptic ulcer disease
   d. Excessive cuff pressure in ventilation tubes

89. The "lambda" (or A-frame) airway deformity is commonly recognized as a sign of which of the following?
   a. Posttracheostomy airway stenosis
   b. Idiopathic airway stenosis
   c. Prolonged intubation airway stenosis
   d. Chemically induced airway stenosis

90. Idiopathic laryngotracheal stenosis usually affects which of the following?
   a. Any ring between the cricoid and carina
   b. The first and second tracheal rings only
   c. The second and third tracheal ring
   d. None of the above

91. Which of the following has *NOT* been recognized as a potential treatment for vocal cord reinnervation?
   a. Ansa cervicalis to recurrent laryngeal nerve
   b. Ansa cervicalis to thyroarytenoid neuromuscular pedicle
   c. Single division of phrenic to posterior cricoarytenoid
   d. Vagus to recurrent laryngeal nerve

92. Treatment for bilateral vocal cord immobility includes the following *EXCEPT*:
   a. Posterior arytenoidectomy
   b. Suture lateralization
   c. Type V cordotomy
   d. Aryepiglottoplasty

93. The following are causes of cricoarytenoid joint fixation *EXCEPT*:
   a. Tracheostomy tubes
   b. Rheumatoid arthritis
   c. Wegener granulomatosis
   d. Interarytenoid scarring

94. What percentage of patients with active granulomatosis with polyangiitis (Wegener granulomatosis) will have a negative cytoplasmic ANCA (cANCA) at presentation?
   a. 5%
   b. 10%
   c. 20%
   d. 30%

95. Which of the following statements is true regarding mitomycin C?
   a. It acts by producing oxygen-free radicals creating DNA strand breaks.
   b. It is not a prodrug.
   c. It acts on the basement membrane to reduce intracellular cohesion.
   d. Randomized control trials have proven its efficacy in the human airway.

96. Which of the flow volume loops in Figure 15-1 would be indicative of fixed airway obstruction?
   a. A
   b. B
   c. C
   d. D

97. Which of the following statements is true regarding laryngeal amyloidosis?
   a. It causes dysfunction by perineural invasion.
   b. Beta-pleated sheets are pathognomonic.
   c. It preferentially affects women.
   d. It is treated with intralesional proteases.

98. Which of the following is true of spasmodic dysphonia?
   a. Adductor spasmodic dysphonia is more common.
   b. It can be cured by injection of botulinum toxin into the larynx.
   c. Adductor spasmodic dysphonia presents with a breathy, weak voice.
   d. In 80% of patients a causal emotional factor can be identified.

99. Which of the following *CANNOT* be assessed on fiberoptic endoscopic evaluation of swallowing?
   a. All the phases of swallowing
   b. Vocal cord adduction
   c. Laryngeal penetration
   d. Laryngeal sensation

100. Which of the following is true of vocal fold polyps?
   a. They are commonly bilateral.
   b. They arise from the vocal cord ligament.
   c. They are best assessed on stroboscopy.
   d. They always require surgery for resolution.

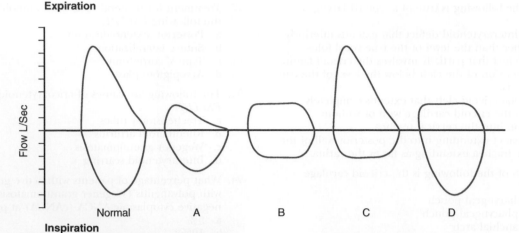

FIGURE 15-1 Flow volume loops.

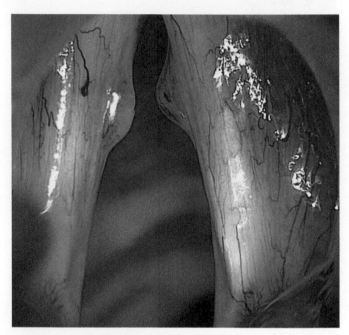

FIGURE 15-2 Vocal cord nodules.

CORE KNOWLEDGE SECTION

VOCAL CORD NODULES

- These are bilateral benign nodules commonly seen in the middle of the membranous vocal cord (Figure 15-2).
- They are more common in boys and women.
- Vocal cord nodules are the most common cause of school-aged hoarseness.
- The mainstay for treatment is speech therapy and, in children, behavioral therapy.
- There is very little benefit from pharmacological treatment.
- Surgery should be considered only in those recalcitrant to definitive speech therapy.
- In the prepubertal patient the disease usually resolves spontaneously following vocal cord lengthening due to hormonal changes.

RESPIRATORY PAPILLOMATOSIS

- Respiratory papillomas are the most common benign neoplasms affecting the larynx (Figure 15-3) and are due

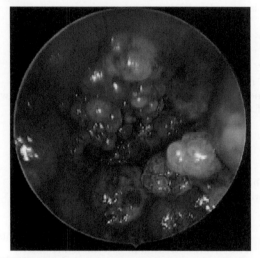

FIGURE 15-3 Recurrent respiratory papillomatosis of the larynx.

to infections with the human papillomavirus, subtypes 6 and 11 commonly, but also 16 and 18.
- In the infected larynx, the increased potential for malignant transformation to squamous cell carcinoma, as compared with the normal population, is marginal.
- The risk of children born of mothers with active genital papillomatosis developing juvenile-onset respiratory papillomatosis is less than 0.5%.
- Congenital respiratory papillomatosis is due to ascending uterine infection; caesarean section is not protective.
- The principle of surgery is not to disrupt the lamina propria because this is an exophytic disease arising from squamous epithelium.
- After confirmation of the diagnosis, surgery is indicated only on lesions causing dysphonia or dyspnea.
- During a surgical intervention the trachea and bronchi must be inspected for spread of disease. Tracheobronchial infection occurs in association with squamous metaplasia of the respiratory epithelium, and in these circumstances there is an increased risk of malignant transformation.

REINKE EDEMA

- This is a description of the polypoid degeneration of the vocal fold, in which there is an accumulation of fluid within the superficial lamina propria (Figure 15-4).

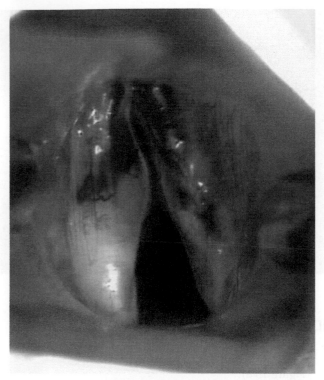

FIGURE 15-4 Reinke edema.

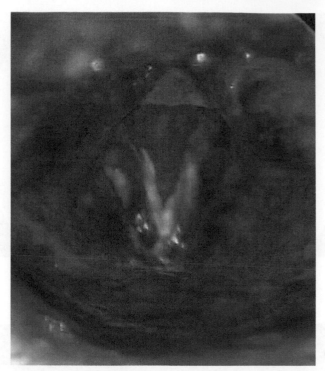

FIGURE 15-5 Laryngeal dysplasia.

- The most common cause is smoking, but laryngopharyngeal reflux, voice abuse, and hypothyroidism are also potential causes.
- In smokers it is thought to be due to damage to collagen.
- It is more prevalent in females.
- Reinke edema commonly results in lowering of the fundamental frequency.
- Treatment comprises a combination of smoking cessation and voice therapy. Surgery is indicated if the diagnosis is in doubt or the patient wishes to have a more "normal" voice.

LARYNGEAL DYSPLASIA

- The World Health Organization (2005) classification of laryngeal dysplasia (Figure 15-5) is as follows:
  - Squamous cell hyperplasia: increased cell numbers in basal layer of epithelium but no cell atypia
  - Mild dysplasia: cell atypia limited to lower third of epithelium
  - Moderate dysplasia: cell disturbance to middle third, prominent nucleoli but no abnormal mitoses
  - Severe dysplasia: atypia and cell disturbance high up in the epithelium
  - Carcinoma in situ: full thickness architectural abnormalities, pronounced atypia, atypical mitotic figures, and abnormal mitoses but basement epithelium intact
- The risk of transformation of dysplasia from premalignant to malignant is 10.6% for mild/moderate dysplasia. However, severe dysplasia carries a 30.4% risk of malignant transformation.

LARYNGOTRACHEAL STENOSIS

- There is no period of endotracheal intubation below which no airway injury occurs and above which injury is inevitable.

- Airway resistance is dictated by the diameter of the airway and by the density of the inspired gas. This is represented by Poiseuille's law:

$$R = \frac{8nl}{\pi r^4}$$

- Neither flexible bronchoscopy nor rigid bronchoscopy allows prolonged access or endoscopic surgery on the larynx or subglottis. Suspension laryngoscopy allows binocular vision, depth of field perception, two hands free for instrumentation, and the use of the laser with a "line-of-sight" technique.
- Prolonged spontaneous breathing techniques are difficult in adult patients as they tend to lighten from anesthesia more rapidly and have an increased risk of laryngospasm.
- Potential risk factors for laryngotracheal stenosis following a period of ventilation include oversized endotracheal tubes, excessive cuff pressures, local infection, duration of intubation, reduced patient immunity, and patient agitation.
- The incidence of laryngotracheal stenosis (Figure 15-6) is similar whether endotracheal tubes or tracheostomies are used. However, an endotracheal tube may injure the glottis. Postintubation impairment of normal glottic movement from posterior glottis scar and cricoarytenoid joint ankylosis is far more difficult to repair than subglottic or tracheal stenosis.
- Risk factors for posttracheostomy stenosis include an oversized tracheal fenestration or significant damage to the tracheal rings. Later scarring and contracture at the stoma site can draw in the lateral ring remnants, leading to a "lambda-shaped" (also called an "A-frame") stenotic deformity. The lesion usually extends over one to two tracheal rings with normal proximal and distal trachea.
- To prevent ischemic damage, the cuff should not exceed a pressure greater than the capillary perfusion pressure of

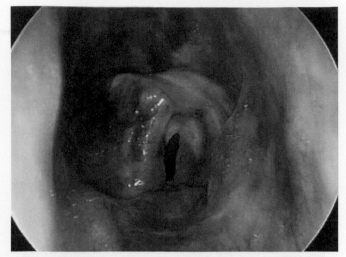

FIGURE 15-6 "Lambda"-shaped posttracheostomy stenosis.

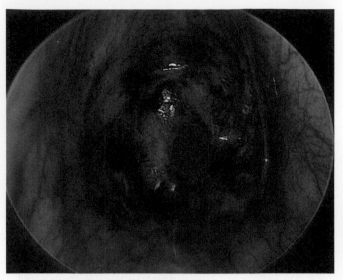

FIGURE 15-8 Grade 3 idiopathic subglottic stenosis.

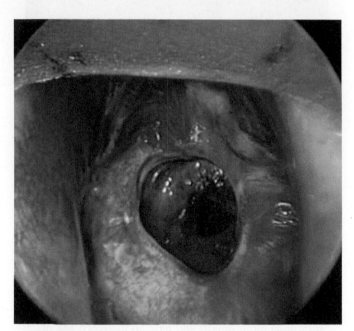

FIGURE 15-7 Stenosis at proximal and distal end of a wire tracheal stent.

the mucosa. The recommendation is that the cuff inflation pressure should not exceed 30 cm H_2O.

- Postintubation airway injury is characterized by two phases: an early phase with mucosal ulceration and perichondritis, followed by the formation of exophytic granulation tissue.
- In the late phase, granulation tissue is gradually replaced with mature fibrotic tissue, and the wound contracts, giving rise to the classical picture of mature airway scar.
- Uncovered or hybrid metal stents (Figure 15-7) should be used only in a select group of patients with a short life expectancy or where the plan is for the stent to be removed. If not removed within the first few weeks of deployment, they become a permanent fixture in the airway.
- There is a high incidence of bacterial colonization of all stents, which can lead to granular tissue formation. The most common organisms are *Staphylococcus aureus* and *Pseudomonas aeruginosa.*

IDIOPATHIC SUBGLOTTIC STENOSIS

- Idiopathic subglottic stenosis is a rare, slowly progressive, fibroinflammatory process of unknown cause (Figure 15-8).
- The stenosis is found in the subglottic region and usually involves the first and second tracheal rings.
- The fibroinflammatory process appears to be confined to the mucosa and does not involve the underlying cartilage.
- Long-term tracheostomy is not a solution for idiopathic subglottic stenosis because the airway above the tracheostomy will scar and close down, leading to aphonia.
- Aggressive endoscopic resection of the stenosis or laser ablation will lead to worse restenosis. The mainstay of treatment is interval dilation. Cricotracheal resection has been advocated as a permanent treatment.
- It is almost exclusively a disease of postpubertal women; however, there have been a few reports in men. The disease appears to be more common in women of European ancestry.

Diagnostic Criteria for Idiopathic Subglottic Stenosis
See Table 15-1.

GRANULOMATOSIS WITH POLYANGIITIS

- Between 17% and 25% of patients who suffer from granulomatosis with polyangiitis (Wegener granulomatosis) (Figure 15-9) may develop airway stenosis.
- Airway inflammation and narrowing in granulomatosis with polyangiitis does not uniformly respond to systemic immunosuppressives and may persist despite adequate disease control in other organ systems. Localized laryngotracheal stenosis may occasionally be the only presenting feature, hence making it difficult to justify the use of systemic corticosteroids and cytotoxic drugs.
- Intralesional corticosteroid injections, radiate lesion cuts, and dilation will treat the majority of new stenoses involving the larynx, trachea, and bronchi due to granulomatosis with polyangiitis (Wegener granulomatosis).

SARCOID

- Sarcoidosis (Figure 15-10) is a rare multisystem immune-mediated disease with strong environmental influences. It

Table 15-1 **Diagnostic Criteria for Idiopathic Subglottic Stenosis**	
Clinical Features	**Serum Biochemistry**

• Female patient (males very rare)
• No history of laryngotracheal injury
  • No endotracheal intubation or tracheotomy/no occurrence of exertional dyspnea within 2 years of intubation/tracheotomy
  • No thyroid/anterior neck surgery
  • No neck irradiation
  • No caustic or thermal injuries
  • No significant anterior neck trauma (blunt or penetrating)
• No history of autoimmunity
  • Negative history for vasculitis, formally ascertained through a vasculitis-specific systemic enquiry and semi-quantified using the Birmingham Vasculitis Activity Scale
  • No history to suggest sarcoidosis or amyloidosis
	• Negative titers for:
	  • Angiotensin-converting enzyme
	  • Antinuclear antibody
	  • Rheumatoid factor
	  • Antineutrophil cytoplasmic antibody
	
	Gross Lesion Morphology
	• The stenosis must include the subglottis.
	
	Histopathology*
	• Exclusion of other pathological entities (e.g., tumors, vasculitides, amyloidosis)
	• Fibrosis restricted to lamina propria with normal perichondrium/cartilage
	• Mixture of granulation and fibrosis with a prominence of keloidal fibrosis

*This is established with a deep endoscopic biopsy at the time of first treatment.

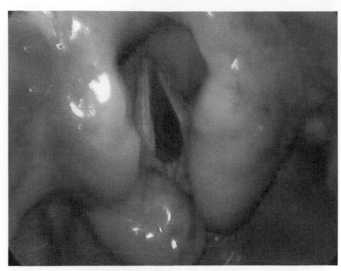

FIGURE 15-10 Laryngeal sarcoidosis.

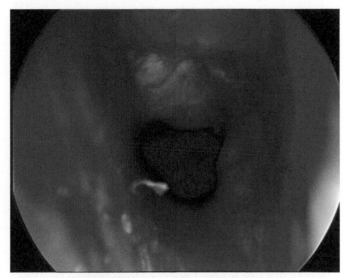

FIGURE 15-11 Amyloidosis of the subglottis.

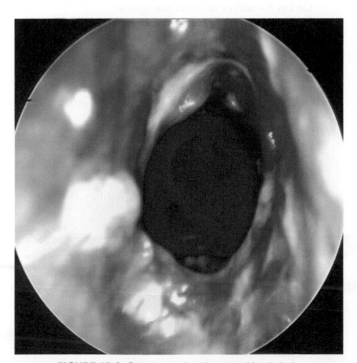

FIGURE 15-9 Granulomatosis with polyangiitis subglottis.

is more common in women and those of Afro-Caribbean origins.
• Otolaryngologists will most commonly see nasal manifestations of sarcoidosis. The larynx is involved in 1% of cases.
• The diagnosis of laryngeal sarcoidosis depends on the presence of typical clinical features and noncaseating granulomatous inflammation on biopsy with the exclusion of other known causes of granulomas, including tuberculosis, leprosy, syphilis, and fungal disease.
• Laryngeal sarcoid has a predilection for the supraglottic region, particularly the epiglottis, aryepiglottic folds, and arytenoid mucosa. The tissue in these areas may appear "swollen," causing narrowing of the supraglottic airway. Surgical tissue reduction may become necessary in symptomatic cases.
• In cases of suspected laryngeal sarcoid, investigations should include serum calcium, serum angiotensin-converting enzyme levels, and inflammatory markers. A chest radiograph is important to exclude hilar lymphadenopathy or other pulmonary involvement. An electrocardiogram may also be necessary to exclude cardiac involvement.

AMYLOID

• Amyloidosis (Figure 15-11) is the abnormal accumulation of protease-resistant proteins in the extracellular space.

- Progressive organ dysfunction is due principally to volumetric expansion with associated pressure effects on local healthy tissues.
- In general, amyloidosis preferentially affects males rather than females by 2:1, typically between their fifth and sixth decades.
- Serum amyloid P component scanning is recommended to determine whether the disease is primary or secondary.
- Laryngotracheal involvement is treated, when symptomatic, with surgical reduction, using cutting instruments or the laser.

MUCOUS MEMBRANE PEMPHIGOID

- Mucous membrane pemphigoid is a relapsing, remitting, autoimmune disease that can present with life-threatening involvement of the upper airways and aerodigestive tract.
- Fiberoptic assessment may reveal hyperemia, subepithelial blisters, or evidence of strictures or scarring of the supraglottis, subglottis, or vocal cords directly.
- The mainstay of treatment is long-term systemic immunosuppression in combination with chemotherapeutics and antibiotics.
- Surgical intervention is controversial because it can lead to further scarring, especially at the level of the larynx.

ISSHIKI THYROPLASTY

- Type I: medialization of the cord by using an implant via a window in the thyroid cartilage.
  - Indication for surgery is dysphonia or aspiration secondary to failure of the cords to meet in the midline.
  - The vocal cord runs parallel to the inferior border of the thyroid cartilage.
  - This is the most common laryngeal framework surgery.
- Type II: the vocal cord is lateralized by inserting a spacer following the creation of a laryngofissure.
  - This technique can be used for adductor spasmodic dysphonia.
  - Lateralization results in a more breathy voice.
- Type III: the vocal cord length is shortened by dividing the thyroid cartilage on either side of the midline and then setting this free segment posterior to its original position.
  - Reducing the tension on the vocal fold causes the pitch to be lowered.
  - Type III surgery can be considered in puberphonia.

- Type IV: lengthening of the cord is achieved by eliminating the gap between the cricoid and thyroid cartilages.
  - Cricothyroid approximation leads to pitch elevation.
  - This is most commonly used in voice feminization.

LARYNGEAL TRAUMA

- When considering penetrating trauma, the neck is divided into zones (Table 15-2).

CLASSIFICATION OF LARYNGEAL TRAUMA (SCHAEFER-FUHRMAN)

- The Schaefer-Fuhrman classification system acts as a guide in the management of laryngeal trauma.
- Group 1
  - Minor laryngeal hematomas or lacerations
  - No detectable fracture
- Group 2
  - Edema
  - Hematoma
  - Minor mucosal disruption without exposed cartilage
  - Nondisplaced fracture
- Group 3
  - Massive airway edema
  - Significant mucosal lacerations
  - Exposed cartilage
  - Displaced fractures
  - Vocal cord immobility
- Group 4
  - Group 3 + severe mucosal disruption
  - Or Group 3 + disruption of anterior commissure
  - Or Group 3 + unstable fracture (two or more fracture lines)
- Group 5
  - Complete laryngotracheal separation
- Management of laryngeal fracture is dependent on the severity of the injury and stability of the laryngeal framework.
- Grades 1 and 2 can be managed conservatively in the majority of cases.
  - Admit with serial nasoendoscopy
  - IV corticosteroids
  - IV proton-pump inhibitors
  - If there is mucosal breech, then IV antibiotics

Table 15-2	**Zones of the Neck**		
Zone	**Inferior Border**	**Superior Border**	**Contents**
1	Clavicle and sternal notch	Horizontal plane of cricoid	Common carotid Vertebral and subclavian arteries Subclavian, innominate, and jugular vein Recurrent and vagus nerve Esophagus Thoracic duct
2	Horizontal plane of cricoid	Horizontal plane through the angle of mandible	Internal and external carotid Jugular and vertebral veins, pharynx, proximal trachea, and larynx Recurrent laryngeal and vagal nerves Spinal cord
3	Horizontal plane through the angle of mandible	Skull base	Extracranial carotid and vertebral arteries Jugular veins Spinal cord Cranial nerves IX-XII Sympathetic trunk

- Grade 3, 4, and 5 require surgical intervention to stabilize the larynx.
- Laryngeal surgery following trauma should ideally occur within 12 hours of the event and no later than 24 hours. Delays in treatment can result in granulation, scarring, and complete laryngotracheal stenosis in severe cases.

CRICOARYTENOID DISLOCATION

- Posterior dislocation is usually caused by extubation, with the vocal fold on the affected side tending to lie in a higher plane.
- Anterior dislocation is usually due to injury from the tip of the anesthetic laryngoscope at intubation. The vocal fold tends to lie in a lower plane on the side of the injury.

ANSWERS

TRUE OR FALSE QUESTIONS

1. T	14. F	27. T	40. T
2. T	15. F	28. F	41. F
3. F	16. T	29. F	42. T
4. F	17. F	30. T	43. F
5. F	18. F	31. F	44. T
6. T	19. F	32. T	45. T
7. T	20. F	33. F	46. F
8. T	21. T	34. F	47. F
9. F	22. F	35. T	48. T
10. T	23. T	36. F	49. F
11. F	24. T	37. T	50. F
12. T	25. T	38. F	
13. T	26. F	39. T	

SINGLE BEST ANSWER QUESTIONS

51. c	64. c	77. d	90. b
52. c	65. b	78. a	91. d
53. c	66. c	79. c	92. d
54. d	67. a	80. b	93. a
55. a	68. c	81. c	94. b
56. d	69. c	82. c	95. a
57. d	70. b	83. c	96. b
58. a	71. d	84. d	97. b
59. c	72. b	85. a	98. a
60. b	73. a	86. b	99. a
61. d	74. c	87. d	100. c
62. c	75. b	88. d	
63. a	76. b	89. a	

SUGGESTED READINGS

1. Bhojani RA, Rosenbaum DH, Dikmen E, et al. Contemporary assessment of laryngotracheal trauma. *J Thorac Cardiovasc Surg.* 2005;130:426-432.
2. Casper JK, Clark WR, Kelley RT, et al. Laryngeal and phonatory status after burn/inhalation injury: a long-term follow-up study. *J Burn Care Rehabil.* 2002;23:235-243.
3. Danic D, Prgomet D, Sekelj A, et al. External laryngotracheal trauma. *Eur Arch Otorhinolaryngol.* 2006;263:228-232.
4. Erdoğan E, Eroğlu E, Tekant G, et al. Management of esophagogastric corrosive injuries in children. *Eur J Pediatr Surg.* 2003;13:289-293.
5. Esteller-Moré E, Ibañez J, Matiñó E, et al. Prognostic factors in laryngotracheal injury following intubation and/or tracheotomy in ICU patients. *Eur Arch Otorhinolaryngol.* 2005; 262:880-883.
6. Minrad G, Kudsk KA, Croce MA, et al. Laryngotracheal trauma. *Ann Surg.* 1992;58:181-187.
7. Nouraei SAR, Ghufoor K, Patel A, et al. Outcome of endoscopic treatment of adult postintubation tracheal stenosis. *Laryngoscope.* 2007;117:1073-1079.
8. Nouraei SAR, Singh A, Patel A, et al. Early endoscopic treatment of acute inflammatory airway lesions improves the outcome postintubation airway stenosis. *Laryngoscope.* 2006;116:1417-1421.
9. Pennington CL. External trauma of the larynx and trachea: immediate treatment and management. *Ann Otol Rhinol Laryngol.* 1972;81:546-554.
10. Ramasamy K, Gumaste VV. Corrosive ingestion in adults. *J Clin Gastroenterol.* 2003;37:119-124.

16 | Aspiration and Swallowing

David M. Hogan | Tara Ramachandra | David J. Brown

TRUE OR FALSE QUESTIONS

T/F 1. The oral preparatory phase of swallowing including mastication to produce a swallow-ready bolus is not usually seen in children until after the age of 6 months.

T/F 2. The three phases of swallow—namely, oral, pharyngeal, and esophageal—are all under entirely voluntary control.

T/F 3. In children who aspirate episodically, upper gastrointestinal series, videofluoroscopic swallow studies (VFSS), and fiberoptic endoscopic evaluation (FEES) of swallowing reliably diagnose aspiration.

T/F 4. Upper gastrointestinal series provides only anatomical assessment of the esophagus, stomach, and duodenum.

T/F 5. In a child at risk of aspiration, liquid barium may be administered via nasogastric tube to enable examination of the gastrointestinal tract below the upper esophageal sphincter.

T/F 6. Modified barium swallow studies can be conducted on all children regardless of the cause of their dysphagia.

T/F 7. Laryngopharyngeal sensation thresholds have been documented as decreased in those children presenting with recurrent pneumonia, gastroesophageal reflux, or neurological disorders.

T/F 8. For children with recurrent aspiration, diagnostic evaluation of their respiratory status, including chest radiographs, bronchoscopy, and pulmonary function testing, can help establish the degree of existing lung injury.

T/F 9. Abnormalities of the nasopharynx directly affect the esophageal phase of swallowing secondary to nasal obstruction.

T/F 10. The impact of nasopharyngeal abnormalities on swallowing is similar regardless of whether the condition is unilateral or bilateral.

T/F 11. A child with unilateral congenital nasal obstruction most commonly presents at birth with cyclical respiratory distress and later develops failure to thrive.

T/F 12. All three phases of swallowing can be affected by anomalies in the oral cavity or oral pharynx.

T/F 13. Functional swallowing and breathing coordination is essential for airway protection.

T/F 14. Cleft lip and/or palate may reduce the efficiency of the child's suck by disrupting the generation of negative pressure in the oral cavity as well as the maintenance of a seal around the nipple.

T/F 15. The correction of feeding and swallowing disorders should take priority above all else to ensure appropriate growth and development of the child.

T/F 16. All children with cleft lip, despite the size, will have difficulty in oral feeding that will not resolve until surgical cleft repair.

T/F 17. Craniofacial syndromes associated with cleft lip and palate do not interfere with aspects of feeding distal to the oral cavity or oropharynx.

T/F 18. In children with isolated Pierre Robin sequence, dysphagia often resolves after airway intervention.

T/F 19. Children with Beckwith-Wiedemann syndrome often present with dysphagia secondary to macroglossia and hypotonia.

T/F 20. Pharyngeal diverticula are a commonly identified cause of dysphagia in children.

T/F 21. A plain radiograph of the neck will often identify a vallecular cyst if present.

T/F 22. The most common cause of failure to thrive, stridor, respiratory distress, or dysphagia in a child is a vallecular cyst.

T/F 23. Diagnosis of laryngomalacia is best achieved with direct laryngoscopy and bronchoscopy under general anesthetic.

T/F 24. Once diagnosed with laryngomalacia, the vast majority of children do not require surgical intervention as long as they are gaining weight and not aspirating.

T/F 25. There is an association between vallecular cyst development and gastroesophageal reflux.

T/F 26. Emesis, choking while feeding, and failure to thrive can be seen in severe laryngomalacia.

T/F 27. Supraglottoplasty is not recommended in children who have failure to thrive or respiratory distress.

T/F 28. Successful supraglottoplasty will also resolve feeding difficulty and choking in children postoperatively.

T/F 29. Evidence of aspiration or penetration of the larynx may be determined through the use of VFSS or FEES.

T/F 30. Infants with deletions of chromosome 22q11 can have associated laryngeal webs.

T/F 31. Open laryngofissure and stent placement should be used for all cases of thin laryngeal webs.

T/F 32. Incomplete formation of the septum between the esophagus and the airway results in formation of laryngeal webs.

T/F 33. VFSS are the test of choice for the diagnosis of subglottic stenosis.

T/F 34. Gastric acid and pepsin have been linked to subglottic stenosis and vocal fold granulomas.

T/F 35. Laryngeal sensation can be affected by gastroesophageal reflux.

T/F 36. Food impaction may be an indication of eosinoophilic esophagitis.

T/F 37. Eosinophilic esophagitis is confluent and therefore requires a single biopsy for diagnosis.

T/F 38. Food allergies play an important role in the pathogenesis of eosinophilic esophagitis.

T/F 39. Continuous positive airway pressure is used to treat children with symptomatic tracheomalacia.

T/F 40. The majority of children with congenital tracheal stenosis can be managed without surgical intervention.

T/F 41. VFSS yield the same diagnostic information as FEES.

T/F 42. After infancy, there is no further maturation of swallowing function.

T/F 43. An upper gastrointestinal series can be used to rule out aspiration.

T/F 44. FEES can rule out aspiration.

T/F 45. In addition to being diagnostic, the VFSS can also help determine therapeutic maneuvers.

T/F 46. VFSS can be useful in children who have food aversions and who refuse to swallow.

T/F 47. One purpose of the VFSS is to determine if the coordination and function of the aerodigestive tract supports safe bolus passage.

T/F 48. Both the VFSS and flexible laryngoscopy can evaluate vocal fold function.

T/F 49. Brainstem imaging is sometimes necessary to determine the etiology of dysphagia.

T/F 50. Nonsurgical treatment is an acceptable initial treatment for type 1 posterior laryngeal clefts.

SINGLE BEST ANSWER QUESTIONS

51. In children with tracheomalacia, which of the following presenting symptoms is the most *UNLIKELY*?
    a. Dysphonia
    b. Dysphagia
    c. Expiratory stridor
    d. Cough

52. Which of the following is *NOT* a cause of tracheomalacia?
    a. Vascular rings
    b. Innominate artery anomalies
    c. Tracheoesophageal fistula
    d. Laryngomalacia

53. Cases of tracheomalacia secondary to weak tracheal cartilages often resolve by the time the child has reached what age?

a. 6-12 months
b. 2-3 years
c. 9-10 years
d. 5-6 years

54. In a child with congenital tracheal stenosis, what percentage of children are estimated to be managed without surgery?
    a. 60%
    b. 90%
    c. 10%
    d. 40%

55. Which of the following is *NOT* required for the diagnosis of eosinophilic esophagitis?
    a. Consistent clinical symptoms
    b. Biopsies performed only after a 6 to 8 week trial of proton pump inhibition
    c. Normal stomach and duodenal biopsy specimens
    d. Five eosinophils per high-powered field on mucosal biopsy

56. Which of the following treatments is *NOT* effective in the treatment of eosinophilic esophagitis?
    a. Proton pump inhibitors
    b. Implementation of an elemental diet
    c. Systemic steroids
    d. Swallowed topical steroids

57. Symptoms of reflux in children can include all of the following *EXCEPT:*
    a. Regurgitation
    b. Cyanosis
    c. Stridor
    d. Diarrhea

58. Gastroesophageal reflux has been implicated in the etiology of all of the following clinical examination findings *EXCEPT:*
    a. Lingual tonsil hypertrophy
    b. Angioedema
    c. Arytenoid edema
    d. Subglottic edema

59. The diagnostic workup for laryngopharyngeal reflux should include all of the following *EXCEPT:*
    a. pH probe
    b. Barium esophagogram
    c. Vallecula biopsy
    d. Impedance studies

60. Type 3 posterior laryngeal clefts are defined in the Benjamin-Inglis classification by which of the following?
    a. The cleft extending into the intrathoracic trachea
    b. The cleft extending below the true vocal folds and partially through the cricoid cartilage
    c. The cleft extending into the extrathoracic trachea
    d. The cleft lying above the true vocal folds

61. In children with vocal fold paralysis, ensuring adequate nutritional intake can be achieved by all of the following *EXCEPT:*
    a. Placement of a nasogastric tube
    b. Slow-flow nipples
    c. Addition of thickening agents to either breast milk or formula
    d. FEES

62. Which of the following is the most common cause of stridor in infants?
    a. Bilateral vocal cord paralysis
    b. Laryngeal web
    c. Laryngomalacia
    d. Posterior laryngeal cleft

63. Diagnosis of laryngomalacia is best achieved by which of the following?
    a. Awake and upright flexible nasendoscopy
    b. Sleep nasendoscopy
    c. VFSS
    d. Functional magnetic resonance imaging (MRI)

64. Supraglottoplasty is the treatment of choice for severe cases of:
    a. Subglottic stenosis
    b. Laryngomalacia
    c. Posterior laryngeal cleft
    d. Vocal cord paralysis

65. In children presenting with laryngomalacia there is often an association with which other coexistent medical condition?
    a. Gastroesophageal reflux
    b. Central hypoventilation syndrome
    c. Diabetes
    d. Panhypopituitarism

66. Which of the following investigations is *LEAST* likely to reveal the diagnosis of a vallecular cyst?
    a. Lateral soft tissue plain film
    b. Flexible nasendoscopy
    c. MRI
    d. VFSS

67. Which of the following statements regarding vallecular cysts is correct?
    a. They are a common cause of failure to thrive in infants.
    b. They affect the oral preparatory phase of swallowing.
    c. Surgical management requires lateral pharyngotomy for access.
    d. Dysphagia can result from interference with the base of tongue and epiglottic movement.

68. Which of the following is *NOT* thought to contribute to dysphagia in a child with Down syndrome?
    a. Mental retardation
    b. Macroglossia
    c. Hypotonia
    d. Delayed initiation of the oral phase of swallowing

69. Which of the following syndromes has dysphagia secondary to macroglossia?
    a. Cri du chat
    b. Beckwith-Wiedemann
    c. Goldenhar
    d. Treacher Collins

70. Retrognathia and micrognathia are common to all of the following syndromes or sequences as a potential cause for dysphagia *EXCEPT:*
    a. Pierre Robin
    b. Smith-Lemli-Opitz
    c. DiGeorge
    d. Goldenhar

71. Macroglossia can contribute to feeding difficulty by all of the following mechanisms *EXCEPT:*
    a. Restricted tongue movement
    b. Interference with maintenance of adequate lip-tongue and nipple seal
    c. Difficulty controlling food in the oral cavity
    d. Xerostomia secondary to continual open mouth breathing

72. Oral cavity or oropharyngeal anomalies are unlikely to cause difficulty in which of the following phases of swallowing?
    a. Esophageal phase
    b. Pharyngeal phase
    c. Oral phase
    d. Oral preparatory phase

73. Functional swallowing depends on all of the following *EXCEPT:*
    a. Movement of the bolus from the mouth to the stomach
    b. Efficient bolus formation
    c. Glottic closure during the oral phase
    d. Coordination of breathing for airway protection

74. Cleft lip can compromise infant feeding by all of the following mechanisms *EXCEPT:*
    a. Interference with the ability of the lips and tongue to create a seal around the nipple
    b. Interference with the pharyngeal phase of swallowing
    c. Compromise of the compression phase of sucking
    d. Excessive fluid leakage

75. Which of the following syndromes is *NOT* associated with cleft lip and palate?
    a. Stickler
    b. Apert
    c. Treacher Collins
    d. Cri du chat

76. An infant presenting with cyclical cyanosis relieved by crying is likely to have which of the following diagnoses?
    a. Bilateral vocal cord paralysis
    b. Bilateral choanal atresia
    c. Beckwith-Wiedemann syndrome
    d. Pierre Robin sequence

77. If clinically you suspect an infant has congenital nasal pyriform aperture stenosis, which of the following investigations would be most useful in confirming your diagnosis?
    a. Cross-sectional imaging
    b. VFSS
    c. FEES
    d. Arterial blood gas analysis

78. Dysphagia management may include all of the following *EXCEPT:*
    a. Establishing a safe airway
    b. Supplemental nutrition
    c. Alternative feeding routes
    d. Hypoglossal nerve stimulator implantation

79. During the pharyngeal phase of swallowing, which event does *NOT* play a role?
    a. Laryngeal elevation
    b. Cessation of breathing
    c. Vocal fold abduction
    d. Relaxation of the upper esophageal sphincter

80. Which of the following statements about the esophageal phase of swallowing is correct?
    a. It is entirely volitional.
    b. It is the second phase of swallowing.
    c. It begins when the bolus enters the esophagus.
    d. It ends when the bolus passes the cricopharyngeus.

81. Breathing and swallowing share two of which of the following common conduits?
    a. Oral cavity and nasopharynx
    b. Esophagus and pharynx
    c. Oral cavity and pharynx
    d. Esophagus and nasopharynx

82. Which of the following usually provides a diagnosis in children who aspirate episodically?
    a. Upper gastrointestinal series
    b. VFSS

c. FEES

d. None of the above

83. Upper gastrointestinal series do *NOT* provide anatomical or physiological information regarding which of the following anatomic sites?
    a. Stomach
    b. Oral cavity
    c. Esophagus
    d. Duodenum

84. VFSS are useful in evaluating oropharyngeal dysfunction in children because of which of the following?
    a. They simulate functional feeding as closely as possible by impregnating liquids and/or foods with barium contrast material.
    b. They accurately define anatomy distal to the cervical esophagus.
    c. They can be employed in children with behavioral issues or who are unwilling to comply with examination.
    d. They provide important information regarding swallowing physiology despite the lack of anatomic information.

85. FEES is useful in all of the following situations *EXCEPT*:
    a. Children with vocal fold dysfunction
    b. Children with the inability to manage oral secretions
    c. Children with a decreased level of consciousness
    d. Children who are nonoral feeders

86. Standardized evaluation of mucosal responsiveness to sensory input is best achieved using which of the following investigations?
    a. FEES touching the adjacent mucosa
    b. Modified barium swallow
    c. FEES with sensory air pulse testing
    d. VFSS

87. Elevated thresholds of laryngopharyngeal sensation have been documented in all of the following conditions *EXCEPT*:
    a. Recurrent pneumonia
    b. Gastroesophageal reflux
    c. Posterior laryngeal cleft
    d. Neurologic disorders

88. During which phase of swallowing does breathing stop?
    a. Oral preparatory
    b. Oral
    c. Pharyngeal
    d. Esophageal

89. The first priority in evaluating children with aerodigestive disorders is to:
    a. Check for a tongue tie
    b. Rule out laryngomalacia
    c. Assure they have a coordinated suck-swallow-breathe pattern
    d. Ensure a safe airway

90. The common conduit for breathing and swallowing is:
    a. The nasal cavity
    b. The pharynx
    c. The larynx
    d. The nasopharynx

91. Which of the following factors influences swallowing maturation?
    a. Puberty
    b. Sensory inputs
    c. Gastroesophageal reflux
    d. Breastfeeding

92. Which of the following is most likely to increase a child's risk for dysphagia?
    a. Gastroesophageal reflux
    b. Esophageal achalasia
    c. Pyloric stenosis
    d. Trisomy 21

93. Which of the following can help determine the extent of lung injury from chronic aspiration?
    a. High-resolution computed tomography (CT)
    b. Lipid-laden macrophages test
    c. Ciliary biopsy
    d. Impedance testing

94. Infants born with bilateral choanal atresia may have cyclical cyanosis that is alleviated by which of the following?
    a. Placing a 6-Fr suction catheter in the nose
    b. Nasal cannula with oxygen
    c. Suctioning the nose
    d. Crying

95. Before orally feeding a patient with a congenital oral cavity anomaly, which of the following is the most important first step?
    a. Order an MRI of the head and neck.
    b. Order a VFSS.
    c. Request a consultation for a surgical gastric tube.
    d. Address any airway concerns.

96. Isolated cleft palate contributes to dysphagia by which of the following mechanisms?
    a. Not allowing the lips to create a seal around the nipple
    b. Interfering with the compression phase of feeding
    c. Preventing adequate negative pressure
    d. Drainage from the nasal cavity into the oral cavity

97. Which of the following swallowing phases does laryngomalacia alter?
    a. Oral
    b. Oral preparatory
    c. Esophageal
    d. Pharyngeal

98. Which of the following is the mechanism of dysphagia in children with retrognathia?
    a. Abnormal tooth development
    b. Overbite deformity
    c. Retrodisplacement of the tongue
    d. Abnormal dental occlusion

99. Which of the following is correct about laryngomalacia?
    a. It is caused by gastroesophageal reflux disease (GERD).
    b. Ninety percent of children require surgical intervention.
    c. CO_2 laser supraglottoplasty resolves dysphagia associated with laryngomalacia.
    d. Failure to thrive is an indication to perform a supraglottoplasty.

100. A posterior laryngeal cleft is diagnosed by which of the following?
    a. VFSS
    b. FEES
    c. Direct laryngoscopy
    d. Flexible laryngoscopy

CORE KNOWLEDGE

BACKGROUND

- The process of swallowing is generally separated into three phases: oral, pharyngeal, and esophageal.
  - *Oral phase:* Food is converted to a ball, or bolus, that is pushed to the back of the mouth. After 6 months of age, solid foods are chewed during the *oral preparatory phase.*
  - *Pharyngeal phase:* Tongue base and pharyngeal muscles propel boluses through the pharynx to the relaxed upper esophageal sphincter. Simultaneous airway protection is achieved by elevation of the velum, cessation of breathing, elevation of the larynx, and adduction of vocal folds.
  - *Esophageal phase:* The bolus passes through the esophagus and into the stomach.
- The progression from primitive swallowing reflexes of infancy to voluntary biting, chewing, and bolus formation is dependent on appropriate cognitive, sensory, and neurological developments.
- There are two primary functions of swallowing.
  - To protect the airway while directing food, liquid, and oral secretions from the mouth to the stomach
  - To ensure adequate nutrition for normal growth and development

EVALUATION OF INFANTS AND YOUNG CHILDREN WITH SUSPECTED DYSPHAGIA

- Clinical evaluation includes a thorough history and physical examination.
- Instrumental evaluation
  - Upper gastrointestinal series
    - Procedure: Liquid barium is administered orally or by nasogastric tube.
    - Assess anomalies distal to the oropharynx, such as malrotation or gastrointestinal obstruction.
    - Screen for oropharyngeal structure and function.
  - VFSS
    - Also known as *modified barium swallow study*
    - Procedure: Barium-impregnated food or liquid is ingested to simulate functional feeding
    - Evaluation of oropharyngeal dysphagia (oral cavity, pharynx, and cervical esophagus)
      - Anatomy/structure
      - Coordination, safety, and efficiency of bolus passage
    - May also identify strategies to improve efficiency and safety
  - FEES
    - Procedure: Extended nasopharyngolaryngoscopic evaluation
    - Evaluation of nasopharynx, oropharynx, and larynx during active swallowing, spontaneous swallowing, and phonation
    - Useful in children unable to tolerate VFSS, in nonoral feeders, and in those with dysfunctional vocal folds
    - FEES with sensory air pulse testing (FEES-ST) involves calibrated air pulses to assess sensory input responsiveness. Thresholds can be elevated in children with neurologic disorders, GERD, and recurrent pneumonia.
- Additional testing may include skull base or spine imaging, pulmonary function tests, chest radiographs, CT, and gastrointestinal tract endoscopy or bronchoscopy when indicated.

FOUR ANATOMIC SITES OF DYSPHAGIA

- Nose and nasopharynx (Figures 16-1 and 16-2)
  - Obstruction will affect oral and pharyngeal phases of deglutition, resulting in feeding difficulties during infancy.
  - Causes include piriform aperture stenosis, midface hypoplasia, septal deviation, rhinitis, congenital midline nasal masses (nasal dermoid, encephaloceles, and gliomas), nasal tumors, adenoid hypertrophy, and choanal atresia.
  - Bilateral nasal obstruction tends to be more severe than unilateral obstruction and will usually present shortly after birth with respiratory distress with cyclic cyanosis that ends with crying spell. Affected children will often feed ineffectively due to frequent coughing and choking.
  - Unilateral obstruction can present later in life with rhinorrhea or congestion.
  - Clinical assessment usually begins with an attempt to pass a 6-Fr nasal suction catheter or with flexible fiberoptic endoscopy. If preliminary evaluation suggests obstruction, then imaging can be considered.
- Oral cavity and oral pharynx (Figure 16-3; see Figure 16-1)
  - Obstruction may affect oral and pharyngeal phases of swallowing with the possibility of obstructing the upper airway.
  - First, assess and stabilize respiratory issues, then initiate evaluations for suspected dysphagia.
  - Effective swallowing depends on efficient formation of a food bolus, followed by bolus movement from the mouth to the stomach, while breathing is coordinated to protect the airway.

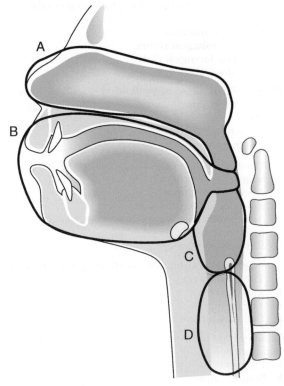

FIGURE 16-1 Four anatomic sites of dysphagia. **A,** Nose and nasopharynx. **B,** Oral cavity and oral pharynx. **C,** Hypopharynx and larynx. **D,** Trachea and esophagus. (Courtesy Johns Hopkins University, Art as Applied to Medicine.)

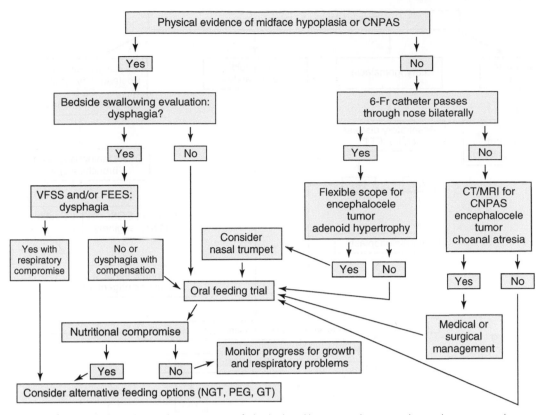

FIGURE 16-2 Evaluation and management of dysphagia with suspected nose and nasopharynx anomaly. *CNPAS,* Congenital nasal piriform aperture stenosis; *CT,* computed tomography; *FEES,* fiberoptic endoscopic evaluation of swallowing; *GT,* gastrostomy tube; *MRI,* magnetic resonance imaging; *NGT,* nasogastric tube; *PEG,* percutaneous endoscopic gastrostomy; *VFSS,* videofluoroscopic swallow studies.

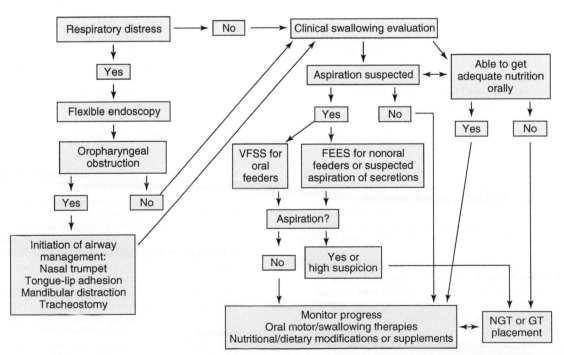

FIGURE 16-3 Evaluation and management of dysphagia with suspected oral cavity and oropharynx anomaly. *FEES,* Flexible endoscopic evaluation of swallowing; *GT,* gastrostomy tube; *NGT,* nasogastric tube; *VFSS,* videofluoroscopic swallow studies.

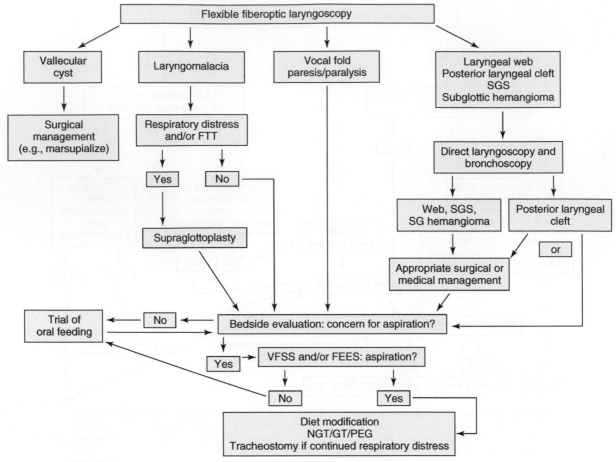

FIGURE 16-4 Evaluation and management of dysphagia with suspected hypopharynx and larynx anomaly. *FEES*, Flexible endoscopic evaluation of swallowing; *FTT*, failure to thrive; *GT*, gastrostomy tube; *NGT*, nasogastric tube; *PEG*, percutaneous endoscopic gastrostomy; *SG*, subglottic; *SGS*, subglottic stenosis; *VFSS*, videofluoroscopic swallow studies.

- Bottle feeding and breastfeeding require compression of the nipple and the creation of enough negative pressure for suction. Compromise of either action can decrease the efficiency of feeding.
  - Cleft lip and palate
    - Cleft lip: Lips and tongue cannot create an adequate seal around the nipple, inhibiting compression and allowing leakage of milk.
    - Cleft palate: The suction phase is affected because the child cannot generate sufficient negative intraoral pressure.
    - Associated syndromes: Stickler, Treacher Collins, Apert, CHARGE (coloboma, heart disease, atresia, retardation, genital hypoplasia, ear anomalies), Pierre Robin sequence, 22q11
  - Retrognathia and micrognathia result in tongue retrodisplacement with potential airway and feeding problems.
    - Associated syndromes: Goldenhar, Treacher Collins, Smith-Lemli-Opitz, and cri du chat
    - In Pierre Robin sequence, palatal and tongue base obstruction arise from elongation of the vellum and pharynx collapse.
  - Macroglossia inhibits appropriate lip-tongue and nipple seal, and it may also restrict tongue movement.
    - Associated syndromes: Down, Beckwith-Wiedemann

- Hypopharynx and larynx (Figure 16-4; see Figure 16-1)
  - Anomalies may affect pharyngeal and esophageal phases of swallowing.
  - Flexible fiberoptic laryngoscopy is usually performed as an initial evaluation.
  - *Vallecular cysts:* Mucous retention cysts that may result in respiratory distress and dysphagia due to retroflexion of the epiglottis. The lateral flow of food may also be inhibited. Management involves marsupialization of the cyst.
  - *Laryngomalacia:* Collapse of epiglottis and/or arytenoids during inspiration is the most common cause of stridor in infants. Associated feeding difficulties include emesis, failure to thrive, and choking episodes. There is a strong association with reflux, leading many clinicians to empirically prescribe antireflux agents. While more than 90% of patients are treated nonsurgically, supraglottoplasty may be indicated for children with respiratory distress or failure to thrive.
  - *Vocal fold paralysis:* After establishing diagnosis with flexible fiberoptic laryngoscopy, VFSS and/or FEES can identify penetration or aspiration. Different feeding methods and liquid viscosities can also be assessed.
  - *Laryngeal webs:* Infants may have hoarseness, a weak cry, distress, aphonia, stridor, or dysphagia. Webs may be managed by simple endoscopic lysis or open laryngofissure with keel placement for thicker webs.

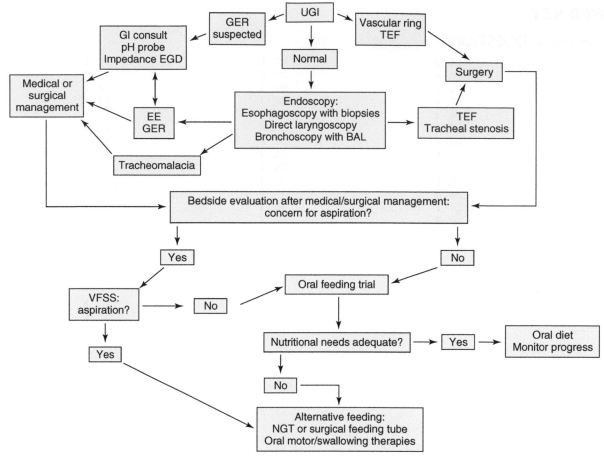

FIGURE 16-5 Evaluation and management of dysphagia as a result of suspected tracheal or esophageal anomaly. *BAL,* Bronchoalveolar lavage; *EE,* eosinophilic esophagitis; *EGD,* esophagogastroduodenoscopy; *GER,* gastroesophageal reflux; *GI,* gastrointestinal; *NGT,* nasogastric tube; *TEF,* tracheoesophageal fistula; *UGI,* upper gastrointestinal series; *VFSS,* videofluoroscopic swallow studies.

- *Posterior laryngeal clefts:* There are four types of clefts, which range in severity from interarytenoid to intrathoracic trachea. Infants present with aspiration, choking, stridor, chronic cough, and failure to thrive. Direct laryngoscopic probing of the interarytenoid area confirms diagnosis. Chest CT can help assess chronic lung damage.
- *Subglottic stenosis:* Increased work of breathing may result in reflux, aspiration, and worsening narrowing. After a stable airway is achieved, bedside swallow, VFSS, or FEES can be performed.
- Trachea and esophagus (Figure 16-5; see Figure 16-1)
  - Anomalies may affect pharyngeal and esophageal phases of swallowing
  - GERD: Up to two-thirds of children experience symptoms, which usually resolve by age 2. Reflux in children under 2 can manifest as stridor, stertor, cyanosis, vomiting, dysphagia, and failure to thrive. GERD can blunt protective reflexes by altering laryngeal sensation.
  - *Laryngopharyngeal reflux:* Workup may include flexible fiberoptic laryngoscopy, pH probe studies, esophagram, and trial of antireflux agents.
  - *Eosinophilic esophagitis:* Inflammation of the esophageal mucosal and submucosal layers. The disease manifests in the form of feeding difficulties in infants and toddlers, abdominal discomfort and vomiting in school-age children, and dysphagia and food impaction in preadolescents. Diagnosis is made by history and by finding >15 eosinophils per high-powered field on histology. Multiple biopsies may be necessary. Food allergies have been implicated in the pathogenesis of eosinophilic esophagitis. Treatments include systemic and topical corticosteroids, elemental diets, and directed and empiric elimination diets.
  - *Congenital tracheal stenosis* may cause dysphagia due to increased work of breathing or vascular compression of the esophagus. MRI and CT along with bronchoscopy confirm the presence of complete tracheal rings and the length of the stenosis. Surgical management is usually necessary.
  - *Tracheomalacia:* Collapse of the trachea in the anterior to posterior dimension due to impaired structural integrity of the trachea. Infants present with expiratory stridor, coughing, wheezing, and occasional dysphagia. The diagnosis is made by either airway fluoroscopy or bronchoscopy. Generally, tracheomalacia from weak tracheal cartilage will resolve spontaneously in 2 to 3 years, as the airway grows. Continuous positive airway pressure may be of benefit to symptomatic infants, and surgical correction of underlying esophageal or vascular anomalies may be indicated.

ANSWER KEY

TRUE OR FALSE QUESTIONS

1. T	14. T	27. F	40. F
2. F	15. F	28. F	41. F
3. F	16. F	29. T	42. F
4. F	17. F	30. T	43. F
5. T	18. T	31. F	44. F
6. F	19. F	32. F	45. T
7. F	20. F	33. F	46. F
8. T	21. F	34. T	47. T
9. F	22. F	35. T	48. F
10. F	23. F	36. T	49. T
11. F	24. T	37. F	50. T
12. F	25. F	38. T	
13. T	26. T	39. T	

SINGLE BEST ANSWER QUESTIONS

51. a	64. b	77. a	90. b
52. d	65. a	78. d	91. b
53. b	66. a	79. c	92. b
54. d	67. d	80. c	93. a
55. d	68. a	81. c	94. d
56. a	69. b	82. d	95. d
57. d	70. c	83. b	96. c
58. b	71. d	84. a	97. d
59. c	72. a	85. c	98. c
60. c	73. c	86. c	99. d
61. d	74. b	87. c	100. c
62. c	75. d	88. c	
63. a	76. b	89. d	

SUGGESTED READINGS

1. Arvedson JC. Assessment of pediatric dysphagia and feeding disorders: clinical and instrumental approaches. *Dev Disabil Res Rev.* 2008;14(2):118-127.
2. Cooper-Brown L, Copeland S, Dailey S, et al. Feeding and swallowing dysfunction in genetic syndromes. *Dev Disabil Res Rev.* 2008;14(2):147-157.
3. Dodrill P, Gosa MM. Pediatric dysphagia: physiology, assessment, and management. *Ann Nutr Metab.* 2015;66(suppl 5):24-31.
4. Gates J, Hartnell GG, Gramigna GD. Videofluoroscopy and swallowing studies for neurologic disease: a primer. *Radiographics.* 2006;26(1):e22.
5. Gisel E. Interventions and outcomes for children with dysphagia. *Dev Disabil Res Rev.* 2008;14(2):165-173.
6. Kuperminc MN, Gottrand F, Samson-Fang L, et al. Nutritional management of children with cerebral palsy: a practical guide. *Eur J Clin Nutr.* 2013;67(suppl 2):S21-S23. Erratum in: *Eur J Clin Nutr.* 2014;68(2):284.
7. Lefton-Greif MA, Okelo SO, Wright JM, et al. Impact of children's feeding/swallowing problems: validation of a new caregiver instrument. *Dysphagia.* 2014;29(6):671-677.
8. Morgan AT, Dodrill P, Ward EC. Interventions for oropharyngeal dysphagia in children with neurological impairment. *Cochrane Database Syst Rev.* 2012;(10):CD009456, doi:10.1002/14651858.CD009456.pub2.
9. Prasse JE, Kikano GE. An overview of pediatric dysphagia. *Clin Pediatr (Phila).* 2009;48(3):247-251.
10. van den Engel-Hoek L, Erasmus CE, van Hulst KC, et al. Children with central and peripheral neurologic disorders have distinguishable patterns of dysphagia on videofluoroscopic swallow study. *J Child Neurol.* 2014;29(5):646-653.

Sleep Apnea and Snoring | 17

Derek J. Lam

TRUE OR FALSE QUESTIONS

DIAGNOSIS OF OBSTRUCTIVE SLEEP APNEA (OSA)

T/F 1. In addition to loud snoring, restless sleep, and daytime somnolence, symptoms of OSA also include memory loss, depression, and nocturnal enuresis.

T/F 2. Dry mouth is a relatively infrequent symptom of OSA.

T/F 3. Headaches are more prevalent in patients with OSA than in the non-OSA population.

T/F 4. Compared with men, women with OSA are more likely to report symptoms of insomnia, heart palpitations, and migraine headaches.

T/F 5. Conditions that should be considered in the differential diagnosis for sleepiness or fatigue include cardiovascular disease, medication side effects, and endocrine dysfunction.

T/F 6. An Epworth Sleepiness Scale (ESS) score of 8 suggests significant daytime sleepiness or fatigue.

T/F 7. Electrooculography, body-position monitors, and chin electromyography are considered a standard part of an in-laboratory nocturnal polysomnogram.

T/F 8. A neck circumference of 15 inches in a nonobese man suggests an increased risk for OSA.

T/F 9. The Mueller maneuver does not reliably facilitate patient selection for surgical intervention for OSA.

T/F 10. Imaging modalities such as cephalometry, computed tomography (CT), and magnetic resonance imaging (MRI) have all been shown to reliably distinguish OSA patients from non-OSA patients.

T/F 11. Differences in craniofacial anatomy between OSA and non-OSA patients are more pronounced in the nonobese population.

T/F 12. In adults, in order to qualify as a hypopnea, a reduction in airflow of >50% must be associated with both an oxyhemoglobin desaturation and an arousal demonstrated on electroencephalography.

T/F 13. All patients undergoing bariatric surgery should have a polysomnogram done as part of a preoperative clinical evaluation.

T/F 14. Upper airway resistance syndrome is characterized by obstructive events that do not quite meet criteria as apneas or hypopneas but do result in significant gas exchange abnormalities.

T/F 15. Modified Mallampati classification class III includes a partial view of the tonsillar pillars and uvula with a full view of the soft and hard palates.

T/F 16. Objective testing is required to establish the severity of OSA.

T/F 17. Home testing with a portable monitor may be used to diagnose OSA only in patients with a high pretest likelihood of moderate to severe OSA.

T/F 18. Unattended portable monitoring may not be used to monitor response to non–continuous positive airway pressure (CPAP) treatments for OSA, including oral appliances, upper airway surgery, and weight loss.

T/F 19. A type III portable monitor cannot distinguish between sleep and awake states.

T/F 20. Based on the 2012 American Academy of Sleep Medicine scoring rules, the Respiratory Disturbance Index and the Apnea-Hypopnea Index (AHI) refer to the same parameter and can be used interchangeably.

T/F 21. In a 50-year-old man, an apnea-hypopnea index of 10 in the absence of daytime sleepiness symptoms or nighttime obstructive symptoms is sufficient for a diagnosis of OSA.

TREATMENT OF OSA

T/F 22. The presence and severity of OSA must be determined before initiating surgical therapy.

T/F 23. Bariatric surgery can significantly improve obesity-related OSA as early as 1 month after surgery.

T/F 24. The most important impact of obesity on the pathophysiology of OSA is the deposition of adipose tissue in the subcutaneous and submucosal tissues in the neck and pharynx.

T/F 25. Weight loss should be recommended for all overweight patients with OSA.

T/F 26. Greater baseline AHI and ESS scores are associated with worse adherence to CPAP treatment.

T/F 27. Autotitrating positive airway pressure (PAP) devices have shown improved adherence rates compared with CPAP devices.

T/F 28. Patients with congestive heart failure or significant lung disease such as chronic obstructive pulmonary disease are not candidates for autotitrating PAP treatment.

T/F 29. Oral appliance therapy is indicated for treatment of mild to moderate OSA in patients who do not respond to CPAP.

T/F 30. Adherence to oral appliance therapy is generally worse than adherence to CPAP.

T/F 31. Oral appliances may aggravate temporomandibular joint disease and may cause changes in occlusion and discomfort.

T/F 32. Modafinil, a central stimulant, has been approved to treat sleepiness in OSA patients who are regular users of CPAP but still experience excessive daytime sleepiness.

T/F 33. The majority of OSA patients have multilevel obstruction.

T/F 34. The anatomic site most commonly identified endoscopically as a site of obstruction is the retroglossal airway.

T/F 35. Any discussion of possible surgical treatment for OSA should also include the possibility of a tracheotomy.

T/F 36. Placement of palatal implants to help stiffen the soft palate is an effective treatment for moderate to severe OSA.

T/F 37. Intracapsular tonsillectomy or tonsillotomy has been shown to result in decreased postoperative pain and rate of postoperative hemorrhage compared with traditional subcapsular techniques.

T/F 38. Uvulopalatopharyngoplasty (UPPP) as a single procedure can reliably normalize AHI or have substantial impact on preoperative AHI values in patients with moderate to severe OSA.

T/F 39. Common complications of genioglossus advancement include numbness of the lower lip, infection, and change in occlusion.

T/F 40. The success rate of maxillomandibular advancement (MMA), often performed after other surgical interventions have failed, approaches 90%.

T/F 41. Although hospitalization is recommended for most OSA patients undergoing airway surgery, the majority of patients undergoing palatal, nasal, or mixed nasal/palatal surgeries are treated in an ambulatory setting.

T/F 42. MMA can improve polysomnography parameters comparable to CPAP in the majority of patients.

T/F 43. Inferior turbinate reduction and tonsillectomy can both reduce CPAP pressure requirements and improve CPAP utilization.

T/F 44. Nasal surgery alone can result in consistent improvement in both AHI and subjective symptoms of OSA and overall quality of life.

T/F 45. Tonsillectomy alone can be considered as a primary surgical treatment for OSA in adults noted to have significant grade 3 or 4 tonsillar hypertrophy.

T/F 46. UPPP can help improve CPAP compliance.

T/F 47. UPPP has a higher rate of success in treating mild OSA than in moderate to severe OSA.

T/F 48. In children with OSA who are treated with adenotonsillectomy, at least 20% will have some degree of residual OSA postoperatively.

T/F 49. Patients who are most likely to benefit from positional therapy tend to be younger, have a lower AHI, and are less obese.

T/F 50. Patients who are observed to have palatal complete concentric collapse during sleep endoscopy would be expected to have no improvement in AHI with hypoglossal nerve stimulation therapy.

SINGLE BEST ANSWER QUESTIONS

51. Major risk factors for OSA in adults include which of the following?
    i. Obesity
    ii. Male gender
    iii. Postmenopausal status
    iv. Age
    a. i
    b. i and ii
    c. i, ii, and iv
    d. All of the above

52. Fujita type III classification of the pattern of upper airway obstruction refers to obstruction at which region?
    a. Retropalatal region
    b. Retrolingual region
    c. Both the retropalatal and retrolingual region
    d. None of the above

53. Which of the following are common questionnaires used to screen for symptoms of OSA?
    a. Berlin questionnaire
    b. STOPBang questionnaire
    c. ESS
    d. All of the above

54. Sequelae of untreated OSA in adults include which of the following?
    i. Insulin resistance
    ii. Increased mortality
    iii. Hypertension
    iv. Dysphagia
    a. ii
    b. ii and iii
    c. i, ii, and iii
    d. All of the above

55. Which of the following muscles is considered most important in maintaining upper airway patency during sleep?
    a. Levator veli palatini
    b. Superior constrictor
    c. Tensor palatini
    d. Genioglossus
    e. No one muscle is clearly more important than the other muscles of the oral cavity and pharynx.

56. Cephalometric characteristics most strongly associated with OSA include all of the following *EXCEPT*:
    a. Decreased pharyngeal length
    b. Inferiorly positioned hyoid bone
    c. Increased soft palate thickness
    d. Longer soft palate
    e. None of the above

57. A standard nocturnal polysomnogram includes which of the following monitors?
    i. Electroencephalogram
    ii. Submental electromyogram
    iii. Tracheal microphone
    iv. Pulse oximetry
    v. Esophageal pressure monitor
    a. i, ii, and iii
    b. i, ii, and iv
    c. i, iii, and iv
    d. i, ii, iii, and iv
    e. All of the above

58. Obstructive sleep apnea syndrome is defined as which of the following?
    i. Five or more respiratory events (apneas, hypopneas, or respiratory event–related arousals) per hour
    ii. 15 or more respiratory events (apneas, hypopneas, or respiratory event–related arousals) per hour
    iii. Associated excessive daytime somnolence, waking with gasping, choking, or breath holding
    a. i only
    b. ii only
    c. i and iii
    d. (i and iii) or ii

59. "Good compliance" with positive airway pressure therapy is typically defined as which of the following?
    a. At least 3 hours per night for 4 nights per week
    b. At least 4 hours per night for 5 nights per week
    c. At least 6 hours per night for 5 nights per week
    d. At least 6 hours per night for 7 nights per week

60. Which of the following is *NOT* considered an indication for surgical treatment of OSA?
    a. Mild OSA with severe obstructing anatomy that is surgically correctable
    b. Failure of CPAP therapy
    c. Failure of positional therapy
    d. Failure of oral appliance therapy

61. Which of the following procedures can be performed in an office-based setting under local anesthetic?
    i. Radiofrequency turbinate reduction
    ii. Placement of palatal implants
    iii. Palatal radiofrequency ablation
    iv. Tongue base radiofrequency ablation
    a. i
    b. i and ii
    c. i, ii, and iii
    d. All of the above

62. Which of the following conditions is *NOT* considered high risk for OSA?
    a. Congestive heart failure
    b. Atrial fibrillation
    c. Nocturnal dysrhythmias
    d. Type 2 diabetes
    e. End-stage renal disease
    f. Preoperative for bariatric surgery

63. A 40-year-old man with a body mass index (BMI) of 35 kg/m^2 and large tonsils is hypertensive despite optimal medical management. He has a history of mild snoring and has an ESS score of 11. Which of the following is the most appropriate next step in management?
    a. Observation
    b. Home sleep testing with portable monitoring
    c. In-laboratory polysomnography
    d. Tonsillectomy followed by objective testing

64. Acceptable portable monitoring should at a minimum include which of the following?
    a. Blood oxygenation
    b. Blood oxygenation and airflow
    c. Blood oxygenation, airflow, and respiratory effort
    d. Blood oxygenation, airflow, respiratory effort, and electroencephalography

65. Which of the following is *NOT* a behavioral treatment option for OSA?
    a. Weight loss
    b. Daytime napping
    c. Avoidance of alcohol and sedatives before bedtime
    d. Positional therapy

66. Normalization of AHI with PAP therapy results in resolution of hypersomnia in all but what percentage of patients?
    a. 10%
    b. 20%
    c. 30%
    d. 50%

67. Which of the following is the minimum average nightly CPAP use necessary to achieve improvement on the Multiple Sleep Latency Test?
    a. 3 hours
    b. 4 hours
    c. 6 hours
    d. 8 hours

68. Indications for use of an oral appliance include which of the following?
    i. Mild to moderate OSA
    ii. Failed CPAP trial
    iii. Failed behavioral measures such as weight loss or positional therapy
    iv. Primary snoring with failed behavioral measures
    a. i
    b. i and ii
    c. i, ii, and iii
    d. All of the above

69. The Friedman staging system for adult OSA is based on assessments of which of the following?
    i. Tonsil size
    ii. Tongue-palate position
    iii. BMI
    iv. Neck circumference
    a. i
    b. i and ii
    c. i, ii, and iii
    d. All of the above

70. The VOTE classification system refers to which type of assessment?
    a. Drug-induced sleep endoscopy
    b. Oral cavity/oropharynx examination
    c. Cephalometry
    d. Cine MRI

71. Which of the following is a potential limitation of drug-induced sleep endoscopy?
    a. Lack of standardized sedation regimen
    b. Variability in classification of findings
    c. Poor approximation of natural sleep
    d. All of the above

72. A 38-year-old patient with a BMI of 38 kg/m^2, neck circumference of 17 inches, grade 3 tonsils, and only the base of the uvula and entire soft palate visible on oral examination is scheduled for a UPPP. According to the Friedman staging system, what is his expected prognosis for surgical success (defined as postoperative AHI <20 with ≥50% reduction from baseline)?
    a. 95%
    b. 80%
    c. 40%
    d. 8%

73. Which of the following procedures is *NOT* intended to improve the retrolingual airway?
    a. Partial midline glossectomy
    b. Lingual tonsillectomy
    c. MMA
    d. Genioglossal advancement
    e. UPPP
    f. Hyoid myotomy and suspension

74. Which of the following procedures is most likely to address dynamic lateral pharyngeal wall collapse?
    a. UPPP
    b. Tonsillectomy
    c. Z-palatoplasty
    d. Expansion sphincter pharyngoplasty

75. Which of the following is *NOT* a potential complication of UPPP?
    a. Stridor
    b. Velopharyngeal insufficiency
    c. Dysphagia
    d. Decreased CPAP compliance

76. Which of the following medical treatments is recommended for the treatment of mild OSA in children?
    a. Protriptyline
    b. Intranasal corticosteroids
    c. Mirtazapine
    d. Paroxetine

77. Regarding tonsillectomy, which of the following statements is true?
    a. As a single therapy, tonsillectomy can be recommended for treatment of OSA in the presence of tonsillar hypertrophy in adults.
    b. Adenotonsillectomy for treatment of pediatric OSA is curative in more than 90% of children.
    c. Clinical examination assessments of tonsil size correlate strongly with OSA severity.
    d. Radiofrequency tonsil reduction is recommended as a single procedure for the treatment of OSA.

78. Which of the following is the strongest risk factor associated with progression of OSA over time?
    a. Increasing age
    b. Male gender
    c. Increasing weight
    d. Severe snoring

79. Compared with CPAP, mandibular advancement devices (MADs):
    a. Are more successful at reducing AHI
    b. Are better at controlling snoring
    c. Do not require a titration procedure to be effective
    d. Show better compliance than CPAP

80. Compared with mouth breathing, unobstructed nasal breathing:
    a. Results in increased ventilation
    b. Increases upper airway dilator muscle activity
    c. Is less common in patients with OSA
    d. All of the above

81. Which of the following has *NOT* been associated with persistent OSA after adenotonsillectomy in children?
    a. Obesity
    b. Male gender
    c. Severe preoperative OSA
    d. Neuromuscular comorbidity

82. A 12-year-old boy presents with a history of heavy snoring, gasping and snorting during sleep, witnessed apneic pauses, and daytime sleepiness. Physical examination findings include a BMI in the 95th percentile for age, 3+ tonsils, modified Mallampati class III, and a large tongue. The next most appropriate step in management is:
    i. Obtain a sleep study
    ii. Nutritionist referral to discuss weight-loss strategies
    iii. Tonsillectomy

iv. CPAP trial
v. Multilevel surgery
    a. i
    b. ii
    c. iii
    d. ii and iii
    e. ii and iv
    f. ii and v

83. In an unselected population of adult patients with mild to moderate OSA, UPPP has a reported success rate (defined as >50% reduction in AHI and AHI <20 events/hour) closest to:
    a. 30%
    b. 50%
    c. 70%
    d. 90%

84. When used optimally and consistently, which of the following treatments has *NOT* demonstrated consistent efficacy in improving snoring, AHI, or sleep quality of life?
    a. Oropharyngeal exercise
    b. Tongue-retaining devices
    c. Nasal dilators
    d. Intranasal steroids

85. Which of the following factors is associated with treatment success in using MADs?
    a. Supine-dependent sleep apnea
    b. Severe OSA
    c. Male gender
    d. Increasing BMI

86. Which of the following statements is true regarding MADs?
    a. Compliance is generally better than with CPAP.
    b. Excessive salivation is a common side effect.
    c. MADs are recommended as a first-line treatment for mild to moderate OSA.
    d. All of the above are true.

87. A 55-year-old man presents with a BMI of 28 kg/m² and an AHI of 50. Drug-induced sleep endoscopy reveals complete multilevel obstruction involving both the retropalatal and retrolingual airways. Despite a patent nasal airway without significant evidence of nasal obstruction, he is intolerant of CPAP. Which of the following is likely to be the most effective surgical treatment in this patient?
    a. UPPP + radiofrequency ablation of the tongue base
    b. UPPP + hyoid suspension
    c. MMA
    d. Radiofrequency ablation of both the soft palate and the tongue base

88. During the examination of the oral cavity and oropharynx of an OSA patient, with the tongue in a relaxed neutral position within the oral cavity, the entire soft palate and the base of the uvula are visible. This corresponds to which modified Mallampati class?
    a. I
    b. II
    c. III
    d. IV

89. Weight reduction in patients with OSA has consistently resulted in which of the following changes?
    a. Reduced AHI
    b. Increased rapid eye movement sleep
    c. Reduced sleepiness
    d. All of the above
    e. None of the above

90. Positional therapy for treatment of OSA:
    a. Has not shown any efficacy in the treatment of OSA
    b. Has demonstrated short-term moderate improvement in AHI
    c. Is equivalent to CPAP therapy when patients are compliant
    d. Is more effective in older, obese patients

91. A 3-year-old girl with significant snoring, witnessed apneic pauses, gasping, and snorting undergoes a sleep study and is found to have an AHI of 4.5 with oxygen saturation nadir of 90%. What is the degree of OSA severity?
    a. Normal
    b. Mild
    c. Moderate
    d. Severe

92. The same 3-year-old girl as in question 91 is found on physical examination to have a BMI in the 99th percentile, chronic mouth breathing with significant nasal congestion and rhinorrhea, 2+ tonsils, and modified Mallampati class III. Which of the following is the next step in management?
    a. Tonsillectomy and adenoidectomy
    b. Adenoidectomy alone
    c. Tonsillectomy alone
    d. CPAP trial

93. In studies of the outcomes of adenotonsillectomy for treatment of OSA in children, what is the lowest reported rate of complete resolution of OSA?
    a. 10%
    b. 25%
    c. 50%
    d. 75%

94. What is the primary functional difference between type III and type IV portable monitors for the diagnosis of OSA?
    a. Ability to distinguish sleep and awake states
    b. Ability to accurately calculate AHI
    c. Ability to distinguish central versus obstructive events
    d. Ability to monitor muscle tone

95. Palatal implants are generally recommended for treatment of isolated palatal collapse in patients with:
    a. Snoring only
    b. Moderate to severe OSA and nonobese body habitus

    c. Mild to moderate OSA and nonobese body habitus
    d. Mild to moderate OSA regardless of body habitus

96. Regarding hyoid myotomy and suspension, which of the following statements is *INCORRECT*?
    a. Hyoid suspension has demonstrated significant improvement in AHI and daytime sleepiness.
    b. Hyoid suspension is not recommended as an isolated procedure in patients who fail CPAP and are found to have significant retrolingual collapse.
    c. Hyoid suspension is recommended in combination with other procedures as part of multilevel surgery that includes the retrolingual airway.
    d. All of the above statements are true.

97. What is the average rate of success (defined as 50% reduction in AHI, postoperative AHI <20) of multilevel surgery in adults with a broad range of OSA severity who have failed conservative treatment including CPAP?
    a. 25%
    b. 50%
    c. 66%
    d. 80%

98. What is the most common complication after MMA?
    a. Velopharyngeal insufficiency
    b. Dysphagia
    c. Malocclusion
    d. Numbness of the lower lip or chin

99. Which of the following is *NOT* a common treatment for Pierre Robin sequence?
    a. Prone positioning
    b. Tracheotomy
    c. Genioglossus advancement
    d. Mandibular distraction osteogenesis
    e. Tongue-lip adhesion

100. Laser-assisted uvuloplasty is generally recommended for treatment of which of the following?
    a. Snoring only
    b. Mild OSA in nonobese individuals
    c. Moderate OSA in nonobese individuals
    d. Laser-assisted uvuloplasty is not generally recommended for treatment of snoring or OSA.

CORE KNOWLEDGE

CLASSIFICATION AND PATHOPHYSIOLOGY OF OBSTRUCTIVE SLEEP APNEA

- Snoring affects at least 40% of men and 20% of women and often accompanies sleep-disordered breathing. However, only 2% of woman and 4% of men older than 50 years of age have symptomatic OSA. In children, the prevalence of habitual snoring has been estimated to affect up to 12% of children, and the prevalence of pediatric OSA has been estimated to range from 2% to 6%.
- Major risk factors for adult OSA include obesity, male gender, postmenopausal status, and increasing age.
- Obesity is a major risk factor for OSA due to the increased fat deposition around the neck and parapharyngeal spaces as well as effects on metabolism, ventilation, and lung volume. The most important impact of obesity is the

reduction in lung volume, which reduces the "tracheal tug" that helps to increase pharyngeal cross-sectional area and stiffens the upper airway. Reduced lung volume also worsens hypoxemia during sleep.
- Significant OSA is present in 40% of obese individuals; 70% of OSA patients are obese.
- Adult OSA is defined by five or more respiratory events per hour—apneas, hypopneas, or respiratory effort–related arousals—in association with excessive daytime somnolence; waking with gasping, choking, or breath holding; or witnessed reports of apneas, loud snoring, or both. The presence of 15 or more obstructive respiratory events per hour of sleep in the absence of sleep-related symptoms is also sufficient for the diagnosis of OSA.

- Pediatric OSA is less well-defined than in adults; however, unlike in adults, an AHI >1 is considered abnormal, particularly in the presence of significant daytime symptoms that in children can include poor concentration, attention deficit, and hyperactivity, in addition to daytime somnolence.
- Obstruction that occurs during OSA is caused by the interaction of easily collapsible upper airway structures and relaxation of the pharyngeal dilator muscles.
- In adults, the three major areas of obstruction are the nasal airway, retropalatal airway, and the retrolingual airway. In children, additional obstruction may be observed in the nasopharynx (due to adenoid hypertrophy) and at the level of the supraglottis due to sleep state–dependent laryngomalacia.
- In adults, untreated OSA has been associated with increased all-cause mortality, cardiovascular disease including hypertension, coronary artery disease, and stroke, neurocognitive difficulties, motor vehicle accidents, and insulin resistance.

OSA DIAGNOSIS

- The most common symptoms of OSA include loud snoring, restless sleep, and daytime hypersomnolence. Other symptoms include witnessed apneas, gasping/choking episodes, nocturia, morning and nocturnal headache, impaired neurocognitive function, and altered or depressed mood.
- In addition to the symptoms listed previously, patients suspected of OSA should be evaluated for secondary conditions including hypertension, stroke, heart disease, cor pulmonale, and a history of motor vehicle accidents.
- The ESS is a commonly used validated screening instrument to assess for excessive daytime somnolence. It is comprised of five daytime situations where patients are asked to score on a 0-3 scale how likely it is that they would fall asleep. A score >10 is considered positive for excessive daytime sleepiness and is suspicious for sleep disturbance.
- Physical examination findings that are associated with OSA include obese body habitus (BMI ≥30 kg/m^2), increased neck circumference (>17 inches in men, >16 inches in women), modified Mallampati score of III or IV, retro-positioned or hypoplastic mandible and maxilla, tonsillar hypertrophy, high-arched/narrow hard palate, elongated soft palate, large tongue, and nasal obstruction due to septal deviation, turbinate hypertrophy, or mucosal edema.
- In-laboratory polysomnography is the gold standard for diagnosis of OSA. This includes a minimum of seven channels including electroencephalography, electrooculography, chin electromyogram, electrocardiography, pulse oximetry, airflow monitors, and thoracic and abdominal respiratory effort monitors.
- Home testing with portable monitors may be used to diagnose OSA in patients with a high pretest likelihood of moderate to severe OSA. It is not indicated in patients with major comorbid conditions including moderate to severe pulmonary disease, neuromuscular disease, or congestive heart failure.
- Portable monitors tend to underestimate the severity of OSA due to (1) inability to detect respiratory event–related arousals that occur in the absence of gas exchange abnormalities and (2) inability to distinguish between periods of wakefulness and sleep, thus generating indices based on recording time and not true sleep time. In individuals with significant insomnia and poor sleep efficiency, this will result in significant underestimation of the apnea-hypopnea index.

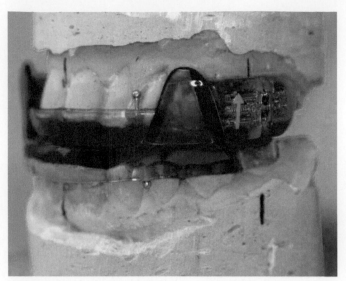

FIGURE 17-1 Mandibular advancement device for mild to moderate sleep apnea.

MEDICAL TREATMENT

- CPAP therapy is routinely recommended as a first-line treatment for OSA in adults. It acts as pneumatic splint that maintains upper airway patency by providing sufficient intraluminal pressure to prevent collapse during sleep. CPAP therapy has been shown to be highly effective in relieving significant upper airway obstruction and reducing the AHI to <5 in the majority of patients, thus improving quality of life and the risk of long-term OSA sequelae. However, up to 50% of adults are noncompliant with the standard CPAP usage recommendation of at least 4 hours per night for 5 to 7 nights per week.
- Weight reduction should be recommended for all overweight OSA patients and should be combined with a primary treatment for OSA because of the low compliance and success rate with dietary programs.
- Positional therapy can be effective in reducing AHI but has poor long-term compliance. It tends to be most effective in younger, less obese individuals with mild OSA.
- MADs reposition the lower jaw forward and downward during sleep, thus widening the upper airways. They are recommended as a first-line treatment for patients with mild to moderate OSA and for patients who do not tolerate CPAP. Although not as efficacious as CPAP, patients generally have higher compliance rates with MADs than with CPAP (Figure 17-1).

SURGICAL TREATMENT

- The most important factor contributing to the success of any surgical intervention for OSA is determination of the location and pattern of obstruction during sleep and careful planning to specifically address these areas. In other words, one must select the correct procedure to perform on the correct patient.
- Physical examination should include an assessment of tonsil size, relative tongue and palate position, shape of the palate and uvula, and degree of oropharyngeal crowding. The modified Mallampati classification system is a common method of categorizing physical examination findings (Figure 17-2). Awake flexible nasopharyngoscopy and drug-induced sleep endoscopy are often used to identify the specific anatomic sites and patterns of obstruction.

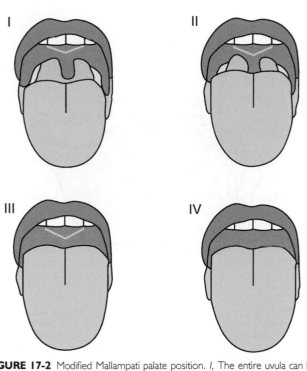

FIGURE 17-2 Modified Mallampati palate position. *I,* The entire uvula can be seen with the tongue at rest. *II,* A partial view of the uvula is seen. *III,* Only the soft and hard palate can be seen. *IV,* Only the hard palate can be seen.

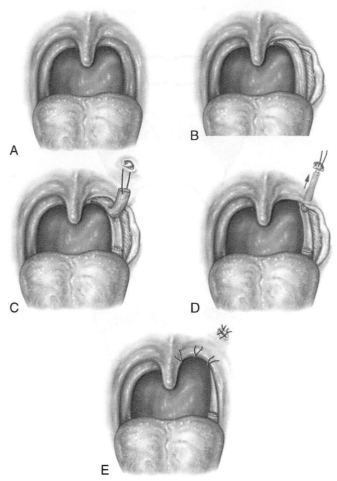

FIGURE 17-3 Expansion sphincter pharyngoplasty technique. **A,** Preoperative view of the oropharynx. **B,** Exposure of the palatopharyngeus (vertical fibers). **C,** Elevation of the palatopharyngeus. **D,** Rotation and tunneling of the palatopharyngeus toward the hamulus. **E,** Suture suspension and approximation. (From Woodson BT, Sitton M, Jacobowitz J. Expansion sphincter pharyngoplasty and palatal advancement pharyngoplasty: airway evaluation and surgical techniques. *Oper Techn Otolaryngol* 2012;23:6.)

- Anatomic targets for surgical treatment include the nasal airway, the palate, the lateral oropharynx, the hypopharynx or base of tongue, and the supraglottis.
- Definitions of surgical success are variable across studies, which is one of the challenges of comparing outcomes of surgical interventions. However, the most commonly described definition of surgical success is a reduction in preoperative AHI by >50% and a postoperative AHI <20 events/hour.
- Nasal procedures commonly used to treat OSA include septoplasty, inferior turbinate reduction, and rhinoplasty or nasal valve surgery. Although nasal surgery alone has not been shown to be curative of OSA, it has demonstrated consistent improvement in subjective symptoms of OSA and quality of life and can also be useful in improving CPAP compliance.
- UPPP traditionally refers to a procedure meant to shorten and elevate the soft palate. However, there have been many variations of the originally described procedure that in general have involved less resection of tissue and more repositioning, all with a goal of increasing the dimension of the retropalatal airway and stabilizing the lateral pharyngeal walls. More recent variations include the Z-palatoplasty, expansion sphincter pharyngoplasty, lateral pharyngoplasty, and palatal advancement. As a single procedure, UPPP works best in patients with primarily retropalatal obstruction and has an overall success rate in unselected populations with mild to moderate OSA of ~50% (Figure 17-3).
- Tonsillectomy with or without adenoidectomy is the recommended first-line treatment in pediatric OSA and is also commonly performed in adult OSA patients with obvious tonsillar hypertrophy. In children, adenotonsillectomy has been shown to be ~80% effective in curing OSA; however, many studies have demonstrated a substantial proportion of patients with residual OSA after adenotonsillectomy.
- There is a wide range of hypopharyngeal procedures, including lingual tonsillectomy, midline posterior glossectomy, genioglossus advancement, genioglossus suspension, hyoid myotomy and suspension, and radiofrequency ablation of the tongue base. As with UPPP, many variations and combinations of these procedures have been described, and they are often used as part of a strategy of multilevel surgery. Success rates for individual procedures vary widely or have been poorly studied, but most of these treatments have demonstrated significant though limited improvements in AHI and subjective symptoms of OSA and tend to be more successful in younger, less obese patients (Figure 17-4).
- MMA and mandibular distraction are two procedures that involve expansion of the bony framework of the upper airway rather than manipulation or ablation of soft tissue. MMA in particular has been shown to be highly effective in treating OSA that is refractory to more conservative medical or surgical treatments, with success rates similar to CPAP (Figure 17-5).
- Tracheotomy is a definitive treatment for OSA, effectively bypassing the upper airway structures that can cause obstruction and thereby eliminating OSA. However, it cannot be used to treat central hypoventilation syndromes without the use of supplemental positive pressure ventilation.

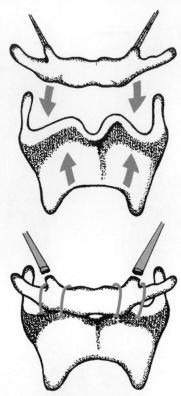

FIGURE 17-4 The modified hyoid myotomy and suspension procedure. (From Riley R, Powell N, Guilleminault C. Obstructive sleep apnea and the hyoid: a revised surgical procedure. *Otolaryngol Head Neck Surg* 1994;111:717.)

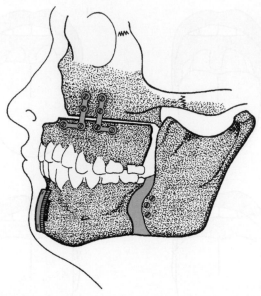

FIGURE 17-5 The maxillomandibular advancement procedure, lateral view. Le Fort I maxillary osteotomy with rigid plate fixation and a bilateral sagittal split mandibular osteotomy with bicortical screw fixation. The advancement is at least 10 mm. A previous genioglossal advancement is shown. (From Powell NB, Riley RW, Guilleminault C. The hypopharynx: upper airway reconstruction in obstructive sleep apnea syndrome. In Fairbanks DNF, Fujita A, eds. *Snoring and Obstructive Sleep Apnea,* 2nd ed. New York: Raven Press; 1994:205.)

ANSWERS

TRUE OR FALSE QUESTIONS

1. T	14. F	27. T	40. T
2. F	15. F	28. T	41. T
3. F	16. T	29. T	42. T
4. T	17. T	30. F	43. T
5. T	18. F	31. T	44. F
6. F	19. T	32. T	45. T
7. T	20. F	33. T	46. F
8. F	21. T	34. F	47. F
9. T	22. T	35. T	48. T
10. F	23. T	36. F	49. T
11. T	24. F	37. T	50. T
12. F	25. F	38. F	
13. T	26. F	39. F	

SINGLE BEST ANSWER QUESTIONS

51. d	64. c	77. a	90. b
52. b	65. b	78. c	91. b
53. d	66. b	79. d	92. a
54. c	67. c	80. d	93. b
55. d	68. d	81. b	94. c
56. a	69. c	82. b	95. c
57. d	70. a	83. b	96. b
58. d	71. d	84. c	97. c
59. b	72. c	85. a	98. d
60. c	73. e	86. d	99. c
61. d	74. d	87. c	100. d
62. e	75. a	88. b	
63. b	76. b	89. d	

SUGGESTED READINGS

1. Randerath WJ, Verbraecken J, Andreas S, et al. Non-CPAP therapies in obstructive sleep apnoea. *Eur Respir J.* 2011;37:1000-1028.

2. Epstein LJ, Kristo D, Strollo PJ, et al. Clinical guideline for the evaluation, management and long-term care of obstructive sleep apnea in adults. *J Clin Sleep Med.* 2009;5(3): 263-276.

3. Aurora RN, Casey KR, Kristo D, et al. Practice parameters for the surgical modifications of the upper airway for obstructive sleep apnea in adults. *Sleep.* 2010;33(10): 1408-1413.

4. Qaseem A, Dallas P, Owens DK, et al. Diagnosis of obstructive sleep apnea in adults: a clinical practice guideline from the American College of Physicians. *Ann Intern Med.* 2014; 161:210-220.

5. Qaseem A, Holty JE, Owens DK, et al. Management of obstructive sleep apnea in adults: a clinical practice guideline from the American College of Physicians. *Ann Intern Med.* 2013;159:471-483.

6. Caples SM, Rowley JA, Prinsell JR, et al. Surgical modifications of the upper airway for obstructive sleep apnea in adults: a systematic review and meta-analysis. *Sleep.* 2010; 33(10):1396-1407.

7. Lin HC, Friedman M, Chang HW, Gurpinar B. The efficacy of multilevel surgery of the upper airway in adults with obstructive sleep apnea/hypopnea syndrome. *Laryngoscope.* 2008;118:902-908.

8. Smith DF, Cohen AP, Ishman SL. Surgical management of OSA in adults. *Chest.* 2015;147(6):1681-1690.

9. Marcus CL, Brooks LJ, Draper KA, et al. Diagnosis and management of childhood obstructive sleep apnea syndrome. *Pediatrics.* 2012;130(3):e714-e755.

10. Marcus CL, Moore RH, Rosen CL, et al. A randomized trial of adenotonsillectomy for childhood sleep apnea. *N Engl J Med.* 2013;368(25):2366-2376.

18 Rhinosinusitis and Functional Endoscopic Sinus Surgery

Adam S. DeConde | Timothy L. Smith

TRUE OR FALSE QUESTIONS

RHINOSINUSITIS

T/F 1. Persistent but improving symptoms 8 days after acute rhinosinusitis (ARS) onset is an indication for antibiotics.

T/F 2. A patient presents with ARS associated with nasal discharge, upper lid edema, and associated facial cellulitis. The patient's extraocular movements, visual acuity, and color vision are all intact. There is no chemosis. This examination suggests this patient will require a surgical intervention in addition to medical therapy.

T/F 3. A patient with suspected acute invasive fungal rhinosinusitis has some pale appearing mucosa. Because there is no frank necrosis of the mucosa, no biopsy is indicated.

T/F 4. The most important prognostic variable in predicting mortality in patients with acute invasive rhinosinusitis is the reversibility of the underlying immune dysfunction.

T/F 5. A patient has thick nasal discharge at baseline, but four times per year gets infections requiring antibiotics. By definition, this patient has recurrent acute sinusitis.

T/F 6. Anatomic variations that are associated with sinus outflow tract contribute to the pathogenesis of recurrent ARS.

T/F 7. Odontogenic infections are marked by Gram-negative bacteria.

T/F 8. All odontogenic infections resolve with effective treatment of the underlying dental disease.

T/F 9. A patient with maxillary molar pain and a periapical lucency of a right third molar tooth root with isolated ipsilateral maxillary disease is best treated with maxillary antrostomy.

T/F 10. Chronic rhinosinusitis (CRS) can have wide-ranging health-related impacts, including on sleep quality and cognitive function.

T/F 11. CRS is a common problem with a prevalence of 2% to 16% in the US population.

T/F 12. The cause of CRS is unknown, but the end result is loss of epithelial barrier integrity, ciliary dysfunction, and dysbiosis.

T/F 13. Presence or absence of nasal polyposis on endoscopy is an important predictor of quality of life gains at 6 months postoperatively.

T/F 14. Polyps in Asians are predominated by eosinophilic cells; Western population polyps are marked by neutrophilic infiltrate.

T/F 15. Objective measures of disease (nasal endoscopy and imaging) do not correlate with subjective measures of disease (disease-specific quality of life instruments).

T/F 16. Asthma and CRS may be linked by a common disease process that can lead to correlation in intensity of sinonasal and pulmonary symptoms.

T/F 17. Sinusitis is almost universally part of the cystic fibrosis (CF) phenotype.

T/F 18. Aspirin-exacerbated respiratory disease (AERD) always manifests both pulmonary and sinonasal symptoms.

T/F 19. Avoidance of aspirin/nonsteroidal antiinflammatory drugs (NSAIDs) can resolve sinonasal and pulmonary manifestations of AERD.

T/F 20. Characteristic radiographic findings are the only finding unique to allergic fungal rhinosinusitis.

T/F 21. Inadvertent retention of allergic mucin during endoscopic sinus surgery for allergic fungal rhinosinusitis (AFRS) may contribute to return of disease.

T/F 22. Pediatric CRS is caused by hypertrophied adenoids.

T/F 23. Adenoidectomy resolves the symptoms in children with medically refractory CRS.

T/F 24. Adenoiditis and CRS in children is straightforward to distinguish clinically.

FUNCTIONAL ENDOSCOPIC SINUS SURGERY

T/F 25. Endoscopic sinus surgery in children is in general more conservative than that in adults.

T/F 26. The natural os of the sphenoid sinus drains laterally to the superior turbinate.

T/F 27. The roof of the maxillary sinus is at the same level as the sphenoid, which is at the same level as the maxillary natural os.

T/F 28. Resection of a destabilized middle turbinate is associated with diminished gains in quality of life.

T/F 29. The posterior wall of the maxillary sinus is a landmark for the plane of the sphenoid face.

T/F 30. The anterior ethmoid artery is protected from inadvertent injury by the bone of the skull base.

T/F 31. In the event of an intraoperative orbital hematoma, do nothing until the oculoplastics team arrives to help.

T/F 32. In the event of an orbital hematoma, lateral canthotomy and cantholysis are always sufficient to relieve intraocular pressures.

T/F 33. The thinnest bone of the skull base is the fovea ethmoidalis, and it is the most vulnerable to injury.

T/F 34. The anterior ethmoid artery must always be identified in sinus surgery through a complete ethmoid dissection.

T/F 35. Lumbar drain is the first-line therapy for an inadvertent cerebrospinal fluid (CSF) leak during endoscopic sinus surgery.

T/F 36. Functional endoscopic sinus surgery (FESS) makes a clinically significant difference in quality of life measures on 70% to 85% of patients who undergo it after failing medical therapy.

T/F 37. Revision surgery is required in <5% of patients undergoing sinus surgery.

T/F 38. Retained ethmoid cells, middle turbinate lateralization, stenosis of prior sinus opening, and bony remodeling leading to stenosis can all result in the need for revision surgery.

T/F 39. Balloon dilation catheters have been tested head-to-head against FESS and deliver comparable outcomes.

T/F 40. The medial extent of the Draf IIa frontal sinusotomy is the nasal septum.

T/F 41. The lateral extent of a Draf III neoostium is the lacrimal sac and periosteum of the radix.

T/F 42. It takes 1 year for Draf III neoostium to stabilize in size.

T/F 43. Pressurized irrigations are an effective way to reach the frontal and sphenoid sinuses in an unoperated patient.

T/F 44. High-volume (>100 cc) irrigations are the most effective mechanism to deliver topical therapies to the frontal recess postoperatively.

T/F 45. Patients who elect surgical therapy over continued medical therapy after having failed a course of medical therapy are approximately three times more likely to resolve facial pain/pressure, thick nasal discharge, and nasal airway obstruction.

T/F 46. Alternating between a transethmoid approach and a transnasal approach to the sphenoid sinus can destabilize the middle turbinate.

T/F 47. Resection of the bottom half of the superior turbinate to access the natural os of the sphenoid spares the olfactory mucosa of the superior turbinate.

T/F 48. Anterograde resection of the uncinate is less likely to lead to inadvertent orbital injury than retrograde resection of the uncinate.

T/F 49. The Draf I procedure entails removal of all cells from the frontal recess.

T/F 50. Aggressive use of the backbiter to bring a maxillary antrostomy can lead to injury of the nasolacrimal duct.

SINGLE BEST ANSWER QUESTIONS

51. Olfactory epithelium is contained in all of the following structures *EXCEPT*:
    a. Superior 1 cm of the septal mucosa
    b. Superior 1 cm of the middle turbinate
    c. Superior half of the superior turbinate
    d. Mucosa covering the fovea ethmoidalis

52. Resection of the middle turbinate is associated with which of the following?
    a. Increased rates of lateralization
    b. Increased rates of synechiae formation
    c. Faster return of nasal polyposis
    d. No difference in quality of life measures compared with patients with no indication for resection

53. All of the following symptoms of patients with CRS who have failed broad-spectrum antibiotics and steroid treatment are more likely to improve compared with patients who continue medical management *EXCEPT*:
    a. Thick nasal discharge
    b. Facial pain/pressure
    c. Olfaction
    d. Nasal airway obstruction

54. All of the following signs and symptoms imply a postseptal orbital infection *EXCEPT*:
    a. Chemosis
    b. Lid cellulitis and edema
    c. Gaze restriction
    d. Diminished perception of color

55. A type 1 diabetic patient presents with diabetic ketoacidosis and nasal congestion and facial pain/pressure. Imaging shows mucosal thickening of the maxillary and ethmoid sinuses. All bone is intact and there are no orbital or neurologic symptoms. On examination there is some pallor to the head of the right middle turbinate. What is the best next step in management?
    a. Serial examinations
    b. Biopsy of questionable tissue with frozen section analysis
    c. Biopsy of questionable tissue with rushed permanent section analysis with fungal staining
    d. Emergency trip to the operating room for exenteration of the sinonasal cavity

56. AFRS potentially overlaps with CRS without nasal polyps (CRSwNP) in all of the following ways *EXCEPT*:
    a. Presence of thick mucus
    b. Presence of polyposis
    c. Characteristic findings on computed tomography (CT) imaging
    d. Presence of fungi on staining

57. A patient with a history of prior endoscopic sinus surgery presents after return of symptoms and failure of broad-spectrum antibiotics and systemic steroids. The patient elects revision surgery. On preoperative imaging all sinuses are open except for bilateral severe osteoneogenesis obstructing the frontal recesses. The most appropriate endoscopic treatment option for this option includes which of the following?
    a. Balloon dilation of the bilateral frontal recesses
    b. Draf I
    c. Draf IIa
    d. Draf IIb
    e. Draf III

58. A patient with facial pain/pressure, nasal airway obstruction, and intermittent clear rhinorrhea presents

for evaluation of sinusitis. The patient has had a CT scan of the sinuses during a recent flare. The scan is remarkable only for a deviated septum and turbinate hypertrophy. The sinuses are clear, but there is a concha bullosa. The patient tolerates nasal endoscopy well. The patient reports having started antibiotics 2 days prior to the CT scan. The patient would like surgery to alleviate the facial pain/pressure and rhinorrhea. The patient is not particularly bothered by the nasal airway obstruction. What is the most appropriate next step?
a. Allergy evaluation and headache evaluation
b. Clinic balloon sinuplasty
c. Balloon sinuplasty in the operating room
d. FESS with septoplasty and inferior turbinate reduction
e. Septoplasty, concha bullosa resection, and bilateral inferior turbinate reduction

59. After total ethmoidectomy clear fluid is issuing from somewhere on the skull base. What is the next best step in management?
a. Pack the ethmoid cavity tightly with Vaseline gauze and call the neurosurgery department to place a lumbar drain intraoperatively.
b. Manage conservatively and see if the postoperative inflammatory response leads to sealing of the leak.
c. Perform a targeted endoscopic repair of the leak.
d. Raise a nasoseptal flap and cover the anterior skull base with it on the side of the leak.

60. During a revision endoscopic sinus surgery the anterior ethmoid artery is inadvertently transected and retracts into the orbit. The patient's ipsilateral eye becomes proptotic, ecchymotic, and tense within minutes. Which of the following interventions should be performed by the sinus surgeon immediately?
a. Lateral canthotomy
b. Lateral cantholysis
c. Endoscopic medial orbital wall decompression if eye continues to be tense after a and b
d. All of the above

61. A patient with CRS undergoes revision endoscopic sinus surgery. The preoperative scan shows nasal polyposis and osteoneogenesis. The final pathology reveals a high degree of tissue eosinophilia (>10/high-powered field). All of the following are risk factors for failure to make an improvement in quality of life EXCEPT:
a. High tissue eosinophilia
b. Presence of nasal polyps
c. Osteoneogenesis on imaging
d. History of prior sinus surgery

62. All of the following have been associated with the need for revision surgery EXCEPT:
a. Retained ethmoid cells
b. Lateralized middle turbinate
c. Retained uncinate process
d. Maxillary antrostomy posterior to the natural os
e. Large antrostomies
f. Stenotic sinusotomies

63. Patients with AERD have presence of asthma without CRS at what frequency?
a. 0% to 10%
b. 30% to 40%
c. 60% to 70%
d. 90% to 100%

64. After adenoidectomy what percentage of children with CRS experience an improvement in CRS symptoms?
a. <5%
b. 50%

c. 75%
d. >95%

65. What percentage of patients with CRSwNP have comorbid asthma/chronic obstructive pulmonary disease?
a. 0% to 10%
b. 30% to 40%
c. 60% to 70%
d. 90% to 100%

66. There is evidence to support culture-directed topical antibiotic therapies in postoperative CRS patients with which of the following?
a. CRSwNP
b. CRSsNP
c. CF-associated CRS
d. AERD with CRS
e. Eosinophilic CRS

67. The anatomic limits of a Draf III neoostium include all of the following EXCEPT:
a. Periosteum of the radix
b. Lacrimal sac
c. Most anterior olfactory fiber
d. Most anterior insertion of the middle turbinate on the skull base

68. What is the Draf IIb medial limit?
a. Middle turbinate
b. Nasal septum
c. Medial wall of the agger nasi
d. Medial wall of the ethmoid bulla

69. Which of the following is a reliable landmark for the anterior ethmoid artery as it emerges from the orbit?
a. The posterior wall of the ethmoid bulla
b. The anterior wall of the ethmoid bulla
c. The ground lamella of the middle turbinate as it inserts laterally
d. None of the above

70. All of the following are important endoscopic landmarks for locating the natural os of the sphenoid EXCEPT:
a. 7 cm from the nasal sill
b. Posterior wall of the maxillary sinus
c. Superior turbinate
d. Height of the maxillary os
e. Floor of the orbit

71. The cardinal symptoms of CRS include all of the following EXCEPT:
a. Thick nasal discharge
b. Nasal obstruction
c. Facial pain/pressure
d. Decreased sense of smell
e. Fever

72. A patient presents with 6 days of thick nasal discharge and facial pain/pressure that was starting to improve 48 hours ago, but now has a fever and increased facial pain/pressure. What would be the next most appropriate step?
a. CT imaging of the sinuses
b. Admit for IV antibiotics
c. Outpatient treatment with oral antibiotics
d. Outpatient treatment with nasal steroid spray and sinus irrigations

73. A patient with CRS and a history of prior sinus surgery years ago presents to the clinic with persistent thick nasal discharge and mild nasal airway obstruction. Endoscopy reveals bilateral total ethmoidectomy, sphenoidotomy, and frontal sinusotomy. There are

remnant ethmoid cells bilaterally that have edema and some discharge. The left frontal recess is without edema or discharge. The right frontal recess is occluded with scar tissue. The patient is not interested in revision surgery; she just wants a refill for her steroid irrigations. In addition to a trial of topical steroids, what else should be recommended at a minimum?
a. Systemic antibiotics
b. Systemic steroids
c. Imaging to rule out mucocele of the right frontal sinus
d. Clinic balloon sinuplasty of the right frontal sinus

74. While performing a maxillary antrostomy, pulsatile bleeding is encountered from the posterior edge of the antrostomy. Packing does not stop the bleeding. What is the next best step in management of this intraoperative bleeding?
a. Suction the monopolar cautery.
b. Pack the nose and send the patient to the interventional neurology suite for internal maxillary artery embolization.
c. Ask the anesthesiology team to lower the mean arterial pressure.
d. Inject the pterygopalatine fossa with 1 cc of 1% lidocaine and 1:100,000 epinephrine.

75. During endoscopic sinus surgery for CRSwNP, a severely degenerated middle turbinate is resected. The stump of the middle turbinate initially has pulsatile bleeding but stops spontaneously. What would be the next best course of action?
a. Proceed to address the next sinus.
b. Place an epinephrine-soaked pledget over the stump to ensure it is hemostatic.
c. Cauterize the proximal stump of the middle turbinate.
d. Perform an endoscopic sphenopalatine artery ligation.

76. Which of the following are safe places to use monopolar cautery in endoscopic sinus surgery for CRS?
a. The anterior ethmoid artery
b. The posterior septal branch of the sphenopalatine artery
c. The posterior ethmoid artery
d. Proximal branches of the sphenopalatine artery
e. b and c
f. b and d

77. A patient with CF-associated sinusitis presents for revision endoscopic sinus surgery. The patient has previously undergone total ethmoidectomy and has no sphenoid disease and no frontal disease. The patient has completely scarred maxillary antrostomies. The surgical intervention should entail which of the following?
a. Frontal sinusotomies
b. Sphenoidotomies
c. Revision maxillary antrostomies
d. Megaantrostomies
e. a, b, and c
f. a, b, and d

78. A patient presents to the clinic reporting six episodes of acute sinusitis over the last year that have all resolved with as many courses of antibiotics. Imaging of the sinuses shows a narrow infundibular width and bilateral Haller cells, but no evidence of mucosal inflammation. What is the next best step in management?
a. FESS targeting the ostiomeatal complex
b. Reimaging the sinuses during the next symptom flare
c. Balloon sinuplasty
d. Long-term macrolide therapy

79. A patient with CRS who has failed medical management asks if endoscopic sinus surgery will "cure" her sinusitis. Which is the most accurate statement about the impact of endoscopic sinus surgery?
a. Less than 5% of patients require revision sinus surgery.
b. More than 85% have complete resolution of sinus-related symptoms.
c. Endoscopic sinus surgery is not an effective intervention for improving quality of life and is reserved for patients with complicated sinusitis.
d. Patients who have failed medical therapy are approximately three times more likely to resolve thick nasal discharge, facial pain/pressure, and nasal airway obstruction compared with patients continuing medical therapy.

80. A transethmoid approach to the sphenoid os is being undertaken for a patient with CRS involving all sinuses. The surgeon is having difficulty identifying the superior turbinate and may have inadvertently resected it at this point. There is a cell that seems quite posterior, but there is concern that this may be a posteriorly pneumatized ethmoid cell and not the sphenoid. The surgeon should do which of the following?
a. Measure 7 cm from the nasal sill via a transnasal route.
b. Confirm accuracy of image guidance on endonasal landmarks to help confirm location.
c. Triangulate the location of the sphenoid face using endoscopic landmarks such as the roof and posterior wall of the maxillary sinus.
d. Abandon the sphenoidotomy if the surgeon is unable to interpret the endoscopic anatomy.
e. b, c, and d

81. What nerve is at risk during aggressive debridement of maxillary intrasinus polyps?
a. Optic
b. Vidian
c. Nasopalatine
d. Infraorbital

82. A patient with CRS of the bilateral sphenoid sinuses returns after failing prior medical and surgical therapy. CT imaging of the sinuses demonstrates bony thickening throughout the recalcitrant sphenoid sinuses, and nasal endoscopy shows a completed occluded sphenoidotomy with scar tissue and a severely stenotic sphenoidotomy draining mucopurulence. What is the next best step in management?
a. Revision sphenoidotomies
b. Balloon sinuplasty
c. Allergy referral
d. Extended sphenoidotomy

83. An Onodi cell results from an exaggerated posterior pneumatization of which of the following cells?
a. Ethmoid bulla
b. Agger nasi
c. The most posterior ethmoid
d. Sphenoid sinus

84. The quality of the endoscopic visual field in general is a function of which of the following?
a. Rate of bleeding
b. Degree of polyposis
c. Volume of the sinus cavities into which blood can drip
d. Degree of osteoneogenesis
e. a and c
f. a, b, and c

85. What is the most anterior ethmoid cell called?
    a. Agger nasi
    b. Onodi
    c. Ethmoid bulla
    d. Frontobullar cell
    e. Suprabullar cell

86. The anterior ethmoid artery is best identified on coronal CT imaging of the sinuses by which of the following?
    a. The plane just posterior to the globe
    b. The "nipple sign" as the artery emerges from the lamina
    c. The point where the superior oblique and medial rectus muscles come into the same plane
    d. All of the above

87. During endoscopic sinus surgery in a surgery center for CRSwNP there is a 500 cc estimated blood loss and the frontal sinuses have yet to be addressed. The patient's past medical history is otherwise unremarkable. What is the next best step in management?
    a. Work faster to decrease blood loss.
    b. Abort the surgical plan, obtain hemostasis.
    c. Balloon any remaining unaddressed sinuses to save time.
    d. Curette out as many remnant ethmoids as possible for 15 minutes more and then obtain hemostasis.

88. A patient with CRSsNP who has failed medical management elects endoscopic sinus surgery. The patient has bilateral ethmoid disease and bilateral frontal disease. What is the most appropriate frontal sinusotomy?
    a. Draf I
    b. Draf IIa
    c. Draf IIb
    d. Draf III
    e. Balloon sinuplasty

89. A patient who has failed multiple prior surgeries for CRS, including an obliteration of the frontal sinuses, presents with frontal pain/pressure and a frontal mucocele with surrounding fat on imaging. The patient's anteroposterior distance from the frontal beak to the skull base is quite wide (2 cm). What is the next best operation in this situation?
    a. Reobliteration via a coronal approach
    b. Riedel's procedure with reconstruction of the frontal bone after the infection is clear
    c. Unobliteration of the frontal sinuses via Draf III
    d. "Above and below" coronal and Draf III approach

90. A patient with CRS and a history of bilateral Caldwell-Luc procedures many years ago presents with bilateral isolated maxillary disease. The patient currently irrigates twice daily with high-volume (100 cc) normal saline irrigations. What is the next best step in management?
    a. Bilateral megaantrostomies
    b. Long-term macrolide therapy
    c. Increase irrigation frequencies and volumes
    d. Allergy referral

91. A patient with prior CRS and a history of prior surgery presents with persistent anosmia and thick nasal discharge. On examination there is a large septal perforation that extends up to the posterior two-thirds of the cribriform plate. There has also been a complete resection of the bilateral middle and superior turbinates to the cribriform plate. There is persistent frontal disease with undissected bilateral frontal recesses. What is the likelihood the patient regains the sense of smell from a revision surgery?

    a. <1%
    b. 20%
    c. 80%
    d. >99%

92. The nasoseptal flap is based off which artery and nerve?
    a. The internal maxillary artery and greater palatine nerve
    b. The posterior septal artery and the nasopalatine nerve
    c. The greater palatine artery and the vidian nerve
    d. The posterior ethmoid artery and the posterior ethmoid nerve

93. A patient with CRS who has failed prior surgical therapy has persistent symptoms despite broad-spectrum antibiotics and systemic steroids. The patient is not happy with the degree of symptomatic control. A CT scan of the sinuses demonstrates retained ethmoid cells. The patient was told that she has a dysbiosis of her sinuses and intense inflammation of the sinuses. What is the next best step in management?
    a. Add baby shampoo to irrigations.
    b. Add manuka honey to irrigations.
    c. Add xylitol to irrigations.
    d. Increase volume of irrigations to 500 cc.
    e. Perform a completion ethmoidectomy.

94. What is the likelihood that endoscopic sinus surgery completely resolves facial pain/pressure in patients with CRS?
    a. 10%
    b. 40%
    c. 60%
    d. 90%

95. What is the likelihood that endoscopic sinus surgery completely resolves thick nasal discharge in patients with CRS?
    a. 10%
    b. 40%
    c. 60%
    d. 90%

96. What is the likelihood that endoscopic sinus surgery completely resolves nasal airway obstruction in patients with CRS?
    a. 10%
    b. 40%
    c. 60%
    d. 90%

97. What is the likelihood that a patient with medically refractory CRS makes a clinically significant improvement in quality of life after endoscopic sinus surgery?
    a. 25%
    b. 50%
    c. 75%
    d. >95%

98. Nationwide, what is the likelihood that a patient undergoing endoscopic sinus surgery experiences an orbital injury?
    a. 1:100,000
    b. 1:10,000
    c. 1:1000
    d. 1:100

99. Nationwide, what is the likelihood that a patient undergoing endoscopic sinus surgery experiences an inadvertent CSF leak?
    a. 1:100,000
    b. 1:10,000
    c. 1:1000
    d. 1:100

100. Nationwide, what is the likelihood that a patient undergoing endoscopic sinus surgery requires a blood transfusion from endoscopic sinus surgery?
    a. 1:100,000
    b. 1:10,000
    c. 1:1000
    d. 1:100

CORE KNOWLEDGE

RHINOSINUSITIS

Acute Rhinosinusitis

- ARS is defined by thick nasal discharge with nasal obstruction and/or facial pain/pressure that lasts for <4 weeks. The key to management of acute rhinosinusitis is differentiating between acute bacterial rhinosinusitis, which benefits from antimicrobial therapy, and viral acute rhinosinusitis, which is not impacted by antimicrobial therapy. No reliable symptoms or physical examination findings can effectively differentiate between a viral and bacterial etiology. Therefore, antibiotic treatment should be instituted if the symptoms of acute rhinosinusitis do not begin to improve after 7 days or after improving the symptoms begin to worsen again (a "double worsening").

- Although the vast majority of cases of ARS will resolve spontaneously, ARS is defined by extension of the infection beyond the anatomy of the sinuses and is a medical emergency. The original Chandler classification described the spread of disease through progressive stages, each with graver consequences, and included preseptal cellulitis, orbital cellulitis, subperiosteal abscess, orbital abscess, and cavernous sinus thrombosis. Early recognition of infection that extends posterior to the orbital septum is critical, because vision- or life-threatening infection may progress despite maximal medical therapy. Signs and symptoms of chemosis, proptosis, gaze restriction, decreased visual acuity, color vision defect, and afferent pupillary defect all imply a postseptal infection. Forehead swelling is associated with extension of disease through the anterior table (Figure 18-1), and neurologic signs, meningismus, and/or decreased consciousness are signs of intracranial extension. In all cases of spread of infection beyond the sinuses, with the exception of a preseptal cellulitis, management likely will require surgical drainage of the sinuses as a part of the intervention.

- Acute invasive fungal rhinosinusitis can manifest in immunosuppressed patients and uncontrolled diabetics.

Symptoms are similar to ARS and complicated ARS and characteristically progress rapidly. Delay in diagnosis of acute invasive fungal rhinosinusitis worsens the prognosis. An aggressive diagnostic approach including early nasal endoscopy with biopsy of pale or nonviable tissue can lead to earlier diagnosis and surgical intervention, which may improve prognosis. Rapid correction of the underlying immunosuppression (if feasible) and tight control of blood glucose in diabetics is also critical and likely the most important factor in determining patient outcomes.

- Recurrent acute rhinosinusitis is defined by more than four episodes of acute rhinosinusitis in a given year. By definition, these patients have complete resolution of symptoms between acute episodes of sinusitis. Recurrent acute rhinosinusitis has been associated with anatomical factors that narrow sinus outflow tracts, including concha bullosa, septal deviation, choanal atresia and hypoplasia of the sinuses, and narrowed infundibular widths. Documented objective evidence of disease on imaging and/or endoscopy is important, and evaluating a patient during an acute flare can determine the presence of sinonasal mucosal inflammation.

- Odontogenic sinusitis results from dental sources of infections that involve the sinuses. Unilateral disease and cacosmia (related to the anaerobic bacteria common in odontogenic infections) are characteristic of odontogenic sinusitis, and antibiotic coverage should include coverage of oral flora. Although odontogenic infections always begin in the maxillary sinuses, these infections can ascend to involve other sinuses. Odontogenic sinusitis may resolve with definitive treatment of the underlying dental disease, but spread beyond the maxillary sinus may result in infection and inflammation independent of the dental status. Likewise, persistent maxillary sinusitis despite adequate medical and/or surgical treatment can be associated with a persistent underlying dental disease.

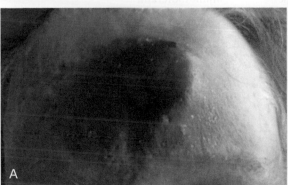 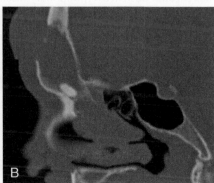

FIGURE 18-1 A, A patient presents with sinusitis and swelling of the forehead. **B,** Imaging demonstrates loss of the anterior table and bony remodeling narrowing the frontal outflow tract.

Chronic Rhinosinusitis

- CRS is defined by >12 weeks of two or more of the following symptoms: mucopurulent drainage, nasal obstruction/congestion, facial pain/pressure/fullness, or decreased sense of smell, along with documented evidence of inflammation of the sinuses on examination (purulence or polyps) or radiography.
- Beyond these local symptoms, the impact of CRS can be broad and potentially include pharyngeal and laryngeal symptoms such as sore throat, dysphonia, and cough as well as general health-related symptoms, including poor sleep quality, fatigue, and decreased cognitive function.
- CRS carries significant health and societal burdens. Epidemiologic studies report a range of prevalence from 2% to 16% depending on methodology. Estimated annual direct costs for CRS in the United States are $4.3 billion.
- The pathogenesis of CRS is in a state of evolution, and there is likely significant heterogeneity and multifactorial mechanisms for any given patient. In truth, CRS is idiopathic, but there are unproven hypotheses that implicate dysregulation of proinflammatory cytokines and defects in the mechanical epithelial barrier and innate immune response. Historically, CRS was thought to be exclusively driven by narrowed anatomy and bacterial overgrowth. CRS is now more broadly recognized as an inflammatory disorder that results from a dysfunctional host-environment interaction. Regardless of the mechanism, the final common pathway results in loss of epithelial barrier integrity, ciliary dysfunction, and dysbiosis.
- CRS is most commonly subdivided by the presence or absence of nasal polyps. CRSwNP is considered an intrinsic mucosal disease with Type 2 helper T cells (T_h2)-skewed immune response with high tissue eosinophilia, whereas CRSsNP emphasizes mechanical obstruction of the ostiomeatal complex or other anatomic bottlenecks with a Type 1 helper T cells (T_h1)-skewed immune response. It should be noted that cytokine skewing is not universal and that Asian polyps skew toward T_h1 with fewer eosinophils than Western polyps. The phenotypic presence of polyps is not a perfect means to stratify the underlying pathogenesis, and these phenotypes likely represent separate but overlapping subtypes of CRS. However, this classification, although convenient and a convention, does not effectively predict quality-of-life outcomes after treatment.
- Objective measures of disease such as nasal endoscopy and radiography do not correlate with subjective symptoms. The role of these diagnostic modalities is to establish the presence of sinonasal mucosal inflammation as well as to identify surgical targets.
- CRS and asthma/chronic obstructive pulmonary disease are often comorbid with up to 60% of patients with CRSwNP reporting asthma. Similarities in cytokine and histopathologic profiles imply that both diseases may be the consequences of eosinophilic degranulation at different sites in the airway. The two diseases have potential to amplify one another via systemic cytokines. Similarly, endoscopic sinus surgery for CRS has been shown to improve pulmonary symptoms in, and reduce pulmonary medication for, bronchial asthma. Asthma has also been associated with diminished outcomes after endoscopic sinus surgery.
- Sinusitis is present in approximately one-third of patients with CF. Sinusitis may be the presenting symptom, and CF should be ruled out in pediatric cases of CRS with bilateral nasal polyposis. A spectrum of CF exists, and CRS may be the presenting symptom in older patients with borderline

sweat testing and CF transmembrane regulator-heterozygotes. The observation that bronchoalveolar lavage and sinus cultures in CF patients is correlated has prompted the question about the impact of control of sinus disease on lung function, but the effects have yet to be clearly established due to a paucity of evidence. CF-associated CRS is unique in that it does show improvement with topical dornase alfa and irrigated antibiotics.
- The association of CRSwNP with asthma and hypersensitivity to aspirin or NSAIDs has historically been termed "aspirin triad" or the eponym "Samter triad." Confirmation of aspirin hypersensitivity can be confirmed/excluded with provocation testing with aspirin. Given that the presence of any given portion of the triad may manifest at different time points in a patient's life, the terminology of "aspirin-exacerbated respiratory disease" (AERD) has been adopted. This terminology is more inclusive and accurate, because 30% to 40% of patients with aspirin-sensitive asthma do not have nasal polyposis. AERD CRS is marked by intense eosinophilic inflammation with increased tissue hypertrophy on imaging and endoscopy, rapid return of polyposis, and increased likelihood of revision endoscopic sinus surgery. Avoidance of aspirin/NSAIDs and surgery that maximizes topical steroid distribution is recommended, although the inflammation is independent of aspirin/NSAID exposure, and desensitization to aspirin after surgery may add value for some patients.
- Controversy exists regarding the classification of AFRS as a distinct subset of CRSwNP. Phenotypically, it is marked by nasal polyposis and thick, "peanut-butter" eosinophilic mucin with characteristic radiological findings of differential densities within the sinuses. The original Bent and Kuhn criteria defining AFRS include (1) nasal polyposis, (2) fungi on staining, (3) eosinophilic mucin without invasion, (4) type I hypersensitivity to fungi, and (5) soft tissue densities on CT radiography. The reality is that these features are not unique to AFRS and can be present in CRSwNP, with the exception of the characteristic CT findings. It is unclear if the type I hypersensitivity plays a role in pathogenesis of CRS for these patients. Clinical outcomes are challenging to tease out from CRSwNP given that many studies include AFRS patients in CRSwNP. Limited data exist covering patients with AFRS, and it is not clear if antifungal therapy is of value. Subcutaneous immunotherapy has demonstrated value for 1 to 2 years beyond cessation of therapy. Surgical therapy is geared at removing all mucin, which may require extended sinusotomies in conjunction with aggressive postoperative medical regimens of oral steroid tapers and continued topical steroids, possibly with immunotherapy.
- Pediatric CRS is fundamentally different from adult CRS. The diagnosis is obfuscated by symptoms that can overlap with adenoid hypertrophy, allergic rhinitis, and recurrent viral upper respiratory tract infections, all of which are common in children. Furthermore, the history and examination may be limited in a young child. Symptomatology is similar to adult sinusitis with the exception of an increased prevalence of chronic cough. CT imaging in children demonstrates higher burdens of sinus inflammation in patients without symptoms of CRS, and the imaging must be fit into the context of clinical symptoms. The pathophysiology is likely different in pediatric CRS than in adult CRS. Histopathologic analysis of pediatric CRS demonstrates increased lymphocytes and fewer eosinophilia and epithelial dysfunction compared with adults. The adenoids may contribute to pediatric

CRS, and adenoidectomy is associated with improvement in CRS symptoms in 50% of children postoperatively. Given the overlap in symptoms of adenoiditis and pediatric CRS, it is unknown whether the symptom improvement is the result of improvement in sinus function or resolution of adenoiditis that was misclassified as CRS.

FUNCTIONAL ENDOSCOPIC SINUS SURGERY

- FESS is predicated on relieving obstruction of the sinus outflow tracts to allow for efficient drainage to prevent pooling of secretions and chronic infection and inflammation.
- FESS exploits the natural flow of cilia by augmenting the natural os of the sinuses. This is in contrast to historical techniques, which were predicated on dependent drainage (e.g., inferior meatal window) or radical surgeries that stripped the mucosa of the sinuses (e.g., radical ethmoidectomy or Caldwell-Luc). The larger outflow tracts decrease the risk of anatomic obstruction of sinuses, allowing for uninterrupted mucociliary clearance, and facilitate topical medical therapies.
- Large prospective cohort studies and comparative effectiveness have demonstrated that FESS is effective in achieving a clinically significant improvement in measures of quality of life in patients who have failed prior medical therapy (i.e., broad-spectrum antibiotics and topical or oral steroids) in 70% to 85% of patients. Patients who have failed to make adequate gains in quality of life after "maximal" medical therapy and who have radiographic or endoscopic evidence of sinus inflammation are candidates for surgical therapy. Patients who elect surgical therapy over continued medical therapy are approximately three times more likely to resolve thick nasal discharge, nasal airway obstruction, and facial pain/pressure.
- Secondary surgical interventions are required in approximately 20% of patients who have undergone FESS. Indications for revision include retained ethmoid cells, middle turbinate lateralization, stenosis of prior sinus openings, bony remodeling causing sinus stenosis (osteoneogenesis), and scar band formation (Figure 18-2). In revision surgery, a more extensive surgical approach is advocated and may entail extended sinusotomies (e.g., megaantrostomies and frontal and/or sphenoid Draf III) (Figure 18-3). Osteoneogenesis is associated with high rates of tissue eosinophilia, increased rates of revision surgery, and diminished postoperative gains in quality of life (Figure 18-4).
- The extent of surgery is tailored to the extent of disease as seen on preoperative imaging and intraoperative endoscopy. Particularly in primary surgery, there is a bias toward surgical conservatism. Balloon dilation catheters are a new technology that has yet to be effectively compared with traditional FESS.
- Although controversy exists over the size of openings of each sinus, each sinus opening has some fundamental limits. The maxillary antrostomy is limited anteriorly by the nasolacrimal duct, superiorly by the floor of the orbit, posteriorly by the posterior wall of the maxillary sinus, and inferiorly by the top of the inferior turbinate. A megaantrostomy is an extended sinusotomy that involves resection of the middle portion of the inferior turbinate with inferior extension of the maxillary antrostomy to the floor of the nasal cavity. The ethmoid cavity is limited by the lamina papyracea laterally and the fovea ethmoidalis superiorly with the lateral lamella of the cribriform and middle turbinate medially. The fovea ethmoidalis is approximately ten times thicker than the lateral lamella of

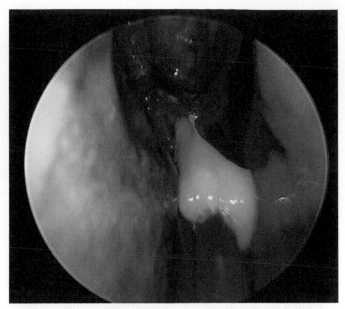

FIGURE 18-2 A right middle turbinate has lateralized postoperatively secondary to scar bands that have pulled it to the lateral nasal wall. As a result, the patient has developed a right-sided sinus infection as evidenced by the mucopurulence suction from the posterior aspect of the maxillary antrostomy.

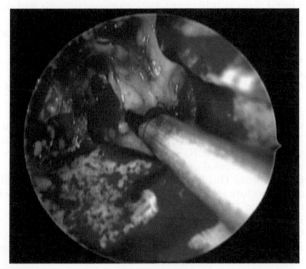

FIGURE 18-3 Intraoperative view of a newly created left megaantrostomy is shown in a patient with Kartagener syndrome who has failed prior surgery.

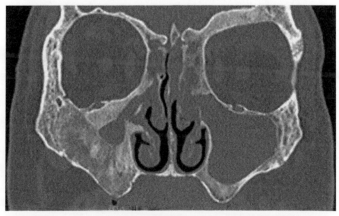

FIGURE 18-4 Severe osteoneogenesis has remodeled much of this patient's sinuses. Osteoneogenesis is associated with increased tissue inflammation and revision surgery.

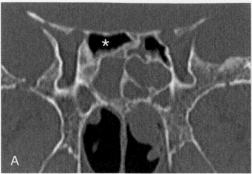 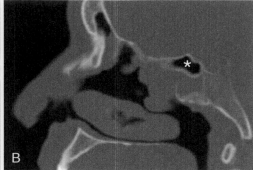

FIGURE 18-5 A, A coronal, bone-window, computed tomography scan of a patient's sphenoid sinuses. The *asterisk* marks the right Onodi cell superior to the right sphenoid sinus. **B,** A sagittal view clearly shows the Onodi cell pneumatized (*asterisk*) superiorly to the sphenoid sinus.

the cribriform. Skull base dissection should be biased laterally to exploit this anatomical difference to diminish the risk of inadvertent CSF leak. The sphenoid sinus is limited laterally by the lamina papyracea, medially by the septum, and superiorly by the sphenoid planum. The inferior extent is typically kept above the posterior septal branch to avoid bleeding, but in salvage surgery the floor can be removed as well as the intersinus septum. The frontal sinus is at high risk for iatrogenic sinusitis and does not tolerate stripped mucosa, given the fundamentally narrowed limits between the orbit, skull base, and frontal beak. Extreme caution and meticulous dissection is required in this anatomy. A Draf I procedure is defined as removal of the bottom portion of the agger nasi and ethmoid bulla. A Draf IIa procedure involves removal of all frontal recess cells between the lamina and middle turbinate in a coronal plane and the frontal beak and skull base in a sagittal plane. A Draf IIb extends the Draf IIa by taking out the floor of the frontal sinus to the septum. A Draf III involves bilateral Draf IIB with the additional removal of the intersinus septum and the frontal beak. This bone is quite thick and requires a drill and therefore exposes bone. Thus, a maximalist approach to the Draf III cavity is advocated with the fundamental limits achieved: periosteum anteriorly, periosteum/lacrimal sac laterally, and first olfactory fiber posteriorly. Recovery from Draf III is significantly longer and requires more and closer postoperative debridement to prevent closure. By 1 year, neoostiums typically have stabilized in size.

- Anatomic variations of each sinus need to be recognized on preoperative scanning by the surgeon. Anatomic variations can lead to increased rates of failure (e.g., Haller cells can lead to synechiae within a maxillary antrostomy) and can increase risk. The Onodi cell is marked by posterior pneumatization of the most posterior ethmoid cell and exposes the optic and carotid artery to risk within the ethmoid bed in extreme cases (Figure 18-5). Presence of an Onodi cell also displaces the sphenoid medially and inferiorly.
- Olfactory neuroepithelium is distributed across the top 1 cm of the septum, superior turbinate, and middle turbinates.
- Topical therapy depends on the delivery mechanism to place the drug into contact with the sinus mucosa. Less

than 3% of nebulized medications, pressurized sprays, and irrigated therapies land within the sinuses, and the frontal and sphenoid sinuses are essentially unreachable prior to FESS. A general trend is observed in cadaveric studies of increased distribution with increased sinus openings. High-volume (>100 cc) irrigation is the most effective means of distribution.
- Middle turbinate resection is associated with longer time to recurrence of polyposis in patients with CRSwNP. Partial middle turbinate is associated with fewer adhesions and fewer revisions. Patients who have undergone middle turbinate resection have quality-of-life outcomes comparable to those of patients who have preserved middle turbinates. In short, whether to perform a middle turbinate resection is a judgment made by the surgeon and may benefit patients when there is an indication (e.g., unstable turbinate, polypoid degeneration, paradoxical turbinate). There is no evidence implicating middle turbinate resection with diminished gains in quality of life.
- Iatrogenic CSF leak can occur when inadvertent violation of the skull base occurs during FESS. The fovea ethmoidalis is the frontal bone's contribution to the ethmoid roof that is 10 times thicker than the lateral lamella of the cribriform plate, which constitutes the medial aspect of the ethmoid roof. High medial dissection, therefore, can result in CSF leak without meticulous dissection under direct visualization. Recognition of a CSF leak should prompt an attempt at repair by identifying the leak, circumferentially exposing 1 cm of bone, and placing a mucosal-free graft. Nationwide, this complication is reported in approximately 1 in 1000 cases.
- Orbital injuries can occur from direct violation of the lamina papyracea and the underlying structures such as the orbital fat and extraocular muscles. Orbital hematoma can result from inadvertent injury to the anterior ethmoid artery, which can retract laterally into the orbit. This is a surgical emergency and requires immediate action by the sinus surgeon, including a lateral canthotomy and cantholysis, and possibly a medial decompression as well if the eye remains tense. Failure to relieve elevated intraorbital pressures results in permanent loss of vision. Nationwide, orbital complications are reported in approximately 1 in 1000 cases.

ANSWERS

TRUE OR FALSE QUESTIONS

1. F	14. F	27. T	40. F
2. F	15. T	28. F	41. T
3. F	16. T	29. T	42. T
4. T	17. F	30. F	43. F
5. F	18. F	31. F	44. T
6. T	19. F	32. F	45. T
7. F	20. T	33. F	46. T
8. F	21. T	34. F	47. T
9. F	22. F	35. F	48. F
10. T	23. F	36. T	49. F
11. T	24. F	37. F	50. T
12. T	25. T	38. T	
13. F	26. F	39. F	

SINGLE BEST ANSWER QUESTIONS

51. d	64. b	77. d	90. a
52. d	65. c	78. b	91. a
53. c	66. c	79. d	92. b
54. b	67. d	80. e	93. e
55. b	68. b	81. d	94. b
56. d	69. d	82. d	95. b
57. e	70. a	83. c	96. b
58. a	71. e	84. e	97. c
59. c	72. c	85. a	98. b
60. d	73. c	86. e	99. c
61. b	74. a	87. b	100. d
62. e	75. c	88. b	
63. b	76. f	89. c	

SUGGESTED READINGS

1. Rosenfeld RM, Andes D, Bhattacharyya N, et al. Clinical practice guideline: adult sinusitis. *Otolaryngol Head Neck Surg.* 2007;137(suppl 3):S1-S31.

2. Fokkens WJ, Lund VJ, Mullol J, et al. European position paper on rhinosinusitis and nasal polyps 2012. A summary for otorhinolaryngologists. *Rhinology.* 2012;50(1):1-12.

3. Smith TL, Kern R, Palmer JN, et al. Medical therapy vs surgery for chronic rhinosinusitis: a prospective, multi-institutional study with 1-year follow-up. *Int Forum Allergy Rhinol.* 2013;3(1):4-9.

4. DeConde AS, Mace JC, Alt JA, et al. Comparative effectiveness of medical and surgical therapy on olfaction in chronic rhinosinusitis: a prospective, multi-institutional study. *Int Forum Allergy Rhinol.* 2014;4(9):725-733.

5. DeConde AS, Mace JC, Alt JA, et al. Investigation of change in cardinal symptoms of chronic rhinosinusitis after surgical or ongoing medical management. *Int Forum Allergy Rhinol.* 2015;5(1):36-45.

6. Naidoo Y, Bassiouni A, Keen M, Wormald PJ. Long-term outcomes for the endoscopic modified Lothrop/Draf III procedure: a 10-year review. *Laryngoscope.* 2014;124(1):43-49.

7. Wu AW, Ting JY, Platt MP, Tierney HT, Metson R. Factors affecting time to revision sinus surgery for nasal polyps: a 25-year experience. *Laryngoscope.* 2014;124(1):29-33.

8. Chaaban MR, Kejner A, Rowe SM, Woodworth BA. Cystic fibrosis chronic rhinosinusitis: a comprehensive review. *Am J Rhinol Allergy.* 2013;27(5):387-395.

9. Thomas WW, Harvey RJ, Rudmik L, Hwang PH, Schlosser RJ. Distribution of topical agents to the paranasal sinuses: an evidence-based review with recommendations. *Int Forum Allergy Rhinol.* 2013;3(9):691-703.

10. Rudmik L, Hoy M, Schlosser RJ, et al. Topical therapies in the management of chronic rhinosinusitis: an evidence-based review with recommendations. *Int Forum Allergy Rhinol.* 2013;3(4):281-298.

19 | Allergy and Immunology of the Upper Airway

Philip D. Knollman | Fuad M. Baroody

TRUE OR FALSE QUESTIONS

INNATE AND ADAPTIVE IMMUNITY

T/F 1. The innate immune system consists of host defense mechanisms that are encoded in the germline genes of the host, including barrier mechanisms, soluble proteins, small bioactive antimicrobial defense molecules, mediators of inflammation, and activated immune cells such as neutrophils, monocytes, and macrophages.

T/F 2. Antimicrobial peptides, such as cathelicidins and defensins, participate in the innate immune response through direct killing of pathogens, recruitment of cellular immune responses, and promotion of tissue inflammation.

T/F 3. The two major effector arms of the adaptive immune response are humoral and cellular.

T/F 4. The adaptive immune system manifests specificity for target antigens, primarily through antigen-specific toll-like receptors.

T/F 5. The majority of T-cell development occurs within the bone marrow, prior to circulating in the bloodstream and populating lymphoid and epithelial tissues throughout the body.

T/F 6. CD8-positive T cells are cytotoxic effector cells, with major cytotoxic activity against cells infected with intracellular pathogens.

T/F 7. CD4-positive TH2 cells produce cytokines such as interleukin (IL)-4, IL-5, and IL-13 and facilitate humoral immunity through B-cell antibody-dependent responses to extracellular pathogens.

T/F 8. CD4-positive TH1 cells produce interferon-γ, activate macrophages, and facilitate the clearance of intracellular pathogens and the delayed-type hypersensitivity response.

T/F 9. B cells provide humoral immunity against extracellular pathogens through the production of antibodies that have direct cytotoxic effects.

T/F 10. Natural killer cells possess cytotoxic activity against target cells that display "nonself" antigens on "self" major histocompatibility complex (MHC) molecules, through a process known as MHC-restricted cytotoxicity.

T/F 11. Both mast cells and basophils possess high-affinity receptors for immunoglobulin (Ig) E, which makes them key initiators of immediate hypersensitivity responses mediated through the release of preformed small molecules upon cell degranulation.

T/F 12. Primary lymphoid organs are sites of mature lymphocyte populations where immune responses are generated.

T/F 13. The ratio of CD4-positive T cells to CD8-positive T cells within the lamina propria of mucosal surfaces is approximately 1:1.

T/F 14. Humoral immune responses may be classified as either T-cell dependent or T-cell independent.

IMMUNOPATHOLOGY

T/F 15. Anaphylaxis is an example of an IgE-dependent mast cell–mediated type I hypersensitivity reaction to the presence of sensitizing allergens.

T/F 16. Type II hypersensitivity reactions are immune complex–mediated reactions in which low-solubility IgG and IgM immune complexes are deposited in normal host tissues, inciting an inflammatory response with resultant host tissue injury.

T/F 17. Type IV hypersensitivity reactions are pathologic variants of normal antibody-independent, T cell–mediated immune responses, in which the T-cell response to environmental antigens becomes exaggerated.

ALLERGIC RHINITIS

T/F 18. Allergic rhinitis has an overall prevalence of 10% to 20%, with a lower prevalence in children compared with adults and male predominance throughout childhood and adulthood.

T/F 19. The severity of symptoms associated with allergic rhinitis is relatively constant throughout childhood and adolescence, decreasing with age thereafter.

T/F 20. Individuals with asthma are twice as likely to develop allergic rhinitis compared with the general population.

T/F 21. Evidence supporting the hygiene hypothesis includes an observed increase in the incidence of allergic and autoimmune disease in developing countries and a concomitant decrease in the incidence of many infectious diseases in developing countries since the beginning of the 1970s.

T/F 22. The mean total productivity losses per employee with allergic rhinitis are greater than the losses associated with other prevalent chronic diseases, such as migraine, depression, respiratory infections, diabetes, and coronary artery disease.

T/F 23. In patients with allergic rhinitis, sensitization to allergens occurs when antigen-specific IgE antibodies attach to high-affinity receptors on mast cells and basophils in the nasal mucosa.

T/F 24. The early allergic response occurs when allergens attach to and cross-link adjacent antigen-specific IgE antibodies attached to the surface of mast cells and basophils, resulting in degranulation and release of inflammatory mediators in the vicinity of the nasal mucosa.

T/F 25. The primary inflammatory mediators of the early allergic response are IL-5, IL-6, IL-8, tumor necrosis factor (TNF)-α, and intercellular adhesion molecule 1.

T/F 26. The late allergic response occurs many hours after allergen exposure and is marked by the recurrence of symptoms, particularly nasal congestion, and an increase in inflammatory mediator concentration and inflammatory cell influx.

T/F 27. Central and peripheral nervous system reflexes amplify the allergic response, resulting in inflammatory changes in sites distant from those of antigen deposition, such as the eyes, paranasal sinuses, and lower airway.

T/F 28. The classification scheme for allergic rhinitis introduced during the Allergic Rhinitis and its Impact on Asthma (ARIA) World Health Organization (WHO) workshop categorizes patients according to frequency and duration of symptoms as well as severity of symptoms.

T/F 29. The classification scheme for allergic rhinitis introduced during the ARIA WHO workshop is utilized for defining offending antigens rather than suggesting treatment algorithms.

T/F 30. Presence of physical examination findings such as "allergic shiners," "adenoid facies," and the "allergic salute" confirm the diagnosis of allergic rhinitis.

T/F 31. Skin testing for allergic rhinitis requires application of specific allergen extracts to the skin, application of diluent for the allergen extracts to serve as a negative control, and application of histamine to serve as a positive control.

T/F 32. A positive reaction on skin testing indicates the existence of antigen-specific IgE antibodies attached to the surface of intradermal mast cells.

T/F 33. In vitro IgE testing is more sensitive than skin testing, especially when results are correlated with the clinical presentation of allergic symptoms.

T/F 34. A positive in vitro or skin test result alone confirms the diagnosis of allergic rhinitis, even in the absence of supporting clinical history.

T/F 35. As a single modality of therapy, avoidance measures are typically not effective in reducing symptoms in patients with allergic rhinitis.

T/F 36. First-generation H₁ antihistamines are more lipophilic, more readily cross the blood-brain barrier, and are more commonly associated with sedative and anticholinergic side effects.

T/F 37. Intranasal H₁ antihistamines, such as azelastine and olopatadine, are less efficacious in the treatment of allergic rhinitis when compared with oral H₁ antihistamines.

T/F 38. Both oral and intranasal decongestants have been associated with the occurrence of rhinitis medicamentosa.

T/F 39. Montelukast has been shown to be equally effective in the treatment of all nasal and ocular symptoms of allergic rhinitis when compared with antihistamines.

T/F 40. In nasal allergen challenge models of allergic rhinitis, pretreatment with intranasal steroids results in significant inhibition of the mediators of early- and late-phase reactions.

T/F 41. Several placebo-controlled clinical trials have demonstrated the effectiveness of intranasal steroid preparations in the reduction of all nasal symptoms associated with seasonal and perennial allergic rhinitis.

T/F 42. Systemic steroids are effective in patients with allergic rhinitis but are not routinely prescribed due to the potential for significant side effects.

T/F 43. Both intranasal steroids and immunotherapy have been shown to alter the natural history of allergic rhinitis.

T/F 44. Immunotherapy is typically reserved for patients with allergic rhinitis who have not experienced adequate responses to pharmacologic treatment.

T/F 45. The ability of allergen-specific immunotherapy to maintain beneficial antiinflammatory effects after discontinuation appears to depend on sustained allergen exposure in order to maintain allergen tolerance.

T/F 46. Administration of subcutaneous immunotherapy (SCIT) is associated with an immediate improvement in the symptoms and quality of life of patients with allergic rhinitis, with effect appreciable within 2 to 3 weeks of initiation.

T/F 47. When compared with placebo controls, sublingual immunotherapy (SLIT) to timothy grass allergens improved daily symptom scores in pediatric and adolescent patients by as much as 50%.

T/F 48. When compared with placebo controls, SLIT to timothy grass allergens reduced daily medication use in pediatric and adolescent patients by as much as 80%.

T/F 49. When compared with placebo controls, administration of intranasal steroids is effective in controlling ocular symptoms associated with allergic rhinitis.

T/F 50. Administration of oral antihistamines with intranasal steroids provides no additional benefit over intranasal steroids alone in the treatment of allergic rhinitis.

SINGLE BEST ANSWER QUESTIONS

INNATE AND ADAPTIVE IMMUNITY

51. The adaptive immune system is characterized by which of the following?
    i.   Specificity for target antigens
    ii. Adaptation to changing environments
    iii. Host barrier mechanisms
    iv. Constitutive expression of inflammatory mediators
    v.   Long-standing immunologic memory

a. i and ii
b. i and iv
c. iii and iv
d. i, ii, and v
e. i, iii, and iv
f. All of the above

52. Toll-like receptors are ubiquitously expressed on various cell types, which recognize molecular patterns present on many pathogens. Pathogen-associated molecular patterns recognized by toll-like receptors include which of the following?
    a. Gram-positive cell wall components, such as peptidoglycan
    b. Gram-negative cell wall components, such as lipopolysaccharides
    c. Bacterial virulence factors, such as pneumolysin
    d. Bacterial DNA and viral RNA patterns
    e. All of the above

53. Within the thymic medulla, developing T cells that react too strongly to self-antigens are deleted by apoptosis, through a process known as:
    a. Positive selection
    b. Negative selection
    c. Central tolerance
    d. Affinity maturation

54. What percentage of T cells within the blood and secondary lymphoid organs are CD4 positive?
    a. 30% to 40%
    b. 40% to 50%
    c. 50% to 60%
    d. 60% to 70%

55. B cells facilitate humoral immunity against extracellular pathogens through the production of antibodies, which may act through all of the following mechanisms *EXCEPT*:
    a. Binding and neutralization of pathogens
    b. Opsonization
    c. Direct cytotoxic effects
    d. Activation of complement

56. Dendritic cells play a central role in processing and modulating the immune response to foreign antigens through all of the following mechanisms *EXCEPT*:
    a. Modulation of epithelial cell function and secretion of epithelial-derived inflammatory cytokines
    b. Induction of B-cell differentiation into antibody-secreting plasma cells
    c. Induction of naive CD4 T-cell differentiation into inflammatory TH2 cells
    d. Production of attractant cytokines that facilitate the recruitment of neutrophils and eosinophils
    e. Induction of tolerance or allergic response to inhaled antigens

57. What role do eosinophils play in allergic disease?
    i. Allergen recognition and cross-linking on mast-cell surfaces, resulting in mast-cell degranulation
    ii. Suppression of local tissue response to inflammatory mediators of IgE-mediated hypersensitivity reaction
    iii. Inactivation of products of mast-cell degranulation, such as histamine, platelet-activating factor, and heparin
    iv. Perpetuation of tissue damage through the toxic effects of its own products of degranulation, such as eosinophilic cationic protein and major basic protein
    a. i
    b. iv

c. ii and iii
d. ii, iii, and iv
e. All of the above

58. Which of the following is considered a primary lymphoid organ?
    a. Thymus
    b. Spleen
    c. Lymph node
    d. Palatine tonsil
    e. Peyer patch

59. Protective immunity against *Streptococcus pneumoniae, Haemophilus influenzae,* and meningococcus is mediated by which process?
    a. T cell–dependent response
    b. T cell–independent response
    c. Innate immune response
    d. Delayed-type hypersensitivity response

60. Which of the following immunoglobulins is primarily responsible for secondary or recall immune responses?
    a. IgA
    b. IgD
    c. IgE
    d. IgG
    e. IgM

61. Which of the following immunoglobulins serve as antigen receptors on B cells?
    a. IgA and IgD
    b. IgG and IgM
    c. IgD and IgM
    d. IgE and IgD

62. Which of the following immunoglobulins is the most efficient complement-fixing antibody?
    a. IgA
    b. IgD
    c. IgE
    d. IgG
    e. IgM

63. Which of the following statements is true regarding the complement system?
    a. The complement system is an effector of both the innate and adaptive immune responses.
    b. The complement pathway is activated by microbial structures independent of antigen presentation by immune cells or antibodies.
    c. The complement pathway is activated by interaction with antigen-antibody complexes.
    d. Components of the complement system may function in phagocytosis, chemotaxis, and cytolysis.
    e. All of the above

IMMUNOPATHOLOGY

64. Cell-mediated immunity operates primarily against all of the following *EXCEPT*:
    a. Viral infections
    b. Fungal infections
    c. Bacterial infections
    d. Intracellular infections

65. Type II hypersensitivity reactions are mediated by which of the following antibodies?
    i. IgE
    ii. IgA
    iii. IgG
    iv. IgM

a. i
b. i and iii
c. ii and iv
d. iii and iv
e. All of the above

66. Type II hypersensitivity reactions lead to host cell and tissue destruction through which of the following antibody-dependent mechanisms?
    a. Opsonization
    b. Complement activation
    c. Antibody-dependent cellular cytotoxicity
    d. All of the above

67. Which of the following is an example of a type III hypersensitivity reaction?
    a. Sensitivity to iodide-containing contrast media
    b. Tuberculin sensitivity test, or purified protein derivative test
    c. Immune complex vasculitis associated with systemic lupus erythematosus
    d. Penicillin-induced autoimmune hemolytic anemia

ALLERGIC RHINITIS

68. The likelihood of atopy, or the predisposition to respond to environmental allergens with the production of specific IgE antibodies, among children with one atopic parent or sibling is approximately:
    a. 10%
    b. 30%
    c. 50%
    d. 80%

69. Factors associated with an increased incidence of atopic disease include all of the following *EXCEPT*:
    a. Higher socioeconomic status
    b. Early exposure to antibiotics in childhood
    c. Attendance at daycare in childhood
    d. Living in a farming environment in childhood
    e. Early exposure to domestic pets in childhood

70. Evaluations with various health-related quality-of-life tools reveal that patients with poorly controlled allergic rhinitis experience which of the following?
    a. Sleep disturbance and daytime sleepiness
    b. Learning problems and decreased productivity for children at school
    c. Decreased productivity and increased absenteeism for adults at work
    d. All of the above

71. Typical signs and symptoms of the early response in allergic rhinitis include all of the following *EXCEPT*:
    a. Nasal congestion
    b. Pruritus
    c. Hives
    d. Sneezing
    e. Rhinorrhea

72. Preformed inflammatory mediators released during mast-cell degranulation in the early allergic response include all of the following *EXCEPT*:
    a. Histamine
    b. Prostaglandin 2
    c. Tryptase
    d. Heparin

73. Contributors to the late allergic response include which of the following?
    a. Release of preformed mediators by stimulated mast cells and basophils

b. Release of newly generated inflammatory cytokines, including IL-1β, IL-5, IL-6, IL-8, TNF-α, and granulocyte-macrophage colony-stimulating factor, by stimulated mast cells and TH2 cells
    c. Perpetuation of nasal mucosal inflammation through recruitment and influx of inflammatory cells, particularly eosinophils
    d. All of the above

74. In patients with allergic rhinitis, exposure to allergen is associated with an upregulation of all of the following inflammatory cell subtypes *EXCEPT*:
    a. Basophils
    b. Eosinophils
    c. TH1 cells
    d. TH2 cells
    e. Langerhans cells

75. The phenomenon whereby patients with allergic rhinitis exhibit hyperresponsiveness to presentation with specific stimuli is known as:
    a. Priming
    b. Sensitization
    c. Early allergic response
    d. Late allergic response

76. Which of the following symptoms is most suggestive of allergic rhinitis?
    a. Anterior rhinorrhea
    b. Posterior rhinorrhea
    c. Itching and sneezing
    d. Nasal congestion

77. A patient who exhibits symptoms of allergic rhinitis for more than 2 hours per day for more than 9 months of the year when exposed to allergens such as dust mites, molds, and animal dander may be classified as having which of the following?
    a. Seasonal allergic rhinitis
    b. Perennial allergic rhinitis
    c. Episodic allergic rhinitis
    d. None of the above

78. A patient with allergic rhinitis who describes his/her symptoms as troublesome, associated with sleep disturbance, and occurring most days during the week over the course of the past 2 months would be classified as having which of the following?
    a. Mild intermittent allergic rhinitis
    b. Mild persistent allergic rhinitis
    c. Moderate to severe intermittent allergic rhinitis
    d. Moderate to severe persistent allergic rhinitis

79. A patient with typical symptoms of allergic rhinitis, particularly with nasal allergen challenge, but without evidence of systemic atopy by skin and serologic testing, would be classified as having which of the following?
    a. Local allergic rhinitis
    b. Episodic allergic rhinitis
    c. Mild intermittent allergic rhinitis
    d. Nonallergic rhinitis
    e. None of the above

80. Which physical examination finding(s) on anterior rhinoscopy is/are pathognomonic for allergic rhinitis?
    a. Nasal polyposis
    b. Mucosal edema and hyperemia
    c. Normal-appearing mucosa with thin secretions
    d. Inferior turbinate mucosal edema and pallor with thin secretions
    e. All of the above
    f. None of the above

81. Total serum IgE levels are elevated in what percentage of patients with allergic rhinitis?
    a. 10%
    b. 30%
    c. 50%
    d. 80%
    e. 100%

82. According to the National Health and Nutrition Examination Survey, the prevalence of positive skin testing or in vitro testing among the study population was:
    a. 10%
    b. 20%
    c. 50%
    d. 75%

83. According to the National Health and Nutrition Examination Survey, the prevalence of full expression of allergic disease among the study population was:
    a. 10%
    b. 20%
    c. 50%
    d. 75%

84. Which of the following oral antihistamines is associated with the highest likelihood of sedating side effects?
    a. Cetirizine
    b. Fexofenadine
    c. Diphenhydramine
    d. Loratadine

85. Administration of oral antihistamines is typically associated with improvement in all of the following symptoms *EXCEPT*:
    a. Nasal congestion
    b. Sneezing
    c. Nasal pruritus
    d. Eye tearing
    e. Rhinorrhea

86. Sedative side effects occur in approximately what percentage of patients taking first-generation oral H_1 antihistamines?
    a. 10%
    b. 20%
    c. 50%
    d. 75%

87. Topical decongestants, such as phenylephrine and oxymetazoline, are recommended only for short-term use due to the association with which of the following side effects?
    a. Epistaxis
    b. Sedation
    c. Septal perforation
    d. Rhinitis medicamentosa

88. Administration of intranasal anticholinergics, such as ipratropium bromide, is typically associated with improvement of which of the following symptoms?
    a. Nasal congestion
    b. Sneezing
    c. Nasal pruritis
    d. Eye tearing
    e. Rhinorrhea

89. Which of the following classes of medications is considered the most efficacious for the treatment of allergic rhinitis?
    a. Intranasal steroids
    b. Oral antihistamines
    c. Intranasal antihistamines
    d. Leukotriene receptor antagonists

90. Various studies have shown that the administration of intranasal steroids is associated with a significant reduction in which of the following?
    i. Inflammatory cell influx into nasal mucosa and nasal secretions
    ii. Production of TH1-type cytokines in nasal mucosa and nasal secretions
    iii. Antigen-induced hyperresponsiveness to subsequent antigen challenge
    iv. Antigen-induced hyperresponsiveness to histamine provocation
    a. i, ii, and iii
    b. i, ii, and iv
    c. i, iii, and iv
    d. All of the above
    e. None of the above

91. What is the most common side effect associated with consistent use of intranasal steroids?
    a. Growth suppression
    b. Epistaxis
    c. Local nasal irritation
    d. Mucosal atrophy
    e. Septal perforation
    f. *Candida* overgrowth

92. Which of the following has been shown to change the natural course of allergic rhinitis?
    a. Intranasal steroids
    b. Intranasal antihistamines
    c. Leukotriene receptor antagonists
    d. Immunotherapy

93. Allergen-specific immunotherapy induces significant immune modulation through which of the following mechanisms?
    a. Desensitization of allergen-specific IgE-bearing mast cells and basophils
    b. IL-10 and transforming growth factor β–mediated T-cell tolerance and deviation toward a regulatory T-cell response
    c. Decrease in allergen-specific IgE serum levels
    d. Increase in allergen-specific IgG4 serum levels
    e. All of the above

94. The typical duration of subcutaneous immunotherapy (SCIT) is:
    a. 1 to 2 years
    b. 2 to 3 years
    c. 3 to 5 years
    d. 5 to 7 years

95. Disadvantages of SCIT include all of the following *EXCEPT*:
    a. Slow onset of action
    b. Long duration of therapy
    c. Decreased effectiveness over the course of therapy
    d. Need for high degree of patient compliance
    e. Potential for local and systemic adverse reactions

96. What is the estimated rate of systemic reactions associated with SCIT injections?
    a. <1%
    b. 2%
    c. 5%
    d. 10%
    e. 15%

97. Which of the following is an advantage of SLIT as compared with SCIT?
    a. Greater number of allergen extracts available
    b. Ease of administration

c. No risk of local or systemic reactions

d. Greater efficacy of treatment

e. Longer duration of treatment effect

98. Which of the following statements regarding the treatment of ocular symptoms associated with allergic rhinitis is correct?

    a. Intraocular antihistamines are associated with equivalent rates of sedation and dry eyes as first-generation oral H_1 antihistamines.

    b. Coadminstration of intraocular antihistamines and intranasal steroids produces a synergistic effect in controlling ocular symptoms.

    c. Intranasal steroids have equivalent efficacy in controlling ocular symptoms when compared with H_1 antihistamines.

    d. Coadministration of intranasal steroids and intranasal antihistamines produces an additive benefit in controlling ocular symptoms.

99. Which combination therapies have been shown to have a clear additive benefit in the treatment of allergic rhinitis?

    a. Intranasal antihistamines and intranasal steroids

    b. Oral antihistamines and intranasal steroids

    c. Oral leukotriene modifiers and oral steroids

    d. Oral antihistamines and oral steroids

    e. All of the above

100. All of the following medications are considered safe during pregnancy (category B agents) *EXCEPT:*

    a. Budesonide

    b. Fluticasone

    c. Loratadine

    d. Cetirizine

    e. Levocetirizine

CORE KNOWLEDGE

INNATE AND ADAPTIVE IMMUNITY

- The immune system protects the host organism from infectious microbes while avoiding responses that produce damage to host tissues.
- The immune system is divided into the innate and adaptive systems.
- The innate immune system includes all aspects of host defense, including barrier mechanisms (epithelium, mucous layer, and mucociliary transport) and soluble bioactive molecules (complement, antimicrobial peptides, cytokines, lipid mediators of inflammation, and bioactive amines and enzymes).
- The adaptive immune system manifests specificity to target antigens, adapts to changing environments, and provides immunologic memory. The adaptive immune system is further divided into cell-mediated and humoral immune responses.
- Primary lymphoid organs are sites of lymphocyte differentiation and maturation into effector cells. These organs include the bone marrow and thymus.
- Secondary lymphoid organs facilitate the interaction between antigen-bearing antigen-presenting cells and antigen-specific T and B cells. These include the systemic immune system, which includes the spleen and lymph nodes, and the mucosal immune system, which includes the tonsils, Peyer patches, and lamina propria of mucosal tissues.
- Lymphoid stem cells differentiate into three cell populations: T cells, B cells, and natural killer cells.
- Myeloid stem cells differentiate into various granulocytes, megakaryocytes, and erythrocytes.
- T-cell development occurs within the thymus, with differentiation into two primary effector cell types, which are specified by the presence of particular T-cell receptors and coreceptors: CD4-positive T cells and CD8-positive T cells.
- CD8-positive T cells are cytotoxic effector cells, with major cytotoxic activity against cells infected with intracellular microbes and against tumor cells. They secrete cytotoxic proteins (perforin and granzymes) at the point of contact with target cells, produce proinflammatory cytolytic cytokines (TNF), and participate in Fas-mediated cytotoxicity.
- CD4-positive T cells are generally designated as helper T cells, and they work to activate both cellular immune responses and humoral immune responses.
- CD4-positive T cells are divided into various subsets and are classically viewed in the context of the TH1/TH2 paradigm, though other subsets of CD4-positive T cells have been described.
- TH1 cells specialize in macrophage activation by interferon-γ, playing a role in intracellular pathogen clearance and delayed-type hypersensitivity.
- TH2 cells produce cytokines such as IL-4, IL-5, and IL-13 and facilitate humoral immunity through B-cell antibody-dependent responses to extracellular pathogens.
- CD4-positive T cells can also differentiate into regulatory T cells, which are characterized by the ability to suppress T-cell responses and prevent autoimmunity.
- B cells develop in the bone marrow and mature within peripheral lymphoid organs.
- B cells provide humoral immunity against extracellular pathogens through the production of antibodies (immunoglobulins) that neutralize pathogens and toxins, facilitate opsonization, and activate complement.
- B-cell responses may be orchestrated with the help of T cells and their cytokines through a process termed T cell–dependent B-cell responses.
- B-cell responses may also occur independent of T-cell stimulation, via direct binding of large antigens that compose the capsule and/or cell walls of bacteria, through a process termed T cell–independent B-cell responses.
- IgG is principally involved in secondary or recall immune responses and is the only immunoglobulin that can cross the placenta, thus protecting the neonate.
- IgM is the major immunoglobulin expressed on the surface of B cells, serving as their earliest antigen receptor and predominating in the early humoral response. It is the most efficient complement-fixing antibody.
- IgA is a secretory immunoglobulin that plays a major role in mucosal immunity through neutralization of foreign substances in order to prevent their systemic access.
- IgE cross-linking on basophil and mast-cell surfaces through antigen binding triggers the release of mediators of allergic, or immediate hypersensitivity, reactions.
- Monocyte-derived cells include Langerhans cells within the epidermis, Kupffer cells in the liver, microglial cells in the central nervous system, and dendritic cells dispersed throughout most tissues of the body. These cells all serve as antigen-presenting cells.

- Follicular dendritic cells reside in B cell–rich follicles of the lymph nodes and spleen. They facilitate the generation and maintenance of memory B cells.
- Tissue dendritic cells engulf and process antigen in situ, then travel to T cell–rich areas of the lymph nodes or spleen to present antigen to resting T cells in order to induce proliferation and differentiation.
- Both foreign and self proteins are processed within antigen-presenting cells by hydrolytic cleavage. Resultant oligopeptide antigens are bound to cell surface MHC molecules for presentation to various effector cells.
- MHC class I molecules bind and present antigens derived from intracellular proteins (e.g., tumor antigens and intracellular viruses).
- MHC class II molecules bind and present antigens derived from extracellular proteins (e.g., extracellular bacteria and nonreplicating vaccine antigens).
- Neutrophils account for 60% to 65% of circulating leukocytes. Neutrophils play a major role in the clearance of microbial pathogens and repair of tissue injury.
- Eosinophils are prominent cells in most allergic responses. Eosinophils serve to suppress local tissue response to inflammatory mediators of IgE-mediated hypersensitivity reactions, and they inactivate products of mast-cell degranulation, such as histamine, platelet-activating factor, and heparin. However, eosinophils may also perpetuate tissue damage through the toxic effects of their own products of degranulation, such as eosinophilic cationic protein and major basic protein.
- Mast cells and basophils are key initiators of immediate hypersensitivity reactions, as these cells respond to the antigen cross-linking of surface-bound IgE antibodies with the release of preformed and newly synthesized mediators of tissue inflammation.
- The complement system is an important effector of the innate and adaptive immune responses. It consists of myriad plasma and cell-surface proteins that are sequentially activated to interact with one another, with antibodies, and with cell membranes. These then mediate functions such as immune adherence, phagocytosis, chemotaxis, and cytolysis.
- Cytokines are a diverse group of small, secreted proteins that mediate interactions among various effector cells. Each cytokine may have multiple activities on different effector-cell types. Cytokines serve as mediators of effector-cell chemotaxis, activation, differentiation, growth, and proliferation, and as mediators of inflammation and immune regulation.

IMMUNOPATHOLOGY

- Humoral and cell-mediated immune responses of the adaptive immune system are extremely efficient when directed to eliminate pathogens; however, these same immune mechanisms may cause host-tissue destruction and therefore lead to disease states.
- Hypersensitivity reactions are immunopathologic reactions of the immune system characterized by host-tissue destruction. They are divided into four types.
  - Type I hypersensitivity includes mast cell–mediated reactions, whereby mast cells and basophils release mediators of inflammation in response to the presence of sensitizing allergens. Type I hypersensitivity responses can be IgE-dependent (e.g., allergy, anaphylaxis) or IgE-independent (sensitivity to iodide contrast media).
  - Type II hypersensitivity includes cytotoxic antibody-mediated reactions, whereby IgG or IgM antibodies attach to antigens on the surface of target host cells

or tissues, resulting in destruction of these host cells or tissues through opsonization, complement activation, or cell lysis. An example is penicillin-induced autoimmune hemolytic anemia.
  - Type III hypersensitivity includes immune complex–mediated reactions, whereby IgG or IgM antibodies form soluble immune complexes around target antigens, deposit on normal host tissues, and activate neutrophil-mediated inflammatory responses that inflict host tissue injury as a result. An example is serum sickness and immune complex vasculitis.
  - Type IV hypersensitivity, also known as delayed-type hypersensitivity, includes antibody-independent T cell–mediated reactions, whereby T-cell responses to environmental antigens become exaggerated, resulting in host tissue destruction. An example is the cutaneous reaction to purified protein derivative administration in patients previously infected by or vaccinated against *Mycobacterium tuberculosis*.

ALLERGIC RHINITIS

- Allergic rhinitis is a clinical hypersensitivity of the nasal mucosa to foreign antigens mediated through IgE antibodies (Figure 19-1).
- The prevalence of allergic rhinitis is between 10% and 20%, affecting 20 million to 40 million individuals in the United States annually.
- The prevalence of seasonal allergic rhinitis is higher in children and adolescents. In childhood, boys are affected more frequently than girls. In adulthood, the prevalence among men and women is approximately equal.
- The likelihood of atopy, which is the predisposition to respond to environmental allergens with the production of specific IgE antibodies, in a child of two parents unaffected by atopic disease is approximately 15%. The likelihood of atopy in a child of one affected parent or with one affected sibling is approximately 30%. The likelihood of atopy in a child of two affected parents is approximately 50%.
- Allergic rhinitis is four to six times more likely to develop in individuals with asthma as compared with the general population.
- Epidemiologic data provide strong evidence of a steady rise in the incidence of allergic and autoimmune diseases in developed countries since the 1970s.
- The hygiene hypothesis suggests that the decrease in infectious diseases as a result of antibiotic administration, vaccination, and improved hygiene is causally linked to the increase in the incidence of allergic disease.
- A significant impairment of quality of life in patients with allergic rhinitis has been documented by using generic and disease-specific quality-of-life tools.
- Poorly controlled allergic rhinitis contributes to sleep disturbance and daytime sleepiness, learning difficulty in school, decreased productivity at work, and increased absenteeism from work.
- The annual health costs related to allergic rhinitis in the United States range from $2 billion to $5 billion.
- Sensitization is the process through which low-dose exposure to particular foreign antigens leads to the production of antigen-specific IgE antibodies that bind to the surfaces of mast cells and basophils at sites of allergic reactions.
- During the early allergic response, reexposure to allergens in sensitized individuals leads to antigen binding and cross-linking of antigen-specific IgE molecules on the surfaces of mast cells and basophils, resulting in degranulation and release of inflammatory mediators.

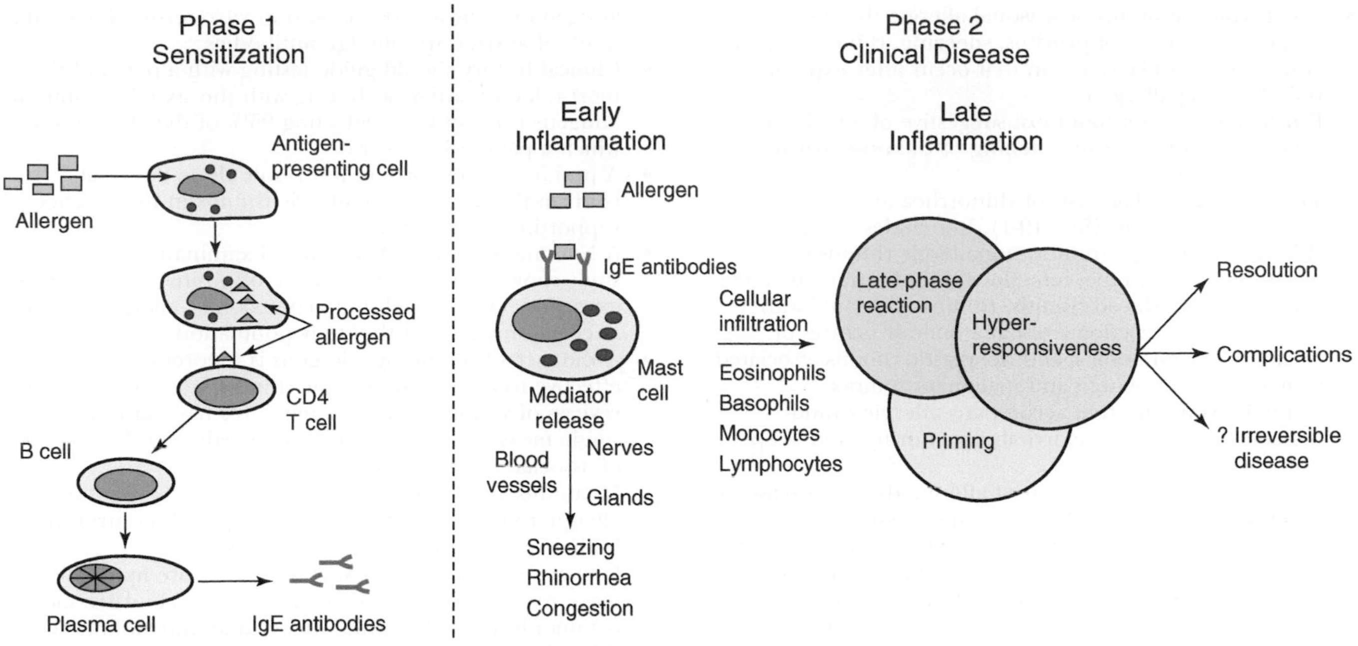

FIGURE 19-1 Pathophysiology of allergic rhinitis.

Box 19-1   DIFFERENTIAL DIAGNOSIS OF RHINORRHEA AND NASAL OBSTRUCTION

Allergic Rhinitis

Seasonal/perennial/episodic or intermittent/persistent

Local Allergic Rhinitis

Negative skin/radioallergosorbent testing but positive nasal allergen challenge

Nonallergic Rhinitis

Perennial (vasomotor): constant symptoms of profuse, clear rhinorrhea and nasal congestion without correlation to specific allergen exposure or signs of atopy

Cold air–induced: nasal congestion and rhinorrhea on exposure to cold, windy weather; occurs in both allergic and nonallergic individuals

Nonallergic Rhinitis with Eosinophilia Syndrome

Most often seen in adults; characterized by eosinophilia on nasal smears and with negative test results for specific allergens

Infectious Rhinitis

Bacterial, viral, fungal

Granulomatous Rhinitis

Sarcoidosis, Wegener granulomatosis

Drug-Induced Rhinitis

Oral contraceptives, reserpine derivatives, hydralazine hydrochloride, topical decongestants (rhinitis medicamentosa), beta-blockers (eye drops)

Rhinitis from Mechanical Obstruction

Septal deviation: common; might exacerbate nasal obstruction in allergic rhinitis

Foreign body: unilateral purulent nasal discharge is the usual manifestation of a foreign body; resolves after removal

Choanal atresia or stenosis: bilateral choanal atresia is usually diagnosed early in life, but unilateral choanal atresia or stenosis can go unnoticed for several years; it is easily diagnosed by nasal endoscopy and axial computed tomography of the midfacial skeleton

Adenoid hypertrophy: common cause of nasal obstruction in children

Others: encephaloceles, lacrimal duct cysts, dermoids

Neoplastic Rhinitis

Benign: polyps, juvenile angiofibroma, inverted papilloma

Malignant: adenocarcinoma, squamous cell carcinoma, esthesioneuroblastoma, lymphoma, rhabdomyosarcoma

---

- The preformed mediators released during mast-cell degranulation include histamine, heparin, and tryptase. Newly synthesized mediators include prostaglandins and leukotrienes.
- Preformed and newly synthesized inflammatory mediators stimulate nerves, glands, and blood vessels, resulting in the clinical manifestations of the early allergic response, which include pruritus, sneezing, rhinorrhea, and nasal congestion.
- The late allergic response may occur 4 to 10 hours after allergen exposure and is characterized by a recurrence of symptoms, most notably nasal congestion.
- The events of the late allergic response are accompanied by the release of preformed inflammatory mediators by mast cells and basophils, influx of inflammatory cells such as TH2 cells and eosinophils, and secretion of inflammatory cytokines by mast cells and TH2 cells.
- The nasal response to allergens is accompanied by ocular, pulmonary, and sinus responses, which are due in part to a neural reflex with contributions from the sympathetic and parasympathetic nervous systems and neuropeptides.
- Priming is a phenomenon characterized by an increase in the severity of clinical symptoms and inflammation upon repeated exposure to relevant allergens.
- Increased reactivity to irritant stimuli is often reported by patients with allergic rhinitis, through a phenomenon of nonspecific hyperresponsiveness, in which the inflamed nasal mucosa of patients with allergic rhinitis presents an exaggerated response to these stimuli.

- The classic symptoms of seasonal allergic rhinitis are recurrent episodes of pruritus, sneezing, rhinorrhea, nasal congestion, and lacrimation that occur after exposure to the offending allergen.
- Pruritus is the symptom most suggestive of an allergic etiology. This may involve itching of the nose, palate, throat, eyes, and ears.
- The differential diagnosis of rhinorrhea and nasal obstruction is broad (Box 19-1). It includes allergic rhinitis, nonallergic rhinitis, nonallergic rhinitis with eosinophilia syndrome, infectious rhinitis, granulomatous rhinitis, drug-induced rhinitis, rhinitis associated with mechanical obstruction from anatomic structures or retained foreign bodies, and neoplastic rhinitis associated with a variety of benign and malignant tumors.
- Systemic symptoms that accompany allergic rhinitis include malaise, fatigue, irritability, snoring, and sleep disturbance.
- The traditional classification of allergic rhinitis is seasonal, perennial, or episodic. An additional classification system was proposed at the ARIA WHO workshop, which divides allergic rhinitis into intermittent and persistent disease.
- Seasonal allergic rhinitis is defined by symptoms that occur during exposure to seasonal allergens such as tree pollens, grasses, ragweed, and others.
- Perennial allergic rhinitis is defined by duration of nasal symptoms for more than 2 hours per day for more than 9 months of the year, typically in association with exposure to house dust mites, indoor molds, animal dander, and cockroaches.
- Episodic rhinitis refers to symptoms on exposure to allergens not normally present in the patient's environment, such as a pet at a relative's house.
- Intermittent allergic rhinitis refers to symptoms present for less than 4 days per week or for less than 4 consecutive weeks.
- Persistent allergic rhinitis refers to symptoms present for more than 4 days per week or for more than 4 consecutive weeks.
- In the ARIA classification, severity of disease is gauged by its influence on a patient's quality of life.
- Mild allergic rhinitis refers to symptoms that are present but not troublesome to the patient. Moderate to severe allergic rhinitis refers to symptoms that are present, troublesome, and associated with one or more of the following: sleep disturbance, impairment at school, impairment at work, or impairment at daily activities.
- Local allergic rhinitis is a clinical phenotype of rhinitis that is characterized by typical symptoms of allergic rhinitis, a positive response to nasal challenge, but skin or serologic allergy testing results that are negative.
- Diagnosis of local allergic rhinitis can be confirmed by detection of nasal allergen-specific IgE, a positive nasal provocation response, or both in the absence of systemic atopy.
- Physical examination findings may be suggestive of allergic rhinitis but they do not confirm the diagnosis. Typical findings may include "allergic shiners," "adenoid facies," and the "allergic salute."
- The nasal mucosa in patients with allergic rhinitis may appear pale, bluish, and edematous, coated in thin, clear secretions; however, no appearance of the nasal mucosa is pathognomonic for allergic rhinitis.
- Physical examination findings are useful in identifying or ruling out other problems as well, such as rhinosinusitis, nasal polyposis, prior trauma, systemic disease, mechanical obstruction due to foreign body, and/or mass lesions.
- Two common tests are utilized to confirm the diagnosis of allergic rhinitis: skin testing with application of specific antigen extracts to the skin and in vitro testing for serum levels of antigen-specific IgE antibodies.
- Clinical history should guide testing with a panel of the most relevant antigens. Testing with the six most common antigens is effective in detecting 95% of the allergens to which a patient is sensitive.
- A positive in vitro or skin test result alone does not confirm the diagnosis of allergic rhinitis in the absence of supporting clinical history.
- A National Health and Nutrition Examination Survey study showed that the prevalence of positive allergy testing exceeded 50%, though full expression of allergic disease affected only 20% of the study population.
- Avoidance of offending allergens is theoretically an effective treatment for allergic rhinitis; however, systematic reviews of various avoidance measures have shown that single measures are not effective in reducing the severity of associated symptoms.
- H_1 antihistamines are effective agents for the treatment of allergic rhinitis, but they do not completely control the bothersome symptom of nasal congestion
- First-generation H_1 antihistamines are more lipophilic, more readily cross the blood-brain barrier, and are more commonly associated with sedative and anticholinergic side effects.
- Intranasal H_1 antihistamines, such as azelastine and olopatadine, are at least as efficacious in the treatment of allergic rhinitis as oral H_1 antihistamines.
- Leukotriene receptor antagonists are effective in controlling the symptoms of allergic rhinitis, and their efficacy parallels that of oral antihistamines.
- Topical decongestants, such as phenylephrine and oxymetazoline, are recommended for use for short duration only due to the association with rhinitis medicamentosa.
- Administration of intranasal anticholinergics, such as ipratropium bromide, is typically associated with improvement in rhinorrhea.
- Intranasal steroids are potent antiinflammatory agents that control almost all aspects of allergic nasal inflammation.
- Intranasal steroids are superior in efficacy to antihistamines and leukotriene receptor antagonists in controlling symptoms of the disease and improving quality of life.
- The most common side effect associated with consistent use of intranasal steroids is local nasal irritation (10%). Other common side effects include epistaxis (8%), septal perforation (rare), and *Candida* overgrowth (rare). There is no consistent evidence of growth retardation or interference of the hypothalamic-pituitary axis.
- Immunotherapy is an effective treatment of allergic rhinitis and is the only therapy known to alter the natural course of the disease.
- Immunotherapy is typically reserved for patients who have not experienced adequate responses to pharmacologic treatment.
- Allergen-specific immunotherapy induces significant immune modulation through desensitization of allergen-specific IgE-bearing mast cells and basophils, induction of T-cell tolerance and deviation toward a regulatory T-cell response, decrease in allergen-specific IgE serum levels, and increase in allergen-specific IgG4 serum levels.
- Immunotherapy may be administered by SCIT or SLIT.
- For patients receiving SCIT, symptom improvement begins within 12 weeks and continues over a period of 1 to 2 years after treatment. The duration of SCIT is typically 3 to 5 years.
- SCIT is associated with local and systemic adverse reactions. The rate of serious systemic reactions, including

death, is far less than 1%; however, given the concern for potential systemic reactions, it is recommended that patients receive SCIT in a supervised medical facility, with monitoring for 30 minutes after every injection.

- The advantages of SLIT over SCIT include ease of administration, usefulness in children who dislike injections, and avoidance of the need to go to the doctor's office to receive the treatment.
- Local side effects of SLIT include itching and swelling of the lips and oral cavity. Systemic anaphylactic reactions have been described but are extremely rare.
- Ocular symptoms associated with allergic rhinitis may be attributed to both the direct deposition of allergen onto the conjunctiva and to the nasocular reflex.
- Multiple medication preparations are effective in controlling ocular symptoms associated with allergic rhinitis, including antihistamine ophthalmic drops, intranasal antihistamines, oral antihistamines, and intranasal steroids.
- Intranasal steroid administration alone is as effective as intranasal antihistamine administration in controlling ocular symptoms, likely related to a reduction in intranasal inflammation and inhibition of the nasocular reflex.
- Multiple combination therapies have been proposed and administered in the treatment of allergic rhinitis. Studies have shown an additive benefit or superior control of symptoms with combinations such as intranasal steroids with intranasal antihistamines and intranasal steroids with intranasal decongestants, when compared with placebo and monotherapy treatments.
- The authors' general guidelines for the management of allergic rhinitis include the following: for mild disease, treatment with as-needed intranasal steroids is recommended; for moderate to severe disease, regular use of intranasal steroids with or without intranasal antihistamines is recommended; for patients who are unwilling to use an intranasal medication or who are bothered by local irritation, treatment with oral antihistamines is recommended.
- Follow-up after initiation of therapy is recommended at 2 weeks in order to assess response to therapy. If a response is partial, residual complaints are assessed and additional agents are added to target those symptoms. Residual ocular symptoms may be treated with the addition of intraocular antihistamines. Residual nasal congestion may be treated with the addition of intranasal antihistamines. Residual rhinorrhea may be treated with the addition of ipratropium bromide. If no response to maximal medical therapy is observed, alternative diagnoses should be considered. For significant disease with no response to maximal medical therapy, immunotherapy should be considered.

ANSWERS

TRUE OR FALSE QUESTIONS

1. T	14. T	27. T	40. T
2. T	15. T	28. T	41. T
3. T	16. F	29. F	42. T
4. F	17. T	30. F	43. F
5. F	18. F	31. T	44. T
6. T	19. T	32. T	45. T
7. T	20. F	33. F	46. F
8. T	21. F	34. F	47. F
9. F	22. T	35. T	48. T
10. F	23. T	36. T	49. T
11. T	24. T	37. F	50. T
12. F	25. F	38. F	
13. F	26. T	39. T	

SINGLE BEST ANSWER QUESTIONS

51. d	64. c	77. b	90. c
52. e	65. d	78. d	91. c
53. b	66. d	79. a	92. d
54. d	67. c	80. f	93. e
55. c	68. b	81. b	94. c
56. b	69. c	82. c	95. c
57. d	70. d	83. b	96. a
58. a	71. c	84. c	97. b
59. b	72. b	85. a	98. c
60. d	73. d	86. b	99. a
61. c	74. c	87. d	100. b
62. e	75. a	88. e	
63. e	76. c	89. a	

SUGGESTED READINGS

1. Bousquet J, Schünemann HJ, Samolinski B, et al. Allergic Rhinitis and its Impact on Asthma (ARIA): achievements in 10 years and future needs. *J Allergy Clin Immunol.* 2012; 130(5):1049-1062.

2. Meltzer EO, Gross GN, Katial R, Storms WW. Allergic rhinitis substantially impacts patient quality of life: findings from the Nasal Allergy Survey Assessing Limitations. *J Fam Pract.* 2012;61(suppl 2):S5-S10.

3. Burks AW, Calderon MA, Casale T, et al. Update on allergy and immunotherapy: American Academy of Allergy Asthma and Immunology/European Academy of Allergy and Clinical Immunology/PRACTALL consensus report. *J Allergy Clin Immunol.* 2013;131:1288-1296.

4. Radulovic S, Calderon MA, Wilson D, Durham S. Sublingual immunotherapy for allergic rhinitis. *Cochrane Database Syst Rev.* 2010;(12):CD002893, doi:10.1002/14651858. CD002893.

5. Heederick D, von Mutius E. Does diversity of environmental microbial exposure matter for the occurrence of allergy and asthma? *J Allergy Clin Immunol.* 2012;130:44-50.

6. Lloyd CM, Saglani S. T cells in asthma: influences of genetics, environment, and T-cell plasticity. *J Allergy Clin Immunol.* 2013;131:1267-1274.

7. Akdis CA, Akdis M. Mechanisms of allergen-specific immunotherapy. *J Allergy Clin Immunol.* 2011;127:18-27.

8. Rondon C, Campo P, Togias A, et al. Local allergic rhinitis: Concept, pathophysiology, and management. *J Allergy Clin Immunol.* 2012;129:1460-1467.

9. Simons FER, Simons KJ. Histamine and H1-antihistamines: celebrating a century of progress. *J Allergy Clin Immunol.* 2011;128:1139-1150.

10. Carr W, Bernstein J, Lieberman P, et al. A novel intranasal therapy of azelastine with fluticasone for the treatment of allergic rhinitis. *J Allergy Clin Immunol.* 2012;129(5): 1282-1289.

11. Wallace DV, Dykewicz MS, Bernstein DI, et al. Joint Task Force on Practice; American Academy of Allergy, Asthma & Immunology; American College of Allergy, Asthma and Immunology; Joint Council of Allergy, Asthma and Immunology. The diagnosis and management of rhinitis: an updated practice parameter. *J Allergy Clin Immunol.* 2008;122(suppl 2):S1-S84.

Facial Plastic Surgery | 20

Tara Ramachandra | David M. Hogan

TRUE OR FALSE QUESTIONS

T/F 1. The standard point of reference for positioning a patient for clinical photographs or cephalometric radiographs is the Frankfurt line.

T/F 2. The human face is almost always completely symmetrical when comparing halves through the midsagittal plane.

T/F 3. Facial width is evaluated using the rule of fifths.

T/F 4. When evaluating facial height using the rule of thirds, the upper third of the face is measured from the trichion to the nasion.

T/F 5. The trichion is a fixed landmark that can be used to accurately measure facial height over time.

T/F 6. The human face can be divided into esthetic units and subunits that are useful in planning reconstruction after extirpation.

T/F 7. The upper eyelid crease is created by the insertion of the levator aponeurosis and orbital septum into the epidermis and orbicularis oris.

T/F 8. The upper eyelid normally covers a small portion of the iris and pupil.

T/F 9. Incisions perpendicular to relaxed skin tension lines give the most favorable scars.

T/F 10. The nasofacial angle, measuring the incline of the nasal dorsum in relation to the facial plane, can vary between 30 and 40 degrees, but ideally measures 36 degrees.

T/F 11. A columellar show of between 3 and 5 mm is considered acceptable.

T/F 12. The length of the ear is approximately half its width.

T/F 13. The long axis of the ear roughly parallels the long axis of the nasal dorsum.

T/F 14. Hyperdynamic facial lines are often found on the lower eyelids and cheek.

T/F 15. Hyperdynamic facial lines are caused by skin folding secondary to loss of underlying soft tissue support.

T/F 16. The mentocervical angle should be approximately 80 to 95 degrees and measured between a line through the nasion and the pogonion and the angle it makes with a line through the menton and the cervical point.

T/F 17. When reconstructing large defects on the face and neck, local flap use may result in considerable impairment in form and/or function.

T/F 18. Regarding pivotal flaps, the greater the degree of pivot, the longer the effective flap length.

T/F 19. Rotation flaps are best used to close triangular defects adjacent to the flap.

T/F 20. To reduce flap edema, when designing a rotation flap it is best to have the flap based superiorly.

T/F 21. Facial scars are best camouflaged if placed along the borders of esthetic regions.

T/F 22. Scalp tissue is usually quite elastic.

T/F 23. A standing cutaneous deformity caused during use of a rotation flap can be removed primarily, as it never contributes to the vascularity of the rotation flap.

T/F 24. The abundant vascularity of the skin of the face and neck means that the ratio of flap length to width can often exceed 3:1.

T/F 25. An interpolated flap often requires a second procedure to inset the flap after the development of a local random blood supply.

T/F 26. Advancement flaps rely on primary movement of the surrounding tissue and tissue elasticity of the flap acting as secondary movement to achieve defect closure.

T/F 27. Secondary skin movement in advancement flaps may be detrimental secondary to displacement of facial structures nearby.

T/F 28. Skin cancer most frequently occurs on the nose.

T/F 29. When dividing the pedicle of a paramedian forehead flap, excess pedicle should always be returned to the forehead above the level of the eyebrows.

T/F 30. When considering the esthetic subunits of the lip, the lower lip is generally not divided into separate units, whereas the upper lip is.

T/F 31. When performing a lower lip wedge excision, the wedge should be carried below the mental line only when tumor extirpation dictates.

T/F 32. When constructing an Abbe or Estlander flap, the height of the flap should equal the height of the defect, and the width of the flap should equal the width of the defect.

T/F 33. Microtia is a more common congenital ear abnormality compared with protruding ears.

T/F 34. The inheritance of protruding ears is autosomal dominant with complete penetrance.

T/F 35. The otic placode is first noticeable during the third week of intrauterine growth.

T/F 36. The six hillocks of His fuse by the sixth week of intrauterine growth.

T/F 37. The normal range for the auriculocephalic angle is 25 to 35 degrees.

T/F 38. When cut, cartilage will bend toward the cut side.

T/F 39. A telephone ear deformity results from excessive overcorrection of the mid third of the ear.

T/F 40. Rates of postoperative hematoma following otoplasty are lower in cartilage-cutting techniques.

T/F 41. Persistent or progressive pain after otoplasty is expected and is not an indication to remove the pressure dressing.

T/F 42. The expected loss of correction associated with suture techniques in otoplasty is approximately 40%.

T/F 43. Epidermal inclusion cyst and sebaceous cyst are synonymous.

T/F 44. Proliferating trichilemmal tumors have no malignant transformation potential.

T/F 45. Dermoid cysts result from entrapment of epidermis along lines of embryonic fusion.

T/F 46. An ephelis differs from lentigines in that it consists of an overall increase in the number of melanocytes.

T/F 47. Hypertrophic scarring is defined as a proliferation beyond the margins of the original insult.

T/F 48. Xanthelasma is not found in normolipidemic patients.

T/F 49. The vasculitis associated with chondrodermatitis nodularis helicus can extend deeply and require cartilage excision.

T/F 50. Stevens-Johnson syndrome is characterized by erythema and blistering of the skin and mucous membranes of greater than 30% of body surface area.

SINGLE BEST ANSWER QUESTIONS

51. From which region is the Frankfurt horizontal plane drawn?
    a. Superior aspect of the external auditory canal to the inferior border of the infraorbital rim
    b. Superior aspect of the root of the helix to the inferior border of the infraorbital rim
    c. Inferior aspect of the external auditory canal to the inferior border of the infraorbital rim
    d. Inferior aspect of the root of the helix to the inferior border of the infraorbital rim

52. When examining the width of the face, the width of one eye should equal all of the following EXCEPT:
    a. One-fifth of the total facial width
    b. The intercanthal width
    c. The width of the mouth
    d. The width of the nasal base

53. Which of the following measurements is NOT part of the rule of thirds when evaluating facial height?
    a. Trichion to nasion
    b. Glabella to subnasale
    c. Glabella to trichion
    d. Subnasale to menton

54. The nasofrontal angle formed by a line tangent to the nasal dorsum intersecting a line tangent to the glabella through the nasion should be within which range of angles?
    a. 90 to 110 degrees
    b. 115 to 135 degrees
    c. 70 to 90 degrees
    d. 135 to 145 degrees

55. Which of the following is NOT a major esthetic unit of the face?
    a. Forehead
    b. Eyes
    c. Ears
    d. Nasal vestibule

56. The nasolabial angle formed from the intersection of a line tangent between the labrale superioris and the subnasale and that tangent between the subnasale and the most anterior point of the columella should measure:
    a. 95 to 110 degrees in men
    b. 95 to 110 degrees in women
    c. 75 to 85 degrees in men
    d. 75 to 85 degrees in women

57. When examining nasal tip projection, the ratio between upper lip length and nasal projection should roughly equal:
    a. 1:2
    b. 1:3
    c. 1:1
    d. 1:1.5

58. Using Goode method, the ratio of a vertical line from the nasion to the alar groove with a line perpendicular from the alar groove to the nasal tip should equal:
    a. 0.35 to 0.45
    b. 0.45 to 0.50
    c. 0.55 to 0.60
    d. 0.65 to 0.75

59. When considering the ideal ear, which of the following measurements are most accurate?
    a. The ear protrudes from the skull at an angle of 20 to 30 degrees and has a posterior rotation of 15 degrees from the vertical plane.
    b. The ear protrudes from the skull at an angle of 15 degrees and has a posterior rotation of 20 to 30 degrees from the vertical plane.
    c. The ear protrudes from the skull at an angle of 35 to 40 degrees and has a posterior rotation of 10 degrees from the vertical plane.
    d. The ear protrudes from the skull at an angle of 10 degrees and has a posterior rotation of 35 to 40 degrees from the vertical plane.

60. Which of the following critical factors should NOT be commented on in the clinical notes or to an examiner in vivo when analyzing the facial skin?
    a. Texture
    b. Thickness
    c. Elasticity
    d. Translucence

61. All of the following are examples of hyperdynamic facial lines EXCEPT:
    a. Crow's feet
    b. Melolabial sulcus
    c. Glabella lines
    d. Horizontal forehead creases

62. Using the Fitzpatrick Classification of Sun-Reactive Skin Types, which of the following statements is *INCORRECT*?
    a. Type 1 skin always tans and never burns.
    b. Type 2 skin usually burns and tans with difficulty.
    c. Type 4 skin rarely burns and tans with ease.
    d. Type 5 skin very rarely burns and tans very easily.

63. Of the following, which is *NOT* a classification for cutaneous flaps?
    a. Classification by method of transfer
    b. Classification by blood supply
    c. Classification by skin match
    d. Classification by proximity to the defect

64. Which of the following methods of transfer does *NOT* apply to local cutaneous flaps?
    a. Pivotal
    b. Microsurgical
    c. Advancement
    d. Hinged

65. Which of the following local flaps is an example of a pivotal flap?
    a. Interpolated
    b. Bipedical
    c. V-Y flap
    d. Unipedicle

66. When rotating a pivotal flap through 180 degrees, what is the amount of effective length that may be lost as a result?
    a. 15%
    b. 20%
    c. 30%
    d. 40%

67. Scalp defects are best reconstructed with which of the following types of flap, secondary to the shape of the cranium and relative lack of skin elasticity?
    a. Advancement flap
    b. Transposition flap
    c. Rotation flap
    d. Free flap

68. An interpolated flap can be used as a single-stage reconstruction when which most important condition is met?
    a. The pedicle is de-epithelialized and passed under the intervening skin.
    b. The skin color and texture exactly match between donor and defect sites.
    c. A good random blood supply exists.
    d. The defect is located in close proximity to the base of the flap.

69. Which of the following is *NOT* a feature of advancement flaps for reconstruction?
    a. They have a linear configuration.
    b. Tissue is moved through two vectors.
    c. They depend on tissue elasticity.
    d. They often require undermining of surrounding soft tissue to achieve closure.

70. When reconstructing nasal defects of a convex aesthetic unit, which percentage defect is best repaired first by removing the remaining skin of the subunit?
    a. 5%
    b. 20%
    c. 35%
    d. 50%

71. When raising a paramedian forehead flap based on the supratrochlear artery, the origin of the supratrochlear artery is most commonly found:
    a. 0.5 to 1.0 cm lateral to midline
    b. 1.7 to 2.2 cm lateral to midline
    c. 2.3 to 2.7 cm lateral to midline
    d. 2.8 to 3.1 cm lateral to midline

72. Regarding the Karapandzic flap, which of the following is *INCORRECT*?
    a. It is an innervated reconstructive option for lip defects.
    b. It often results in microstomia.
    c. It is useful for the reconstruction of defects less than one-third of lip width.
    d. It restores a continuous circle of functioning orbicularis oris muscle.

73. Aesthetic goals for repairing forehead defects include all of the following *EXCEPT*:
    a. Avoidance of diagonal scars
    b. Maintenance of eyebrow symmetry
    c. Maintenance of natural frontal hairlines
    d. Planning vertical scars where possible

74. Which of the following will give the *WORST* cosmetic result for the repair of forehead defects generally?
    a. Skin graft
    b. Healing by secondary intention
    c. Primary closure
    d. Local advancement flaps

75. Regarding tissue expansion for defect repair, which of the following is *NOT* a disadvantage?
    a. It is a two-stage procedure.
    b. The end cosmetic result
    c. Tissue expansion must occur prior to defect creation.
    d. There is considerable associated deformity during the expansion.

76. Which of the following is the most common abnormality regarding protruding ears?
    a. Unfurled helix
    b. Deficiency of triangular fossa
    c. Hypertrophic conchal bowl
    d. Loss of antitragus

77. Which of the following is *NOT* a sensory supply to the pinna?
    a. C2 and C3
    b. V_2
    c. VII
    d. X

78. Which of the following pairs is *INCORRECT* in relation to the evolution of the external ear from the hillocks of His?
    a. First hillock → the tragus
    b. Third hillock → the helix
    c. Fifth hillock → the antihelix
    d. Sixth hillock → the lobule

79. Which of the following statements is correct?
    a. By 3 years of age 90% of auricular growth has been completed.
    b. Cartilaginous growth is almost complete by age 5 years.
    c. The vertical dimension of the average adult ear is 7 cm.
    d. The incidence of protruding ears in Caucasians is approximately 15%.

80. Regarding complications following otoplasty, which of the following is *NOT* an early complication?
    a. Perichondritis
    b. Cartilage necrosis
    c. Hematoma
    d. Keloid scar formation

81. Regarding late complications of otoplasty, which of the following is *INCORRECT*?
    a. Keloid scarring is most commonly seen in older, fairer skinned patients.
    b. Foreign body granuloma formation is more often seen when braided sutures are used compared with monofilament sutures.
    c. Recurrent frostbite may occur due to disruption of the auricular blood supply.
    d. Hypoaesthesia after otoplasty is secondary to injury of the greater auricular nerve.

82. Which of the following statements regarding skin malignancies is correct?
    a. Basal cell carcinoma is the most common malignancy, but melanoma causes the most deaths related to skin cancer.
    b. Basal cell carcinoma is the most common malignancy, but squamous cell carcinoma causes the most deaths related to skin cancer.
    c. Squamous cell carcinoma is the most common malignancy, but basal cell carcinoma causes the most deaths related to skin cancer.
    d. Squamous cell carcinoma is the most common malignancy, but melanoma causes the most deaths related to skin cancer.

83. Which of the following human papilloma virus (HPV) subtypes is not typically associated with verruca vulgaris?
    a. HPV 2
    b. HPV 27
    c. HPV 16
    d. HPV 57

84. Which of the following is *NOT* a subtype of melanocytic nevi?
    a. Dysplastic
    b. Compound
    c. Spitz
    d. Intraepidermal

85. Regarding melanocytic lesions of the head and neck, which of the following is *NOT* an indication for biopsy, providing it is not practical to excise the entire lesion?
    a. Variegation in color
    b. Diameter greater than 2 mm
    c. Asymmetry of the border
    d. Evolution of the lesion

86. With respect to lentigines, which of the following statements is *INCORRECT*?
    a. Cryotherapy is effective for solitary lesions, as keratinocytes are preferentially destroyed at low temperatures.
    b. Lentigines are characterized by a proliferation of benign melanocytes at the dermoepidermal junction.
    c. Lentigines are photoinduced and darken on sun exposure.
    d. Clinically, lentigines have more even pigment distribution when compared with melanoma in situ.

87. Of the following, which is *NOT* characteristic for a diagnosis of neurofibromatosis type 1?
    a. Lisch nodules
    b. Café au lait macules
    c. Bilateral vestibular schwannomas
    d. Optic gliomas

88. Regarding congenital bullous diseases, which of the following descriptions is correct for dystrophic epidermolysis bullosa?
    a. Blistering occurs in the epidermis.
    b. Blisters can occur at various levels.
    c. Blistering occurs within the dermis.
    d. Blistering occurs at the dermoepidermal junction.

89. Treatment options of pemphigus and pemphigoid include all of the following *EXCEPT*:
    a. Immunoglobulin infusion
    b. Oral corticosteroids
    c. Monoclonal antibodies
    d. Systemic immunosuppression

90. Regarding Stevens-Johnson syndrome, which of the following statements is *INCORRECT*?
    a. Adult cases are usually infectious in nature.
    b. Fever and malaise are common first symptoms, followed by cutaneous and mucosal lesions.
    c. It is characterized by erythema and blistering of the skin and mucous membranes of less than 10% of body surface area.
    d. Oral corticosteroids used after substantial desquamation have been shown to increase morbidity.

91. Of the following risk factors for development of malignant skin lesions, which of the following is thought most important for the development of squamous cell carcinoma?
    a. Exposure to chemical carcinogens
    b. Cumulative sun exposure
    c. Sunburns
    d. Intense and intermittent sun exposure during childhood

92. Which of the following types of melanoma is most likely to lack a radial growth phase?
    a. Superficial spreading
    b. Lentigo maligna
    c. Nodular
    d. Acral lentiginous

93. Which of the following is the most common variant of basal cell carcinoma?
    a. Infiltrative
    b. Morpheaform
    c. Sclerosing
    d. Nodular

94. Which of the following is *NOT* associated with Gorlin syndrome?
    a. Bifid ribs
    b. Microcephaly
    c. Ovarian fibromas
    d. Basal cell carcinoma

95. Regarding squamous cell carcinoma, which of the following is *NOT* considered a trait associated with increased aggressive behavior?
    a. Increasing differentiation
    b. Perineural invasion
    c. Depth of invasion greater than 4 mm
    d. Lesions greater than 2 cm in diameter

96. Which of the following is *NOT* a risk factor for the development of Merkel cell carcinoma?
    a. Ultraviolet radiation exposure
    b. Arsenic exposure
    c. Immunosuppression
    d. Merkel cell polyomavirus infection

97. Which of the following lesions is most commonly associated with tuberous sclerosis?
    a. Angiofibroma
    b. Acrochordon
    c. Xanthelasma
    d. Sebaceous hyperplasia

98. Which of the following is *INCORRECT* regarding morphea?
    a. It is thought to have an autoimmune cause.
    b. It is usually a self-limiting condition.
    c. It is a systemic manifestation of scleroderma.
    d. Adult onset of the disease is uncommon.

99. Which of the following is correct regarding melanoma?
    a. Survival is not related to tumor thickness.
    b. Patients with atypical nevi are not at increased risk of developing melanoma compared with the general population.
    c. Light skin, hair, and eye color are not risk factors for melanoma.
    d. Tumor ulceration and mitotic rate are important prognostic factors.

100. Keratoacanthomas require removal with adequate margin and depth for histopathologic review because
    a. Not all keratoacanthomas will involute.
    b. They consist of keratinocytes with follicular features.
    c. Frequent mitoses at the base of the lesion and a rapid growth phase are suggestive of squamous cell carcinoma.
    d. Involution may result in scarring.

CORE KNOWLEDGE

AESTHETIC FACIAL ANALYSIS

- Soft tissue reference points are shown in Figure 20-1 and Box 20-1.
- The Frankfurt horizontal line (Figure 20-2) is the standard reference line for patient positioning during photographs. It is drawn from the superior aspect of the external auditory canal to the inferior border of the infraorbital rim. The point of transition between the lower lid and cheek skin forms the soft tissue definition for the infraorbital rim.

Facial Proportions

- Facial symmetry is assessed by comparing halves through a midsagittal plane.
- Facial width is evaluated by dividing the face into equal vertical fifths (Figure 20-3). Each eye should equal one-fifth of total facial width, as should the intercanthal distance or nasal base width.

- Facial height is most commonly assessed by dividing the face into equal thirds (Figure 20-4): from trichion to the glabella, from the glabella to the subnasale, and from the subnasale to the menton.

Subunit Analysis

- The facial aesthetic units are the forehead, eyes, nose, lips, chin, ears, and neck.
- Units are based on skin thickness, texture, color, and contour.
- More favorable scars are achieved when incisions are made parallel to relaxed skin tension lines (Figure 20-5) and within unit or subunit borders.

FOREHEAD

- Boundaries: hairline to the glabella
- Contour: ideally a gentle convexity on profile
- *Nasofrontal angle* (Figure 20-6): intersection of line tangent to glabella through nasion and line of nasal dorsum. Ranges from 115 to 135 degrees.

EYES

- Lateral position of the brow should be at the supraorbital rim in men and above the rim in women.
- Medial edge of the eyebrow lies on a perpendicular line that passes through the lateralmost portion of the nasal ala, around 10 mm above the medial canthus. The highest point of a female's eyebrow arc is at a line drawn tangentially from the lateral limbus.
- The lateral canthus is slightly more superior than the medial canthus, and the eye should be almond shaped.
- The upper lid crease is created by the insertion of the orbital septum and levator aponeurosis into the orbicularis oculi and dermis.

NOSE

- Laterally, the nose begins at the nasion (same level as superior palpebral fold) and ends at subnasale.
- Nine nasal subunits: dorsum, tip, columella, two sidewalls, two soft tissue triangles, two ala

---

Box 20-1   SOFT TISSUE ANATOMIC LANDMARKS

Trichion: anterior hairline in the midline
Glabella: most prominent point of the forehead on profile
Nasion: the deepest depression at the root of the nose; typically corresponds to the nasofrontal suture
Radix: root of the nose, a region and not a point; part of an unbroken curve that begins at the superior orbital ridge and continues along the lateral nasal wall
Rhinion: soft tissue correlate of the osseocartilaginous junction on the nasal dorsum
Sellion: osseocartilaginous junction on the nasal dorsum
Supratip: point cephalic to the tip
Tip: ideally, the most anterior projection of the nose on profile
Subnasale: junction of columella and upper lip
Labrale superius: vermilion border of upper lip
Stomion: central portion of interlabial gap
Stomion superius: lowest point of upper lip vermilion
Stomion inferius: highest point of lower lip vermilion
Labrale inferius: vermilion border of lower lip
Mentolabial sulcus: most posterior point between lower lip and chin
Pogonion: most anterior midline soft tissue point of chin
Menton: most inferior soft tissue point on chin
Cervical point: innermost point between the submental area and the neck

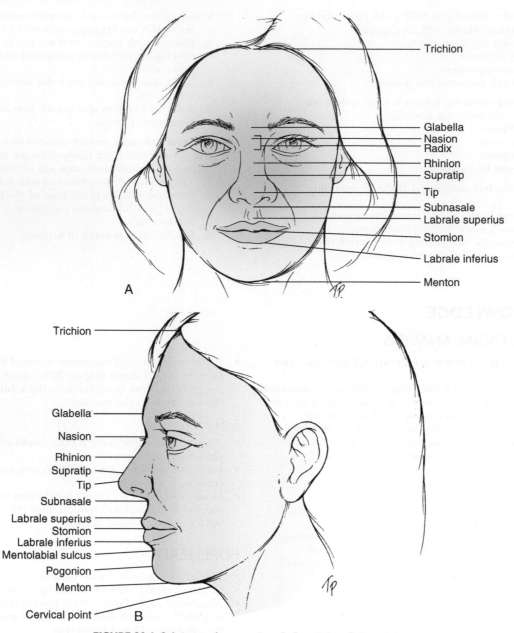

FIGURE 20-1 Soft tissue reference points. **A,** Frontal view. **B,** Lateral view.

NASOFACIAL RELATIONSHIPS

- *Nasofrontal angle:* see Figure 20-6, described previously.
- *Nasolabial angle:* angular inclination of the columella where it meets the upper lip (Figure 20-7). Should be 95 to 110 degrees in women and 90 to 95 degrees in men.
- *Nasofacial angle:* incline of nasal dorsum relative to the facial plane (Figure 20-8). Varies from 30 to 40 degrees.
- *Nasomental angle:* angle formed by a tangent line from the nasion to the nasal tip intersecting with a line from the tip to the pogonion (Figure 20-9). Ranges from 120 to 132 degrees.

Nasal Rotation and Projection

- *Rotation:* occurs along an arc produced by a radius based at the external auditory canal
- *Projection:*
  - Goode method: ratio of distance between alar groove to tip and nasion to tip should be 0.55 to 0.60

(Figure 20-10), creating a nasofacial angle of 36 degrees.
  - 3-4-5 ratio: hypotenuse is the nasal length, and projection is the smallest arm of the triangle.

Alar-Columellar Complex

- Laterally, ala-to-tip/lobular complex ratio is optimal at 1:1.
- On base view, the nose should be triangular and divided into three equal units.
- Between 3 to 5 mm of columellar show is acceptable.

LIPS

- Upper lip: from subnasale to stomion superius
- Lower lip and chin: from stomion inferius to menton
- Subunits of the lip: see Figure 20-11.

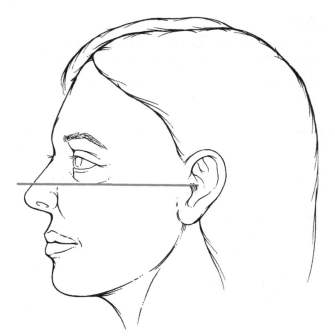

FIGURE 20-2 Frankfurt horizontal plane. A line is drawn from the superior aspect of the external auditory canal to the most inferior aspect of the infraorbital rim.

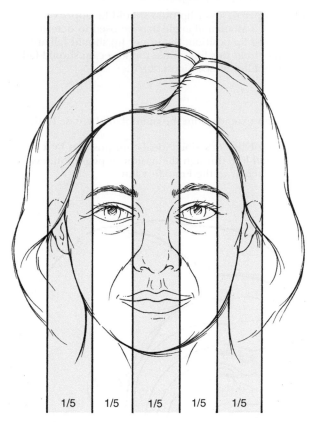

1/5   1/5   1/5   1/5   1/5

FIGURE 20-3 Facial width. The facial width is divided into equal fifths.

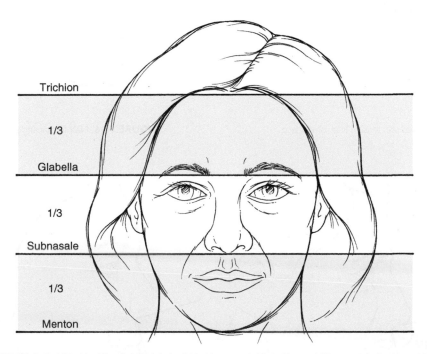

Trichion

1/3

Glabella

1/3

Subnasale

1/3

Menton

FIGURE 20-4 Facial height. The facial height is divided into equal thirds. From trichion to glabella, from glabella to subnasale, and from subnasale to menton.

- Ideal upper to lower lip ratio should be approximately 1:2. The nasomental angle may be used to determine horizontal lip position; the upper lip should fall around 4 mm behind this line, while the lower lip should fall 2 mm behind it (see Figure 20-9).

CHIN

- The chin extends from the mentolabial crease to the menton.
- Gonzalez-Ulloa described ideal chin position by a tangential line through the nasion to pogonion, essentially perpendicular to the Frankfurt line.

NECK

- The ideal neck has a well-defined mandible from the pogonion to the angle of the mandible with an acute mentocervical angle.
- The perception of poor chin projection can result from an obtuse mentocervical angle.

EARS

- The width of the ear is around one-half its length, and ear length should approximate nasal length.
- The long axis of the ear is parallel to the long axis of the nasal dorsum.
- The ear protrudes from the skull at around 20 to 30 degrees. The measurement from the helix to mastoid skin is approximately 15 to 25 mm.

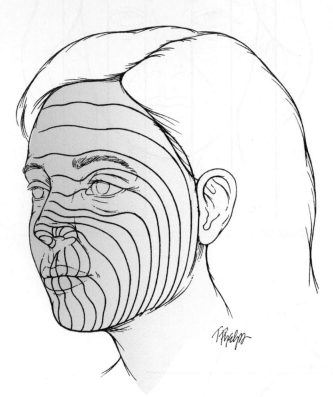

FIGURE 20-5 Relaxed skin tension lines of the face.

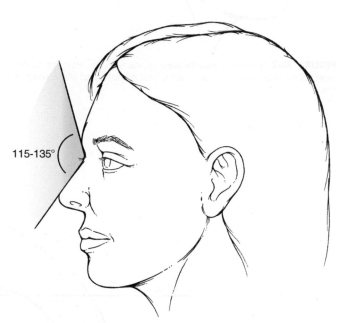

FIGURE 20-6 Nasofrontal angle (115 to 135 degrees).

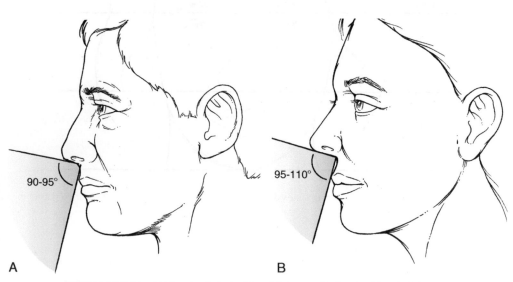

FIGURE 20-7 Nasolabial angle. **A,** Male, 90 to 95 degrees. **B,** Female, 95 to 110 degrees.

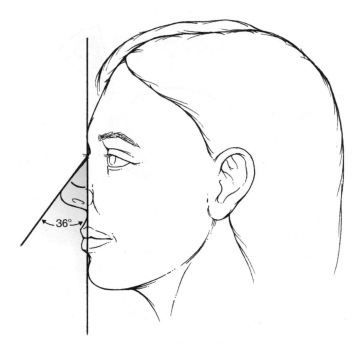

FIGURE 20-8 Nasofacial angle: 30 to 40 degrees.

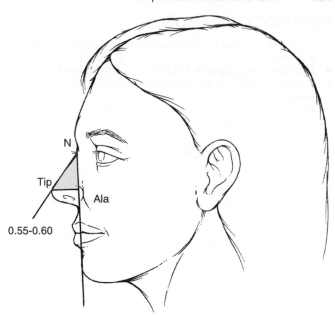

FIGURE 20-10 Goode method of plotting tip projection. *N,* Nasion.

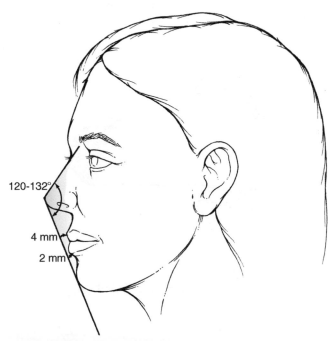

FIGURE 20-9 Nasomental angle: 120 to 132 degrees. The lips should fall just behind this line at a distance of 4 mm for the upper lip and 2 mm for the lower lip.

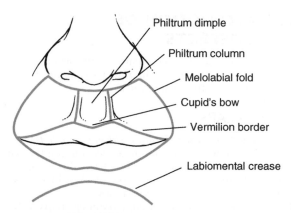

FIGURE 20-11 Lip esthetic subunits.

Table 20-1	**Fitzpatrick Classification of Sun-Reactive Skin Types**	
Skin Type	**Skin Color**	**Characteristics**
I	White	Always burns, never tans
II	White	Usually burns, tans with difficulty
III	White	Sometimes burns, sometimes tans
IV	White	Rarely burns, tans with ease
V	Brown	Very rarely burns, tans very easily
VI	Black	Never burns, always tans

SKIN AND RHYTIDS

- Evaluation of skin texture, thickness, elasticity, and solar damage
- Fitzpatrick skin-type classification (Table 20-1)
- Rhytids, or wrinkles, develop from aging, solar damage, and skin folding due to loss of underlying support.
- Hyperdynamic facial lines, such as horizontal forehead creases, glabellar lines and crow's feet, are caused by long-term facial muscle animation.

BENIGN SKIN LESIONS

EPIDERMAL LESIONS

Seborrheic Keratosis, Verruca Vulgaris

Cysts and Subcutaneous Lesions
- *Epidermal inclusion cyst:* columnar epithelial cells lining a keratin-filled sac
- *Milia:* small (<3 mm), superficial white epidermal inclusion cysts
- *Dermoid cyst:* benign subcutaneous nodules

MELANOCYTIC LESIONS

- *Benign nevus:* may be compound, intradermal, dysplastic, or Spitz
- *Dysplastic nevi:* pigment irregularity and uneven borders
- *Lentigo:* macular hyperpigmented, photoinduced lesions found on the head and neck
- *Ephelis:* freckle (due to increased melanogenesis within normal epidermis)

FIBROADNEXAL LESIONS

- *Skin tags*
- *Keloid and hypertrophic scar*
  - *Keloid scar:* proliferation beyond the margins of the original insult
  - *Hypertrophic scar:* confined to original wound
- *Neurofibroma:* benign proliferation of the peripheral nerve sheath, somewhat pedunculated, flesh-colored papules
- *Angiofibroma:* skin-colored to white papules frequently found on the face
- *Xanthelasma:* accumulation of cholesterol within the dermis of periorbital skin
- *Vitiligo:* patches of depigmentation on the skin

RECONSTRUCTION OF FACIAL DEFECTS

- Reconstructive ladder: secondary intent, primary closure, delayed primary closure, skin graft (partial and full), tissue expansion, flap, free tissue transfer

PIVOTAL FLAPS

- Categorized as *rotational, transpositional,* or *interpolated,* these flaps move toward the defect by rotating the base of the flap around a pivot point. The base of the flap is restricted; therefore, as the degree of pivot increases, the effective length of the flap decreases.
  - (1) *Rotation flaps:* broad-based, curvilinear flaps with reliable vascularity (Figure 20-12)
    - Medial cheek defects near nasal sidewall or nasofacial sulcus
    - Large posterior cheek and upper neck defects can be closed with medial, inferiorly based rotation flaps from the cheek or upper cervical area.
    - Chin reconstruction, glabellar area
    - Well-suited to scalp defects because rotation flaps do not depend on tissue elasticity and the curvilinear incisions conform well to the spherical skull.
    - Disadvantages: require a triangular defect, create a right angle at the distal tip as well as standing cutaneous deformity
  - (2) *Transposition flaps:* linear axis flap that moves around a pivot point, but only the base of the flap needs to be contiguous with the defect. Therefore, skin can be recruited from areas of greater skin elasticity.
    - Small- to medium-sized defects in most locations
    - Example: melolabial transposition flap
  - (3) *Interpolated flaps:* linearly configured pivotal flap with base located away from defect
    - The pedicle must pass under or over intervening tissue, so a second procedure is required to inset the flap. The pedicle may be deepithelialized and tunneled under the skin to avoid a second stage.

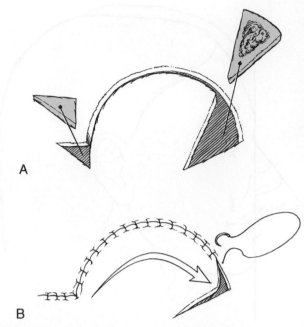

FIGURE 20-12 A, Rotation flaps are pivotal flaps with curvilinear configuration. Removal of a Burow triangle can facilitate repair of the donor site. **B,** Standing cutaneous deformity will form at the base of the flap. Triangle-shaped defects use a portion of this redundant tissue. (From Baker SR, Swanson N. *Local Flaps in Facial Reconstruction.* St Louis: Mosby; 1995.)

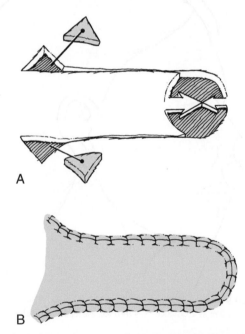

FIGURE 20-13 A, Unipedicle advancement flap is created by parallel incisions, which allow flap tissue to slide in a single vector *(large arrow)* toward the defect. Secondary movement of surrounding skin immediately adjacent to the defect occurs in a direction *(small arrow)* opposite to the direction of flap movement. **B,** Configuration of wound following flap transfer. (Modified from Baker SR, Swanson N. *Local Flaps in Facial Reconstruction.* St Louis: Mosby; 1995.)

- The vertically oriented paramedian forehead flap has excellent vascularity as well as good color and texture match to nasal skin. Its dependable axial blood supply arises from the supratrochlear artery.

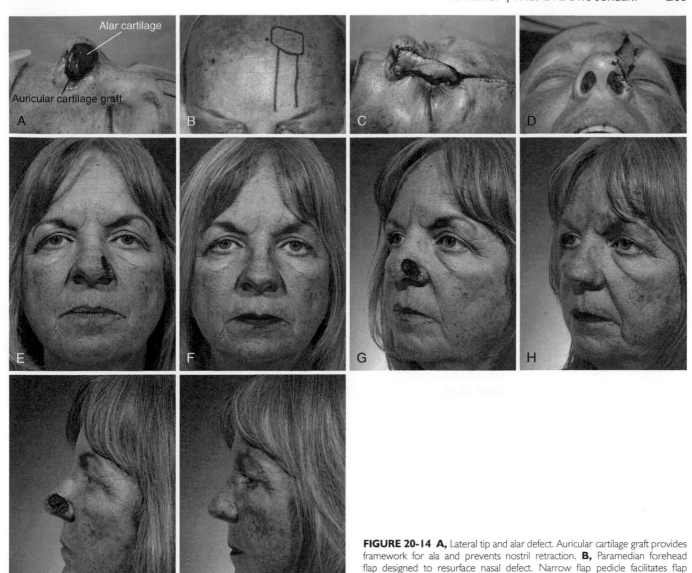

FIGURE 20-14 A, Lateral tip and alar defect. Auricular cartilage graft provides framework for ala and prevents nostril retraction. **B,** Paramedian forehead flap designed to resurface nasal defect. Narrow flap pedicle facilitates flap pivoting and limits size of standing cutaneous deformity at the flap base. **C** and **D,** Interpolated paramedian flap transferred to the nose. **E** to **J,** Preoperative and 6 months postoperative photos.

ADVANCEMENT FLAPS

- Move toward the defect by stretching or recoiling the tissue of the flap.
- Rely on the elasticity of flap tissue (primary movement) and adjacent tissue (secondary movement) for wound closure; therefore, undermining is key.
    (1) *Unipedicle advancement flap:* parallel incisions allow tissue to "slide" in a single vector (Figure 20-13).
        - Standing cutaneous deformities develop on both sides of the base of advancement flaps.
        - Useful near eyebrow, helical rim, upper and lower lips, and medial cheek, vermilion
    (2) *H-Plasty* or *T-plasty:* two unipedicle flaps on opposite sides of a defect
    (3) *Island advancement flap:* segment of skin isolated as an island while protecting the blood supply and subcutaneous tissues
    (4) *V-Y advancement flap:* useful for lengthening or releasing contractures
    (5) *Y-V advancement flap:* used to decrease the redundancy of an area

NASAL DEFECTS

- Small defects are best repaired with a local flap of adjacent nasal skin.
- Larger defects of the nose can be resurfaced using a full-thickness skin graft for shallow wounds or an interpolated paramedian forehead flap or melolabial flap for deeper defects (Figure 20-14).
- Full-thickness nasal defects require external reconstruction with an interpolated flap as well as structural support from cartilage or bone grafts and replacement of internal lining.

FULL-THICKNESS LIP DEFECTS

- Defects less than one-half the lip width: repair primarily or using local flaps.
- Defects from one-half to two-thirds the width of the lip: composite cross-lip flaps from the opposite lip or from the cheek
- Defects greater than two-thirds the width of the lip: regional flaps or microsurgical flaps (Figures 20-15 and 20-16)

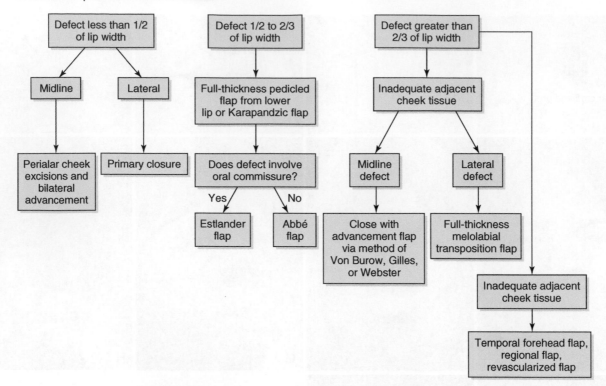

FIGURE 20-15 Algorithm to guide the repair of full-thickness upper lip defects.

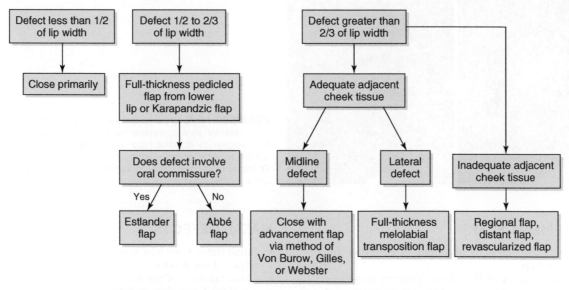

FIGURE 20-16 Algorithm to guide the repair of full-thickness lower lip defects.

OTOPLASTY

- Inheritance: autosomal dominant with variable penetrance.
- Normal auriculocephalic angle: between 25 and 35 degrees
- Normal pinna position: 15 to 20 mm from the helical rim to the scalp.
- Underlying abnormalities: insufficient antihelical fold or deep conchal bowl

OTOPLASTY PROCEDURES

- Cartilage cutting: less frequent loss of correction but higher incidence of cartilage irregularities

- Cartilage sparing: more frequent loss of correction but lower incidence of cartilage irregularities
- Mustardé: suture plication at three points without incision of the cartilage to reestablish the antihelical fold
- Furnas conchal setback: suturing the concha to the mastoid (Figure 20-17)
- Complications: patient dissatisfaction, loss of correction, telephone ear deformity, buckling of the concha, impingement on the external canal

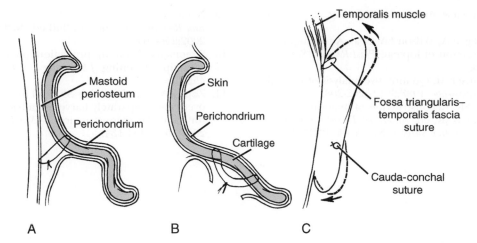

FIGURE 20-17 Suture techniques in otoplasty. **A,** Concha-mastoid sutures. **B,** Scapha-concha sutures. **C,** Effects of fossa triangularis–temporalis fascia and cauda-concha sutures. (Modified from Adamson PA, Tropper GJ, McGraw BL. Otoplasty. In: Krause CJ, Mangat DS, Pastorek N, eds. *Esthetic Facial Surgery*. Philadelphia: JB Lippincott; 1991:721.)

ANSWERS

TRUE OR FALSE QUESTIONS

1. T	14. F	27. T	40. F
2. F	15. F	28. T	41. F
3. T	16. F	29. F	42. T
4. F	17. T	30. T	43. T
5. F	18. F	31. T	44. F
6. T	19. T	32. F	45. T
7. F	20. F	33. F	46. F
8. F	21. T	34. F	47. F
9. F	22. F	35. T	48. F
10. T	23. F	36. F	49. T
11. T	24. T	37. T	50. F
12. F	25. T	38. F	
13. T	26. F	39. T	

SINGLE BEST ANSWER QUESTIONS

51. a	64. b	77. b	90. a
52. c	65. a	78. c	91. b
53. a	66. d	79. b	92. c
54. b	67. c	80. d	93. d
55. d	68. d	81. a	94. b
56. b	69. b	82. a	95. a
57. c	70. d	83. c	96. b
58. c	71. b	84. d	97. a
59. a	72. c	85. b	98. c
60. d	73. d	86. a	99. d
61. b	74. a	87. c	100. c
62. a	75. b	88. c	
63. c	76. a	89. a	

SUGGESTED READINGS

1. Adamson PA, Litner JA. Otoplasty technique. *Facial Plast Surg Clin North Am.* 2006;14:79-87.
2. Baker SR, ed. *Local flaps in facial reconstruction.* 2nd ed. Philadelphia: Elsevier; 2007.
3. Brodsky J. Management of benign skin lesions commonly affecting the face: actinic keratosis, seborrheic keratosis, and rosacea. *Curr Opin Otolaryngol Head Neck Surg.* 2009;17(4):315-320.
4. Burget GC. Aesthetic restoration of the nose. *Clin Plast Surg.* 1985;12(3):463-480.
5. Collar RM, Ward PD, Baker SR. Reconstructive perspectives of cutaneous defects involving the nasal tip:

a retrospective review. *Arch Facial Plast Surg.* 2011;13(2): 91-96.

6. Converse JM, Nigro A, Wilson FA, et al. A technique for surgical correction of lop ear. *Plast Reconstr Surg.* 1955;15:411-418.

7. Crumley RL, Lanser M. Quantitative analysis of nasal tip projection. *Laryngoscope.* 1988;98(2):202-208.

8. Lohuis P, Baker SR. Reconstruction of major nasal defects. In: Thomas JR, ed. *Advanced Therapy in Facial Plastic and Reconstructive Surgery.* New York: PMPA-USA; 2010:665-685.

9. Nachlas NE. Otoplasty. In: Papel ID, ed. *Facial Plastic and Reconstructive Surgery.* 2nd ed. New York: Thieme; 2002:256-269.

10. Simons RL. Nasal tip projection, ptosis and supratip thickening. *J Ear Nose Throat.* 1982;61: 452-455.

11. Zopf DA, Iams W, Baker SR. Full-thickness skin graft overlying a separately harvested auricular cartilage graft for nasal alar reconstruction. *JAMA Facial Plast Surg.* 2013;15(2):131-134.

Rhinoplasty 21

Anthony P. Sclafani | Jonathan Cabin

TRUE OR FALSE QUESTIONS

T / F 1. Modern rhinoplasty was developed about 45 years ago.

T / F 2. Rhinoplasty has progressed from a surgery of reorientation and augmentation to one of tissue reduction.

T / F 3. A nuanced and personalized surgery for each patient is more effective than a lock-step approach.

T / F 4. Thick-skinned patients require relatively more bony-cartilaginous reduction to achieve desirable rhinoplasty results.

T / F 5. The ideal skin type in rhinoplasty is neither thin nor thick, but somewhere in the middle.

T / F 6. Poor tip recoil often goes along with thick alar side walls and skin.

T / F 7. Preoperative examination with nasal speculum is the best way to evaluate the internal nasal valves, including the upper lateral cartilages.

T / F 8. Intraoperative evaluation of nasal anatomy is superior to preoperative evaluation.

T / F 9. If patients do not specifically request alteration of other facial structures, including the chin, these structures should not be addressed during the initial assessment.

T / F 10. A long quadrangular cartilage can interfere with tip rotation.

T / F 11. Black and white photography is preferred in patient photography for the purposes of rhinoplasty.

T / F 12. It is critical for a rhinoplasty surgeon to obtain his/her own photographs, as this crucial part of the patient assessment cannot be trusted to a photographer.

T / F 13. Patient photographs should be taken by first choosing an appropriate focal distance, then gaining focus manually and maintaining this focus throughout to ensure uniform focal distance throughout.

T / F 14. Preoperative computer imaging should provide "best case outcome" for rhinoplasty results.

T / F 15. The need for preoperative laboratory studies in rhinoplasty is patient dependent.

T / F 16. Anticoagulant medications, such as aspirin, must be stopped at least 2 days prior to surgery.

T / F 17. When nasal implants or foreign bodies are suspected, a preoperative computed tomography (CT) scan is recommended to help with localization and analysis.

T / F 18. Local anesthesia should be infiltrated after induction of sedation or general anesthesia.

T / F 19. Proper patient positioning for rhinoplasty involves strict reverse Trendelenburg with no adjustment of head positioning.

T / F 20. Oxymetazoline lowers the seizure threshold.

T / F 21. Lidocaine infiltration typically gives the surgeon 1.5 to 2 hours of anesthetic time.

T / F 22. The amount of local anesthetic required for initial infiltration varies widely, depending on the patient.

T / F 23. If the dorsum becomes distorted during injection, the surgeon is most likely in the wrong plane.

T / F 24. Injection of local anesthetic should be performed directly before beginning rhinoplasty surgery.

T / F 25. Hydrodissection of the septal flaps requires insertion of the needle underneath the perichondrium on either side of the septum.

T / F 26. It is generally recommended to operate on the nasal tip first, as it tends to dictate the required dimensions of the remainder of the nose.

T / F 27. Tip projection generally requires modification in rhinoplasty.

T / F 28. The nasal tripod envisions the nasal tip as having three legs: two legs from each of the lateral crura and a third leg from the combined medial crura.

T / F 29. Radical excision of tip cartilage is frequently required in rhinoplasty surgery.

T / F 30. Complete lower lateral cartilage strips, when compared with interrupted strip techniques, are more risky and generally require more exposure.

T / F 31. Cephalic trimming typically involves interrupting the strip of lateral crus.

T / F 32. To preserve long-term support and natural contouring in tip refinement surgery, it is preferable to leave 6 to 10 mm of uninterrupted lateral crus in the vertical dimension.

T / F 33. When more complex tip work is required, delivery or external approaches are preferred.

T / F 34. In elevation of tissue in the external rhinoplasty approach, it is imperative to stay in a supraperichondrial plane over the cartilages.

T/F 35. Generally speaking, grafting in endonasal rhinoplasty should be achieved with suturing techniques, whereas grafting in external rhinoplasty should be done via "pocket preparation."

T/F 36. When reestablishing the relationship between the tip and the profile line, the goal is for the leading edge of the tip to extend 1 to 2 mm above the cartilaginous profile.

T/F 37. Ideally, women should have a higher tip leading edge than men.

T/F 38. Skin thickness varies little overlying the nose.

T/F 39. Pollybeak deformity can be caused by the underdefinition of the supratip when reducing the cartilaginous dorsum.

T/F 40. The length of the upper lateral cartilages generally plays a large role in the overall length of the nose.

T/F 41. It is recommended to remove only the minimum amount of periosteum from the nasal bones and maxillary ascending processes to facilitate bony reduction.

T/F 42. Excision of redundant soft tissue beneath the dorsal skin is not advised in rhinoplasty.

T/F 43. Expanded polytetrafluoroethylene is the best choice for reconstructing an overreduced bony dorsum, as it is relatively resistant to infection.

T/F 44. The upper lateral cartilages tend to move when lateral osteotomies are performed, because of their intimate anatomic relationship with the nasal bones.

T/F 45. Traumatic infracture is typically necessary when mobilizing the nasal bones.

T/F 46. Disruption of Webster's triangle risks narrowing the patient's airway.

T/F 47. Due to minimal disruption of lateral periosteum, percutaneous osteotomies may be of particular use in patients with significant bony hump reduction where excessive periosteal elevation may have been required medially.

T/F 48. Regardless of whether there is a simple dorsal deviation or there are more complex irregularities, almost all patients require only medial-oblique and lateral osteotomies.

T/F 49. Lateral osteotomies must always be carried out before medial osteotomies are completed.

T/F 50. Despite their popularity, efficacy of postrhinoplasty antibiotics and corticosteroids is largely unproven.

SINGLE BEST ANSWER QUESTIONS

51. Evaluation of skin type for the purposes of rhinoplasty is best performed by which of the following?
    a. Visual inspection of entirely nasal skin
    b. Inspection and palpation of nasal tip
    c. Inspection and palpation of the skin over the nasal skeleton
    d. Inspection and palpation of the skin over key areas of the face

52. Evaluation of all of the following can be performed by preoperative palpation of the nasal vestibule, *EXCEPT:*
    a. Caudal septum twists and angulations
    b. Size and shape of the columella
    c. Quadrangular cartilage length and interference with adequate tip rotation
    d. Location of the rhinion

53. The internal nasal valve is best defined by which of the following structures?
    a. Nasal septum, cephalic margin of the upper lateral cartilages, and the nasal floor
    b. Nasal septum, caudal margin of the upper lateral cartilages, head of the inferior turbinate, and nasal floor
    c. Nasal septum, mid-portion of the upper lateral cartilages, head of the inferior turbinate, nasal floor, and pyriform aperture
    d. Nasal floor, head of the inferior turbinate, and head of the middle turbinate

54. Ideal photographic views of rhinoplasty should include which of the following?
    a. Frontal, lateral, oblique, and basal
    b. Frontal, axial, basal, and lateral
    c. Lateral, basal, medial, and central
    d. Frontal, oblique, basal, and side

55. To minimize local anesthetic needs and distortion of nasal anatomy, which of the following are the best planes for preoperative local anesthetic infiltration?
    a. (1) Supraperiosteal planes lateral and medial to each ascending process of maxilla, (2) supramucoperiosteal and supramucoperichondrial planes of both sides of the septum, and (3) supraperiosteal and supraperichondrial regions over the lower and upper cartilages and nasal bones
    b. (1) Subperiosteal planes lateral and medial to each ascending process of maxilla, (2) submucoperiosteal and submucoperichondrial planes of both sides of the septum, and (3) supraperiosteal and supraperichondrial regions over the lower and upper cartilages and nasal bones
    c. (1) Subperiosteal planes lateral and medial to each ascending process of maxilla, (2) submucoperiosteal and submucoperichondrial planes of both sides of the septum, and (3) subperiosteal and subperichondrial regions over the lower and upper cartilages and nasal bones
    d. (1) Supraperiosteal planes lateral and medial to each ascending process of maxilla, (2) submucoperiosteal and submucoperichondrial planes of both sides of the septum, and (3) supraperiosteal and supraperichondrial regions over the lower and upper cartilages and nasal bones

56. The best form of topical anesthesia is:
    a. 4% cocaine if the patient is sedated and has no cardiac issues, 0.05% oxymetazoline if the patient is under general anesthesia or has cardiac issues
    b. 4% cocaine in all scenarios, unless the patient has cardiac issues
    c. 0.05% oxymetazoline in all scenarios
    d. 4% cocaine if the patient is under general anesthesia and has no cardiac issues, 0.05% oxymetazoline if the patient is sedated or has cardiac issues

57. Which of the following is the recommended local anesthetic for ideal vasoconstriction and anesthesia in rhinoplasty?
    a. 0.05% lidocaine in 1:200,000 epinephrine
    b. 0.05% lidocaine in 1:100,000 epinephrine
    c. 1% lidocaine in 1:100,000 epinephrine
    d. 1% lidocaine in 1:200,000 epinephrine

58. All of the following are *MAJOR* tip support mechanisms *EXCEPT:*
    a. Size, shape, and resiliency of medial and lateral crura
    b. Attachment of the medial crural footplates to the caudal septal cartilage
    c. Upper lateral cartilage attachment to the alar cartilage
    d. Cartilaginous dorsum

59. All of the following are *MINOR* tip support mechanisms *EXCEPT:*
    a. Interdomal soft tissue
    b. Alar cartilage attachment to skin and soft tissue
    c. Vestibular skin
    d. Membranous septum

60. All of the following are components of the lower lateral cartilages *EXCEPT:*
    a. Intermediate crura
    b. Medial crura
    c. Middle lamella
    d. Lateral crura

61. All of the following are valid rhinoplasty incision-approach combinations *EXCEPT:*
    a. Intercartilaginous → retrograde-eversion
    b. Intercartilaginous → tip delivery
    c. Intercartilaginous/marginal → tip delivery
    d. Transcolumellar/marginal → tip delivery (external)

62. All of the following are possible indications for an *OPEN* approach to rhinoplasty *EXCEPT:*
    a. Septal extension grafting
    b. Cleft lip complex deformities
    c. Complex revision rhinoplasty
    d. Mild tip bulbosity

63. In performing narrowing of the lateral crura of the lower lateral cartilages, it is best to maintain a width of at *LEAST:*
    a. 3 to 5 mm
    b. 5 to 7 mm
    c. 7 to 9 mm
    d. 9 to 11 mm

64. Which of the following incision(s) can be used for tip "delivery"?
    a. Intercartilaginous/marginal
    b. Transcartilaginous/marginal
    c. Transcolumellar/marginal
    d. a and c

65. Which of the following incision combinations is used for the open/external rhinoplasty approach?
    a. Intercartilaginous/marginal
    b. Transcartilaginous/marginal
    c. Marginal/transcolumellar
    d. Intercartilaginous/transcartilaginous

66. All of the following are acceptable methods of enhancing tip projection *EXCEPT:*
    a. Spreader grafts
    b. Columellar strut graft
    c. Columellar plumping grafts
    d. Medial crural binding sutures

67. Columellar plumping grafts are appropriate for all of the following *EXCEPT:*
    a. Enhancing tip support
    b. Effacing an acute nasolabial angle
    c. Enhancing tip definition
    d. Treating a retraction or defects in the nasolabial angle

68. Which of the following best describes the components of the cartilaginous vault?
    a. Upper lateral cartilages
    b. Upper lateral cartilages and lower lateral cartilages
    c. Lower lateral cartilages and caudal septum
    d. Upper lateral cartilages and dorsal quadrangular cartilage

69. In which of the following scenarios is it best to perform dorsal reduction first, followed by tip surgery?
    a. Tension nose deformity
    b. Pollybeak deformity
    c. Inverted V deformity
    d. Tip overprojection and underrotation

70. In planning profile alignment, which of the following are the best reference points?
    a. The nasofrontal angle and the tip-defining point
    b. The rhinion and the supratip break
    c. Nasal bony width and dorsal extension
    d. Upper lateral cartilage and nasal bones

71. The nasofrontal angle is best defined as in alignment with which of the following?
    a. Infratarsal crease
    b. Supratarsal crease
    c. Pupils
    d. Lash line

72. After rhinoplasty, "final" nasal appearance is thought to occur how long after the completion of surgery?
    a. 12 to 18 months
    b. 6 to 12 months
    c. 3 to 6 months
    d. 4 to 5 years

73. When evaluating the nasal dorsum, it is important to consider which of the following?
    a. Skin is relatively thick throughout.
    b. Skin is relatively thin throughout.
    c. Skin is relatively thinner over the rhinion than over the supratip area.
    d. Skin is relatively thicker over the rhinion than over the supratip area.

74. In accessing the cartilaginous nasal dorsum, it is best to remain in which of the following?
    a. An immediate subperichondrial plane
    b. An immediate supraperichondrial plane
    c. A subcutaneous plane
    d. A subdermal plane

75. In accessing the bony nasal dorsum, it is best to remain in which of the following?
    a. An immediate subperiosteal plane
    b. An immediate supraperiosteal plane
    c. A subcutaneous plane
    d. A subdermal plane

76. When reducing the cartilaginous dorsum, the removed tissue is best described as which of the following?
    a. Upper lateral cartilage only
    b. Upper and lower lateral cartilages
    c. Upper lateral cartilage and septal cartilage
    d. Quadrangular cartilage only

77. Disruption of the mucoperiosteal flap between the upper lateral cartilages and septum is most likely to cause which of the following?
    a. Nasal airway obstruction
    b. Saddle nose deformity
    c. Increased risk of postoperative hematoma
    d. Pollybeak deformity

78. The use of unilateral spreader grafting versus bilateral spreader grafting is best in all of the following *EXCEPT*:
    a. When there is bilateral nasal valve collapse
    b. When there is dorsal deviation
    c. When there is unilateral nasal valve narrowing
    d. When there is localized disarticulation of the upper lateral cartilage from the nasal bone

79. Disarticulation of the upper lateral cartilage from the nasal bone in isolation can cause all of the following *EXCEPT*:
    a. Dorsal depression
    b. Pollybeak deformity
    c. Nasal valve collapse
    d. A difficult surgical repair

80. All of the following are acceptable surgical tools for bony dorsal reduction *EXCEPT*:
    a. Rubin osteotome
    b. Rasp
    c. Jansen-Middleton forceps
    d. Double-action Becker scissors

81. Which of the following best describes the optimal order for addressing the bony dorsum in rhinoplasty?
    a. (1) Osteotome reduction of hump, (2) rasping of irregularities, and (3) lateral osteotomies
    b. (1) Rasping of irregularities, (2) osteotome reduction of hump, and (3) lateral osteotomies
    c. (1) Lateral osteotomies, (2) osteotome reduction of hump, and (3) rasping of irregularities
    d. (1) Lateral osteotomies, (2) rasping of irregularities, and (3) osteotome reduction of hump

82. Which of the following is *LEAST* ideal in reconstructing an overreduced bony dorsum?
    a. Expanded polytetrafluoroethylene implants
    b. Reimplantation of the removed bony hump
    c. Septal cartilage
    d. Auricular cartilage

83. What is the best explanation for why medial-oblique osteotomies should be performed *prior to* lateral osteotomies?
    a. Lateral osteotomy placement will depend on the placement of the medial-oblique osteotomies.
    b. Medial-oblique osteotomies make the fracture pattern from the subsequent lateral osteotomies more predictable.
    c. Medial-oblique osteotomies are more difficult to make once lateral osteotomies are performed.
    d. Lateral osteotomies are usually not needed once medial-oblique osteotomies are performed.

84. Lateral osteotomies are best performed with a 2 to 3 mm microosteotome because:
    a. There is limited space in the area of the pyriform aperture.
    b. This minimizes the need for periosteal elevation and/or disruption.
    c. The nasal/maxillary bones require a larger force per unit area to successfully break.
    d. This allows micromanipulations as the osteotome is advanced.

85. Which of the following best describes the optimal placement of a low lateral osteotomy entry point?
    a. Below the attachment of the inferior turbinate to the ascending process of the maxilla
    b. Through the attachment of the inferior turbinate to the ascending process of the maxilla
    c. At the pyriform aperture, at or just above attachment of the inferior turbinate to the ascending process of the maxilla
    d. Halfway between the midline and pyriform aperture

86. Which of the following best describes the ideal bony dorsum infracture of older versus younger patients?
    a. The surgeon should aim for complete fractures in all patients, young and old.
    b. The surgeon should aim for incomplete or greenstick fractures in all patients, young and old.
    c. The surgeon should aim for incomplete or greenstick fractures in younger patients and complete fractures in older patients.
    d. The surgeon should aim for incomplete or greenstick fractures in older patients and complete fractures in younger patients.

87. All of the following are acceptable forms of performing lateral osteotomies *EXCEPT*:
    a. Endonasally, through continuous advancement of the osteotome from pyriform aperture to end point
    b. Extranasally, with multiple postage-stamp osteotomies through a single or multiple transcutaneous incisions in horizontal dorsal and vertical nasomaxillary oriented positions
    c. Endonasally, with multiple postage-stamp osteotomies through a single transpyriform incision
    d. Extranasally, with multiple postage-stamp osteotomies through a single or multiple transcutaneous incisions in vertical dorsal and horizontal nasomaxillary oriented positions

88. Intermediate osteotomies are most useful in which of the following scenarios?
    a. Abnormal nasal bony concavities or convexities
    b. Large bony hump
    c. Ethnic nose
    d. Prominent radix

89. Which of the following best describes the relationship between intermediate and lateral osteotomies?
    a. Intermediate osteotomies should always be performed before lateral osteotomies.
    b. Lateral osteotomies should always be performed before intermediate osteotomies.
    c. The sequence of lateral and intermediate osteotomies is not important.
    d. Intermediate osteotomies should always be performed when lateral osteotomies are required.

90. Which of the following is *NOT* a recommended part of aftercare in rhinoplasty?
    a. Splint removal 5 to 7 days postoperatively
    b. Frontal and lateral photos at first postoperative visit
    c. Multiple visits in the first two postoperative years
    d. Nasal massage

91. "Tip recoil" best correlates to which of the following?
    a. The inherent strength and support of the nasal tip
    b. Nasal tip movement with facial expression
    c. The quality and thickness of the skin overlying the nasal tip
    d. The attachments of the intermediate crura of the lower lateral cartilages

92. Which of the following is thought to be the most common cause of postrhinoplasty tip ptosis?
    a. Excessive sacrifice of tip-support mechanisms
    b. Excessive cephalic trimming
    c. Overresection of septal cartilage
    d. Disarticulation of the upper lateral cartilages from the nasal bones

93. All of the following are true about rhinoplasty *EXCEPT*:
    a. Tissue rearrangement and refinement is preferred to tissue reduction and resection.
    b. Individualization based on anatomy is preferred to a lock-step approach.
    c. Tissue healing is generally stable and predictable.
    d. Atraumatic rhinoplasty is achievable by respecting the fairly predictable nasal cleavage planes.

94. All of the following are tip refinement grafting techniques *EXCEPT*:
    a. Columellar strut
    b. Plumping grafts
    c. Shield grafts
    d. Spreader grafts

95. Which of the following are true regarding detachment of the upper lateral cartilage from the nasal bones?
    a. It is difficult to repair.
    b. It can cause nasal airway compromise.
    c. It can cause a visible dorsal depression.
    d. All of the above are true.

96. Spreader grafts can be used for which of the following?
    a. To widen the nasal valve
    b. To straighten a deviation of the cartilaginous dorsum
    c. To refine the nasal tip
    d. a and b

97. Lateral osteotomies most commonly fracture which of the following?
    a. Nasal bone
    b. Maxillary bone
    c. Frontal bone
    d. None of the above

98. An attempt should be made to minimize periosteal disruption over the nasal bones because of which of the following?
    a. The periosteum can serve as a splint to maintain altered bony architecture during recovery.
    b. Increased periosteal disruption can cause increased edema and bleeding.
    c. a and b
    d. None of the above

99. What best describes the role of postoperative corticosteroids and antibiotics in rhinoplasty patients?
    a. Evidence supports antibiotics in preventing postoperative infection, but no evidence exists to support the use of corticosteroids.
    b. Evidence supports corticosteroids in reducing postoperative edema, but no evidence exists to support the use of antibiotics.
    c. Evidence supports the use of corticosteroids in reducing postoperative edema and antibiotics in reducing postoperative infection.
    d. No evidence exists to support the use of postoperative antibiotics or corticosteroids.

100. All of the following are true for dorsal reduction surgery *EXCEPT*:
    a. A rasp can be used for both cartilaginous and bony dorsal reduction.
    b. A rasp can be used to reduce smaller irregularities in the bony dorsum, with a Rubin osteotome preferred for larger humps.
    c. Rasping should always be used after any reduction of the bony dorsum, to smooth out irregularities.
    d. Cartilaginous dorsum is best reduced with sharp dissection, before any reduction of the bony dorsum.

CORE KNOWLEDGE

SURGICAL PHILOSOPHY

- Rhinoplasty is best achieved by conservative techniques based on anatomy encountered and refinement to achieve natural and normal-appearing outcomes.
- Radical departure from time-proven techniques should be considered only in cases of significantly varied anatomy.
- Rhinoplasty has transitioned from an operation of tissue reduction and excision to one of tissue rearrangement and refinement, which coincides with a greater focus on long-term results.
- An approach individualized to the patient, along with atraumatic tissue dissection in proper nasal cleavage planes, is key to successful rhinoplasty.
- The surgically altered nose is continually modified by the healing process and aging phenomena throughout the patient's lifetime, and the immediate or even delayed postoperative outcome never truly represents the "final" anatomic appearance.

PREOPERATIVE EVALUATION

- No single series of maneuvers works for every patient because much depends on a combination of the individual patient's anatomy and the surgeon's skill.
- Patients with minimal deformities are better candidates for a near-perfect result, while patients with larger deformities will generally need to accept minor postoperative imperfections. It is the surgeon's responsibility to balance the wishes of the patient with the limitations of the surgery.

- An experienced surgeon can gain a significant amount of information with preoperative visual and palpatory diagnostic exercises.
- Quality of the skin plays a significant role in potential outcome and should be carefully evaluated preoperatively. "Ideal" skin is not overly thick, thin, or oily.
- Thick skin presents more difficulties in refinement and definition, a higher risk of dorsal overreduction, and more unpredictable postoperative healing.
- Thin, pale, or freckled skin can limit the extent of tissue manipulation, as small irregularities that are generally hidden have the potential to become obvious. Long-term healing is more likely to result in skin retraction and shrinkage.
- The shape, size, asymmetries, resilience, strength, and support of the nasal tip should be evaluated preoperatively. Weak and/or flail tip cartilage is less tolerant of tissue sacrifice and may require more extensive grafting.
- Palpation of the internal vestibules can provide information regarding the columella and septum.
- The following factors should be evaluated because they can interfere with cephalic rotation: (1) the tip-lip complex muscle tethering and length, (2) the length of the quadrangular cartilage, and (3) the nasal spine and caudal septal angle.
- Careful evaluation of the nasal airway is achieved with nasal speculum and fiberoptic camera. The focus should be on the quality and obstructive nature of the bony and

cartilaginous septum, the inferior turbinate, and the internal nasal valve.

- The internal nasal valve is comprised of (1) nasal septum, (2) caudal margin of the upper lateral cartilage, (3) head of the inferior turbinate, and (4) nasal floor.
- Functional evaluation of the valve should always be performed. A curette is introduced endonasally to manually elevate various areas of the upper lateral cartilage, while assessing the patient's airway improvement.
- Notation should be made of the position and inclination of the nasofrontal and nasolabial angles, the shape and size of the ala, the width of the middle and upper thirds of the nose, and the relationship of the nose to other facial features.
- The bony and cartilaginous nasal dorsum should be evaluated for symmetry, position, and contour.
- Facial asymmetries and abnormalities, particularly chin underprojection, should be evaluated preoperatively because they can impact the appearance of the nose. The surgeon may offer improvement of nonnasal structures (i.e., mentoplasty) to enhance rhinoplasty results.
- Use of a three-way mirror and facial photographs are imperative in the preoperative evaluation. Computer imaging may also be used, but care should be taken to present a realistic expectation and not a "best case" scenario.
- Facial photography is important for analysis and documentation. It should be performed in color, and standardized views should be obtained (frontal, lateral, oblique, and basal). Focal distance should be chosen manually, with standardized, preset focus and zoom.
- As in the case of any surgical procedure, consent should be obtained prior to rhinoplasty. The risks, benefits, and alternatives to surgery should be explicitly discussed and all questions should be answered.
- Preoperative laboratory studies should be obtained on a case-by-case basis because it is not required for every patient.
- Aspirin or other medications that enhance anticoagulation should be discontinued at least 2 weeks prior to surgery.
- Routine radiographs are generally not recommended; however, it is reasonable to obtain a CT scan if there is concern about nasal implants or foreign bodies.

ANESTHESIA, ANALGESIA, AND PREPARATION

- Before local infiltration, external nasal markings can be used in areas of intended manipulation and/or critical nasal landmarks. Local anesthetic infiltration and surgical edema can distort anatomy (Figures 21-1 and 21-2).
- There are various anesthesia techniques; however, most employ a combination of intravenous analgesia with local topical and infiltrated anesthesia.
- General endotracheal anesthesia is reasonable and may be utilized according to surgeon and patient preference.
- Local anesthesia should be administered in a comfortable and relaxed patient, after the patient has been sedated with preoperative anesthesia.
- The nose should first be treated with topical anesthetic and decongestant. Four percent cocaine or 0.05% oxymetazoline should be used.
- One percent lidocaine in 1:100,000 epinephrine is preferred for infiltrated anesthesia, providing approximately 1.5 to 2 hours of effective anesthesia and vasoconstriction.
- Injection should be performed 10 to 15 minutes prior to surgical incisions.
- Typically only 5 to 10 mL of local anesthesia is required to achieve adequate vasoconstriction and anesthesia, when

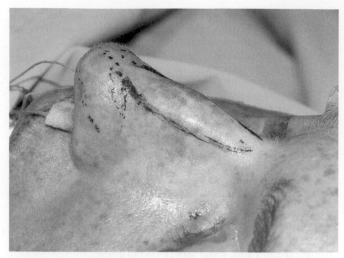

FIGURE 21-1 By palpating the nose internal structures, such as the lower lateral cartilages and a bony-cartilaginous dorsal hump, can be outlined on the skin and surgical resection can be planned.

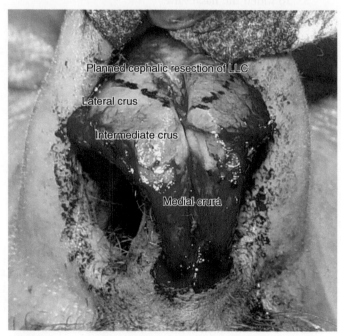

FIGURE 21-2 The external approach affords unparalleled visualization of the lower lateral cartilages (LLC), and asymmetries can be best appreciated. A planned cephalic strip excision is shown here, designed to leave symmetric intact lateral crura.

properly injected into the appropriate surgical planes. If there is septal reconstruction, an additional 3 to 5 mL of local anesthesia can be used for hydrodissection of the septal flaps.
- Four distinct surgical planes exist in the nose, each with minimal amounts of vascular and neural structures: (1) extraperiosteal lateral to ascending process of maxilla, (2) extraperiosteal medial to ascending process of maxilla, (3) submucoperichondrial and submucoperiosteal flanking the nasal septum, and (4) immediate supraperichondrial and supraperiosteal regions over the lower and upper cartilages and nasal bones.
- Infiltration of local anesthesia into the correct surgical planes results in efficient diffusion to the surrounding tissues and the need for relatively less injection for effect.

If done improperly, more injection is typically required, which can cause significant anatomical distortion.

- Infiltration of local anesthetic in the extraperiosteal planes on both sides of the ascending maxilla aids in reducing bleeding with lateral osteotomies.
- "Hydraulic dissection" can be achieved by infiltration of a generous amount of local anesthetic in the submucoperichondrial and submucoperiosteal planes on either side of the septum, with the bevel of the needle pointing toward the cartilage.
- The supraperichondrial and supraperiosteal plane over the upper and lower lateral cartilages and nasal bones is entered in all rhinoplasty operations, and infiltration and operation in the plane produces a virtually bloodless field.
- Depending on the type of intranasal incision used, injection should also be performed in the appropriate area around the lower lateral and/or upper lateral cartilages (intercartilaginous, transcartilaginous, and/or marginal).
- When employing an open approach, injection into the interdomal region, infratip lobule, and columella should be performed.
- Throughout the procedure, the patient should be maintained in the reverse Trendelenburg position with the head elevated, to enhance vasoconstriction and facilitate venous/lymphatic drainage.

SURGICAL REFINEMENT OF THE NASAL TIP

- The nasal tip is typically approached as a distinctive entity, with the objective to construct a defined, stable, properly projecting tip with a triangular shape on base view.
- In most cases it is recommended to operate on the nasal tip first, as it helps with the subsequent alignment and adjustment of the remainder of the dorsum.
- Although the nasal tip anatomy varies widely, there are techniques that can be predictably applied to achieve specific results in the tip (Figure 21-3).

- Minimal cartilaginous resection or disruption is the goal. Conservative cartilaginous strip resection is preferred; however, severe tip deformities may require more aggressive techniques, including division and reestablishment of cartilaginous continuity.
- The major tip support mechanisms are: (1) size, shape, and resiliency of the medial and lateral crura; (2) attachment of the medial crural footplates to the caudal septum; and (3) attachment of the upper lateral cartilage to the cephalic alar cartilage.
- The minor tip support mechanisms are: (1) interdomal soft tissue, (2) cartilaginous dorsum, (3) soft tissue between lateral crus and pyriform wall, (4) alar cartilage attachment to skin and soft tissue, (5) nasal spine, and (6) membranous septum.
- Preservation of tip support mechanisms is key. If disrupted, major tip support mechanisms must be reestablished. Disruption of several minor tip support mechanisms can also cause tip destabilization, ptosis, and deprojection.
- The "nasal tripod" is formed by each of the lateral crura and the combined medial crura, with the nasal tip-defining point at the apex. This concept enables predictable change in tip position with manipulation of any of these tripod "legs."
- The four major incisions for access of tip cartilage are: (1) transcartilaginous, (2) intercartilaginous, (3) marginal, and (4) transcolumellar. An appropriate incision or combination of incisions can be determined once desired tip changes are defined.
- Transcartilaginous incision is made within the cartilage of the upper lateral or lower lateral cartilage.
- Intercartilaginous incision is made between the cartilage of the upper lateral and lower lateral cartilage.
- Marginal incision is made on the caudal edge of the lateral crura.
- Transcolumellar incision is made through the thinnest portion of the columella in the shape of an inverted "V."

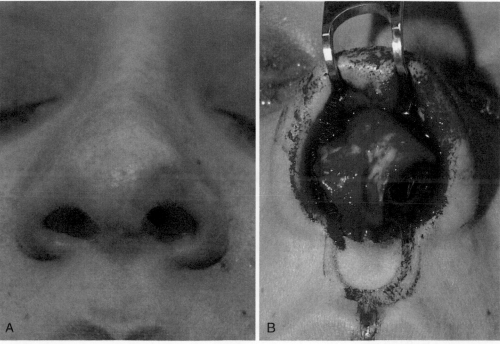

FIGURE 21-3 While appearing grossly symmetric **(A)**, some nasal tips may have significant lower lateral cartilage asymmetries best appreciated during an external rhinoplasty **(B)**.

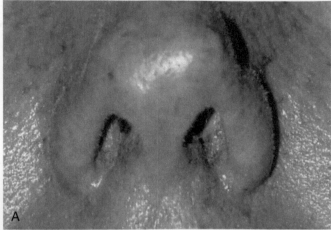

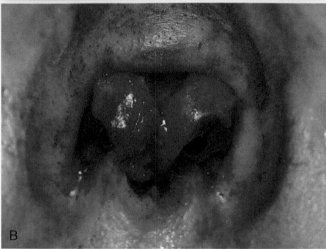

FIGURE 21-4 Open approach rhinoplasty is particularly beneficial in revision rhinoplasty, when bossa **(A)** may be due to gross asymmetries of the shape and orientation of the lower lateral cartilages **(B)**.

- Transcartilaginous or intercartilaginous incisions can be used in isolation when minor nasal tip work is required. These are "nondelivery" incisions, because the majority of the soft tissue envelope is kept undisrupted over the tip.
- Intercartilaginous/marginal or transcolumellar/marginal combinations can be used for more extensive tip work. These combinations can facilitate tip "delivery," which provides full lower lateral cartilage exposure for more extensive tip surgery.
- A transcolumellar/marginal combination is considered an "external" approach, because the tip is exposed in its entirety and externalized. This approach may be necessary in cases of severe tip deformities, extremely thick skin or weak cartilage, revision rhinoplasty (Figure 21-4), extensive grafting needs, or cleft lip nasal deformities.
- In the nondelivery approach, the most useful technique for refinement and rotation is "cephalic stripping," whereby a small strip of cephalic lateral crura is resected. This results in subtle changes, with minimal tissue disruption and scarring.
- In the delivery approach, tip refinement and rotation should be attempted with permanent suturing and conservative cartilage resection. Transdomal and dome-binding sutures can be used to provide tip narrowing and refinement.
- In severe deformities, stripping may be insufficient, and cartilage divisions and/or complete resections, along with repositioning and reestablishment, may be necessary for

refinement and rotation. In these cases, there is a greater risk of asymmetric healing and unpredictable scarring.
- Lateral crura should always maintain a final width of 7 to 9 mm.
- Tip projection is typically ideal preoperatively, although some patients may require tip deprojection or enhancement of projection.
- For deprojection, the nasal tripod theory can be applied to make careful and targeted cartilage repositioning and resection.
- Enhancement of projection can be achieved with grafting (i.e., columellar strut or plump grafting) or through careful reduction of columellar soft tissue and binding medial crural sutures.
- Tip grafting can be used to facilitate refinement or changes in rotation and/or projection by angling native cartilage, reinforcing structure, and/or providing direct subcutaneous refinement.
- Some common tip-grafting techniques include columellar struts, shield grafts, infratip lobule grafts, and plumping grafts, all with specific applications for refinement.
- Columellar struts are placed between the medial crura are used to enhance tip support and tip projection.
- Shield grafts are placed subcutaneously on the domes and are used to enhance projection and refine the tip.
- Infratip lobule grafts are placed subcutaneously slightly more inferior than shield grafts and are used to enhance projection and contour tip anatomy.
- Plumping grafts involve minced cartilage placed subcutaneously at the nasolabial angle. These grafts enhance tip support and efface an acute or retracted nasolabial angle.
- Grafting can be achieved through an external approach or a closed approach. Closed endonasal grafting requires exact tissue pockets for precise placement. Open external grafting typically requires graft suturing.

SURGERY OF THE CARTILAGINOUS VAULT

- The cartilaginous vault is comprised of the dorsal quadrangular (septal) cartilage and related upper lateral cartilages.
- The goal of cartilaginous dorsal reduction is the elimination of irregularities or deformities and the establishment of an esthetically appropriate supratip depression.
- Men typically favor a strong, high, and straight-line profile with a 1 to 2 mm drop in tip-defining point. Women generally prefer a slightly more sloped dorsum with a more prominent tip-defining point of 2 to 3 mm. The patient's individual preference is superior to any textbook ideal.
- The nasofrontal angle and tip-defining point are stable references for dorsal analysis throughout the procedure.
- As skin thickness varies over the dorsum, slightly greater reduction may be required in the areas of thicker skin (i.e., supratip), with slightly less reduction in areas of thinner skin (i.e., rhinion).
- The cartilaginous dorsum is accessed within the supraperichondrial plane along the upper lateral cartilages. Because cartilaginous vault reduction is ideally done with direct visualization of the entirety of the bony and cartilaginous dorsum, elevation of the tissue envelope should continue in a subperiosteal plane over the nasal bones before any reduction is attempted.
- With full exposure, the cartilaginous dorsum should be incrementally reduced with sharp dissection, with inspection and palpation of the profile after each successive reduction (Figure 21-5).

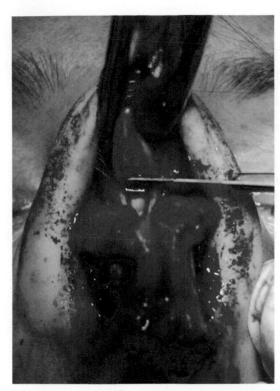

FIGURE 21-5 Dorsal cartilaginous resections should be performed incrementally. Care should be taken to avoid violation of the underlying nasal mucosa. Here the upper lateral cartilages and dorsal septum are seen below the resection.

- Care should be taken to preserve the mucoperiosteum connecting the upper lateral cartilages to the septum, because disruption can adversely affect the internal nasal valve.
- Spreader grafts are placed between the septum and upper lateral cartilage. They are typically used to widen the internal nasal valve but can be applied unilaterally to correct a severe cartilaginous deviation.
- The length of the upper lateral cartilages rarely plays any role in the overall length of the nose, and thus should not require adjustment.
- The attachment between the upper lateral cartilages and the nasal bones should be preserved because cosmetic and airway deformities are almost certain. Repair is difficult but can be attempted with a dorsal onlay graft.

SURGERY OF THE BONY DORSUM

- Once reduction of the cartilaginous dorsum is achieved, the exact degree of bony hump excess is revealed.
- Minimal bony hump reduction can be achieved with a rasp, with larger hump reductions typically requiring a Rubin osteotome. Rasping should always be used for final refinement.
- With rasping, care must be taken to avoid disruption or avulsion of the upper lateral cartilages.
- The final dorsal profile should be aesthetically pleasing and free of irregularities, especially in thin-skinned patients. Running a wet, gloved finger over the dorsum is a useful technique to check for irregularities that are unperceivable to the eye.
- If necessary, conservative excision of redundant subcutaneous soft tissue over the dorsum can also be performed.

- An overresected bony hump can be remedied with replacement of removed hump (if osteotome is used) or with cartilage grafting. Expanded polytetrafluoroethylene alloplastic implants are also an option, but less ideal.

NARROWING OF THE NOSE: OSTEOTOMIES

- Following a reduction of the bony dorsum, narrowing of the nose is typically necessary. This is achieved by osteotome mobilization of the nasal bone and ascending maxillary process complex.
- Medial-oblique osteotomies should first be made on either side of the bony septum, using a small, sharp osteotome. This facilitates a stable fracture pattern for the subsequent lateral, narrowing osteotomies and allows for a less traumatic infracture.
- A lateral osteotomy is typically performed by starting toward the face of the maxilla, eventually coming up to the nasomaxillary junction, and finally intersecting the distal end of the medial-oblique osteotomy.
- Lateral osteotomies are most frequently performed endonasally, through a puncture at the pyriform aperture at or above the inferior turbinate. This positioning preserves Webster's triangle, a small section of bone that is critical for nasal airway patency.
- Endonasally, one can perform a continuous osteotomy or several perforating osteotomies along the line of intended fracture.
- Lateral osteotomies can also be performed in a transcutaneous fashion, making several perforating controlled fractures along the intended lateral osteotomy line, through one or more small skin punctures.
- In any lateral osteotomy, the surgeon should aim to minimize periosteal disruption, as the periosteum can serve as a bony splint, and disruption can cause increased traumatic edema and bleeding.
- Intermediate osteotomies can be used for twisted, asymmetric, or markedly irregular bony architecture, and especially in cases of nasal concavity or convexity. These must be carried out before pursuing lateral osteotomies, as lateral osteotomies cause the nasal bones to be flail, rendering further fracturing near impossible.
- Once all osteotomies are made, careful digital pressure should be used to reduce the bony architecture to the desired width and contour.

POSTRHINOPLASTY CARE

- Postrhinoplasty care is directed toward patient comfort, edema reduction, maintenance of nasal airway patency, and stabilization of refined nasal architecture.
- At the end of the procedure careful taping should be performed to decrease postoperative edema and reinforce cartilaginous positioning. A nasal splint should subsequently be placed to protect and maintain the nasal bony position.
- Corticosteroids and antibiotics can be prescribed, but there is little evidence supporting their use.
- The external splint is removed 5 to 7 days postoperatively, with care taken not to disrupt nasal architecture.
- Facial photographs should be obtained at the first postoperative visit and subsequent visits thereafter.
- After the first postoperative visit, patients should be seen at decreasingly regular intervals to observe postoperative healing and for patient reassurance.
- Longer term (>1 year) follow-ups are advantageous to the surgeon, as he/she can correlate various rhinoplasty techniques to favorable or unfavorable long-term results and continue to refine his/her surgical techniques.

ANSWERS

TRUE OR FALSE QUESTIONS

1. F	14. F	27. F	40. F
2. F	15. T	28. T	41. T
3. T	16. F	29. F	42. F
4. F	17. T	30. F	43. F
5. T	18. T	31. F	44. T
6. F	19. F	32. T	45. F
7. F	20. F	33. T	46. T
8. F	21. T	34. T	47. T
9. F	22. F	35. F	48. F
10. T	23. T	36. T	49. F
11. F	24. F	37. T	50. T
12. F	25. T	38. F	
13. T	26. T	39. T	

SINGLE BEST ANSWER QUESTIONS

51. c	64. d	77. a	90. d
52. d	65. c	78. a	91. a
53. b	66. a	79. b	92. a
54. a	67. c	80. c	93. c
55. d	68. d	81. a	94. d
56. a	69. a	82. a	95. d
57. c	70. a	83. c	96. d
58. d	71. b	84. b	97. b
59. c	72. a	85. c	98. c
60. c	73. c	86. d	99. d
61. b	74. b	87. b	100. a
62. d	75. a	88. a	
63. c	76. c	89. a	

SUGGESTED READINGS

1. Goodman WS, Charles DA. Technique of external rhinoplasty. *Can J Otolaryngol.* 1978;7:13.
2. Gunter JP. Anatomical observations of the lower lateral cartilages. *Arch Otolaryngol.* 1969;89:61.
3. Janeke JB, Wright WK. Studies on the support of the nasal tip. *Arch Otolaryngol.* 1971;93:458.
4. Kridel RWH, Yoon PJ, Koch RJ. Prevention and correction of nasal tip bossae in rhinoplasty. *Arch Facial Plast Surg.* 2003;5:416-422.
5. Sheen JH. Achieving more nasal tip projection by use of small autogenous vomer or septal cartilage grafts. *Plast Reconstr Surg.* 1975;56:35.
6. Sheen JH. Secondary rhinoplasty. *Plast Reconstr Surg.* 1975;56:137.
7. Tardy ME. Rhinoplasty tip ptosis: etiology and prevention. *Laryngoscope.* 1973;83:923.
8. Tardy ME. Transdomal suture refinement of the nasal tip. *Facial Plast Surg.* 1987;4:4.
9. Tardy ME, Hewell TS. Nasal tip refinement: reliable approaches and sculpture techniques. *Facial Plast Surg.* 1984;1:87.
10. Toriumi DM, Mueller RA, Grosch T, et al. Vascular anatomy of the nose and the external rhinoplasty approach. *Arch Otolaryngol Head Neck Surg.* 1996;122:24-34.

Endocrine Surgery

22

Catherine F. Sinclair | Gregory W. Randolph

TRUE OR FALSE QUESTIONS

T/F 1. Differentiation of primitive thyroid tissue into follicles occurs at approximately week 7 of gestation.

T/F 2. The weight of the normal thyroid gland in adults is 25 to 30 g.

T/F 3. The thyroid gland is supplied by three arteries and three veins.

T/F 4. The left recurrent laryngeal nerve (RLN) follows a more medial course in the neck than the right RLN.

T/F 5. In the majority of people, the superior laryngeal nerve divides into an internal and external branch 1 cm above the superior thyroid pole.

T/F 6. Thyroid glands that fail to descend into the neck during embryological development are most commonly located in the lingual region.

T/F 7. Thyroglossal duct cysts (TDCs) are two times less common than branchial cleft remnants.

T/F 8. TDCs are malignant in 1% of cases, and of these, 85% are papillary carcinoma.

T/F 9. The thymus originates from the ventral portion of the same branchial pouch (III) as the inferior parathyroid glands.

T/F 10. Up to 10% of patients may have fewer than four parathyroid glands.

T/F 11. A rise in parathyroid hormone (PTH) levels after intraoperative thyroid lobe palpation may indicate the presence of an intrathyroidal parathyroid gland.

T/F 12. A decrease in thyroid hormone–binding proteins occurs with glucocorticoid and estrogen administration.

T/F 13. In a patient with hyperthyroidism, if the results of a technetium-99m pertechnetate scan do not match the clinical picture, an I-123 scan should be performed.

T/F 14. Serum thyroid-stimulating hormone (TSH) is the diagnostic test of choice for secondary hypothyroidism.

T/F 15. Subclinical hypothyroidism is defined as an elevated TSH with a normal free 3,5,3′,5′-tetraiodothyronine (thyroxine, T4).

T/F 16. First-trimester pregnant patients with a suppressed TSH and slightly elevated free thyroxine index (FT4I) should not be treated for hyperthyroidism.

T/F 17. The optimal timing for surgical intervention in a pregnant woman with uncontrolled Graves disease is early in the third trimester.

T/F 18. Pemberton sign is sensitive in the evaluation of substernal goiter.

T/F 19. Radioiodine may be a useful treatment for nontoxic multinodular goiter and achieves volume reduction and decreased obstructive symptomatology.

T/F 20. Subtotal thyroidectomy for substernal goiter is defined as total lobectomy with a contralateral remnant approximately equivalent to a small normal lobe.

T/F 21. Tracheomalacia is a possible complication after resection of substernal goiter, with rates approaching 10%.

T/F 22. Of the adult population, 5% to 15% may have a clinically significant thyroid nodule warranting evaluation.

T/F 23. Thyroid nodules that have a greater transverse diameter than anteroposterior diameter on transverse ultrasound view are more likely to harbor carcinoma.

T/F 24. Follicular carcinomas <2 cm without invasion are less likely to be associated with metastatic disease.

T/F 25. Patients with multiple thyroid nodules have the same risk of malignancy as those with solitary nodules.

T/F 26. Thyroid nodules with a Bethesda II grading on cytological analysis require no further follow-up.

T/F 27. For cystic nodules, percutaneous ethanol injection for recurrent symptomatic cystic fluid accumulation has an 80% success rate.

T/F 28. Papillary thyroid carcinoma (PTC) represents 0.5% of all cancers.

T/F 29. At presentation with PTC, macroscopic neck metastases will be detected in approximately 30% of patients.

T/F 30. Macroscopic lymph node metastases are associated with decreased recurrence-free survival (RFS) rates.

T/F 31. Prophylactic central neck dissection improves RFS rates in PTC.

T/F 32. Neck imaging is rarely necessary for macroscopic lateral neck lymph node metastases because neck palpation is usually as sensitive for their detection.

T/F 33. Computed tomography (CT) scans of the neck to investigate for lateral neck metastases in thyroid carcinoma should be performed without iodinated contrast.

T/F 34. Ultrasound and CT are complementary in the evaluation of the neck for lymph node metastases in thyroid carcinoma.

T/F 35. Approximately 50% of tall cell variant PTCs express the BRAF mutation, and this may account for their more aggressive phenotype.

T/F 36. BRAF is the most common oncogene in sporadic PTC.

T/F 37. For a patient with stage 3 well-differentiated thyroid cancer, TSH suppression to <0.1 mIU/L improves survival.

T/F 38. I-131 remnant ablation after thyroidectomy for a high-risk patient with well-differentiated thyroid carcinoma can be performed following thyroxine withdrawal but not with recombinant TSH (rhTSH) stimulation.

T/F 39. Routine adjunctive use of chemotherapy in high-risk patients with differentiated thyroid carcinoma improves RFS.

T/F 40. For medullary thyroid carcinoma (MTC), disease staging is not dependent on patient age.

T/F 41. External beam irradiation may be useful in managing patients with well-differentiated thyroid carcinoma >45 years of age with grossly visible extrathyroidal extension at the time of surgery and a high likelihood of microscopic residual disease.

T/F 42. In familial forms of MTC, C-cell hyperplasia is not thought to be a precursor to malignant transformation.

T/F 43. Ten-year survival rates for MTC range from 30% to 50%.

T/F 44. In MTC, 10% to 15% of patients with cervical lymph node metastases will have evidence of distant metastases.

T/F 45. The major histological subtypes and variants of anaplastic carcinoma have no known prognostic significance.

T/F 46. In a normocalcemic patient with a history of nephrolithiasis, ionized serum calcium testing may be diagnostically useful.

T/F 47. Primary hyperparathyroidism (PHPT) should be considered in patients not with high calcium but with normal parathyroid hormone levels.

T/F 48. In a patient with normal calcium but elevated PTH, a course of thiazide diuretic may help distinguish between true PHPT and renal leak hypercalciuria.

T/F 49. Blood for intraoperative parathyroid hormone assays should usually be drawn from the ipsilateral internal jugular vein and placed in an ethylenediaminetetraacetic acid tube.

T/F 50. Parathyroid carcinoma should be suspected when preoperative PTH levels are elevated five to 10 times above the normal range.

SINGLE BEST ANSWER QUESTIONS

51. Approximately what percentage of the population have more than four parathyroid glands?
    a. 1%
    b. 2%
    c. 5%
    d. 10%

52. Pendred syndrome is associated with all of the following *EXCEPT:*
    a. Goiter
    b. Sensorineural hearing loss
    c. Hypothyroidism
    d. Thyroid nodules
    e. All of the above are associated with this syndrome.

53. Circulating hormones are bound to thyroxine-binding protein, transthyretin, and albumin in which of the following approximate ratios?
    a. 6:2:2
    b. 7:1:2
    c. 8:1:1
    d. 7:2:1
    e. 6:1:3

54. Elevated total T4 levels can occur with which of the following?
    i.   High thyroid-binding globulin serum concentrations
    ii. Low thyroid-binding globulin serum concentrations
    iii. Peripheral resistance to T4
    iv. Dehydration
    a. i, ii, and iii
    b. ii and iv
    c. i and iii
    d. All of the above

55. Anomalies in development of the median thyroid anlage can lead to all of the following *EXCEPT:*
    a. Tubercle of Zuckerkandl
    b. Lingual thyroid
    c. Pyramidal lobe
    d. Thyroglossal duct cyst
    e. Thyroglossal duct fistula

56. Nonrecurrence of the right laryngeal nerve is associated with which of the following?
    i.   Absence of a segment of fourth right aortic arch between the origin of the right common carotid artery and right innominate artery
    ii. An absent innominate artery
    iii. A right subclavian artery arising from the ventral aorta
    iv. The right RLN arising from the vagus nerve at mediastinal level
    a. i, ii, and iii
    b. ii and iv
    c. i and iii
    d. All of the above

57. Pregnancy is associated with which of the following?
    a. Increased thyroid-binding globulin levels
    b. Increased protein-bound levels of 3,5,3′-triiodothyronine (T3) and T4
    c. Normal active levels of T4 and T3
    d. Normal serum TSH levels
    e. All of the above

58. Measurement of TSH alone will likely be sufficient for diagnosis of thyroid dysfunction in which of the following?
    a. Third-trimester pregnancy
    b. Suspected hypothalamic dysfunction

c. Presence of thyroid autoantibodies
d. Recent thyrotoxicosis

59. Which of the following statements is *INCORRECT* for a euthyroid patient with high T4-binding proteins?
    a. Total T4 is increased.
    b. Reverse T3 is decreased.
    c. TSH is normal.
    d. All of the above are correct.

60. When ordering a diagnostic I-123 radionuclide scan, a patient should be counseled to avoid all of the following *EXCEPT:*
    a. Seaweed
    b. Propranolol
    c. Amiodarone
    d. Lugol's solution
    e. Iopanoic acid

61. Which of the following is the most sensitive initial imaging modality to investigate a patient with hyperthyroidism?
    a. Magnetic resonance imaging (MRI)
    b. Ultrasound
    c. I-123 radionuclide scan
    d. Technetium-99m pertechnetate scan
    e. CT

62. Symptoms of hypothyroidism include all of the following *EXCEPT:*
    a. Weight gain
    b. Creatine phosphokinase elevation
    c. Hyponatremia
    d. Carpal tunnel syndrome
    e. Hyperkalemia

63. Which of the following increases the risk of postpartum thyroiditis?
    a. Smoking
    b. Neonate gender
    c. Breastfeeding
    d. Neonate birth weight
    e. All of the above

64. Which of the following is/are potential indication(s) for sternotomy with substernal goiter?
    i. Suspected malignancy extending into the mediastinum
    ii. Mediastinal goiter blood supply
    iii. Recurrent substernal goiters
    iv. Long, thin stalk of tissue connecting cervical and substernal portions
    v. Preoperative true superior vena cava syndrome
    a. i, ii, and iii
    b. ii and iv
    c. i and iii
    d. v
    e. All of the above

65. Thyroid storm during surgery for Graves disease is classically associated with all of the following *EXCEPT:*
    a. Tachyarrhythmias
    b. Congestive heart failure
    c. Delirium
    d. Pulmonary edema
    e. Fever

66. Increasing thyroid nodule prevalence over the past decade is attributed to all of the following *EXCEPT:*
    a. Environmental factors
    b. Increasing median age of industrialized populations
    c. Increased thyroid nodule detection
    d. Increased use of CT and MRI scans

67. Fine needle aspiration (FNA) of subcentimeter nodules:
    a. Should never be performed
    b. Should never be performed for patients without a family history of thyroid carcinoma
    c. Should be performed only for patients with a history of ionizing radiation exposure
    d. Should be performed for positron emission tomography (PET)-positive nodules
    e. None of the above

68. Ultrasound characteristics suggestive of benign thyroid nodule histology include which of the following?
    i. Spongiform appearance
    ii. Calcifications
    iii. Pure cystic nodules
    iv. Irregular borders
    v. Internal vascularity
    a. i, ii, and iii
    b. ii and iv
    c. i and iii
    d. v
    e. All of the above

69. Risk factors for thyroid cancer include which of the following?
    i. Male gender
    ii. Age >60 years
    iii. Age <30 years
    iv. Family history of MEN-1
    a. i, ii, and iii
    b. i and ii
    c. ii and iv
    d. i and iii
    e. All of the above

70. Findings that predict malignancy include all of the following *EXCEPT:*
    a. BRAF
    b. Epidermal growth factor receptor
    c. Galactin-3
    d. RAS
    e. PAX8/PPARγ

71. Histological features of PTC include all of the following *EXCEPT:*
    a. Intranuclear inclusions
    b. Nuclear grooves
    c. Empty nuclei
    d. Psammoma bodies
    e. Encapsulation

72. When PTC spreads to the lateral neck, it most commonly affects which of the following levels?
    a. II, III, IV, and V
    b. I, II, and III
    c. II, III, and IV
    d. III, IV and VI
    e. I, II, III, IV, and V

73. Ultrasound characteristics of lymph nodes with thyroid carcinoma metastases include which of the following?
    i. Absence of a fatty hilum
    ii. Round shape
    iii. Calcification
    iv. Chaotic vascularity
    a. i, ii, and iii
    b. ii and iv
    c. i and iii
    d. All of the above

74. Boundaries of the central neck compartment include all of the following *EXCEPT*:
    a. Innominate artery
    b. Subclavian vein
    c. Hyoid bone
    d. Medial aspect carotid sheath
    e. Deep layer of deep cervical fascia

75. A follicular carcinoma that has grown slightly outside the thyroid gland into nearby tissues has a tumor stage in the TNM staging system of which of the following?
    a. T1b
    b. T2
    c. T3
    d. T4a
    e. T4b

76. A 50-year-old woman has PTC of 4.1 cm in size with macroscopically involved paratracheal and level IV lymph nodes. No distant metastases can be identified. Which of the following is her stage grouping?
    a. Stage 2
    b. Stage 3
    c. Stage 4A
    d. Stage 4B
    e. Stage 4C

77. A 44-year-old woman has PTC of 5.2 cm in size with macroscopically involved paratracheal and level IV lymph nodes and pulmonary metastases. Which of the following is her stage grouping?
    a. Stage 2
    b. Stage 3
    c. Stage 4A
    d. Stage 4B
    e. Stage 4C

78. Which of the following directly increase(s) the risk for developing PTC?
    i. Male gender
    ii. Radiation for childhood cancer
    iii. Exposure to polybrominated diphenyl ethers
    iv. Family history of thyroid cancer
    v. All of the above
    a. i, ii, and iii
    b. ii and iv
    c. i and iii
    d. v

79. Which of the following is/are correct regarding familial nonmedullary thyroid cancer?
    i. It is defined by the presence of three or more first-degree relatives with well-differentiated thyroid cancer
    ii. It follows an autosomal recessive inheritance pattern.
    iii. It exhibits incomplete penetrance.
    iv. It generally behaves less aggressively than sporadic well-differentiated thyroid carcinoma of comparative stage.
    a. i, ii, and iii
    b. ii and iv
    c. i and iii
    d. None is correct.
    e. All are correct.

80. All of the following are correct regarding the diffuse sclerosing variant of PTC *EXCEPT*:
    a. It represents approximately 5% of all PTCs.
    b. It is more frequent in children with Chernobyl radiation exposure.
    c. Bilaterality is common.
    d. Lymph node metastases occur in 20%.
    e. Distant metastasis rate is higher than for classic PTC.

81. Which of the following is the most common site of distant metastatic disease in PTC?
    a. Bone
    b. Lung
    c. Lung and bone
    d. Liver
    e. Other tumor sites

82. Postoperative radioiodine remnant ablation with I-131 following surgery for well-differentiated thyroid carcinoma is intended to:
    a. Remove normal residual thyroid tissue
    b. Facilitate follow-up with thyroglobulin
    c. Destroy residual microscopic lymph node metastases
    d. All of the above

83. Which of the following is/are possible complications of I-131 ablative therapy?
    i. Xerostomia
    ii. Dental caries
    iii. Nasolacrimal duct obstruction
    iv. Leukemia
    a. i, ii, and iii
    b. ii and iv
    c. i and iii
    d. None of the above
    e. All of the above

84. Which of the following is correct regarding Hürthle cell tumors?
    a. They account for 15% to 20% of all thyroid cancers.
    b. They are composed mainly of Hürthle cells with a predominance >25% of the cell population.
    c. Evidence of vascular and/or capsular invasion distinguishes malignant from benign lesions.
    d. They have a lower rate of distant metastases than papillary and follicular thyroid carcinomas.
    e. All of the above are correct.

85. Which of the following statements is *INCORRECT* regarding the RLN and differentiated thyroid carcinoma?
    a. If the RLN is encased by tumor and ipsilateral vocal fold paresis or paralysis is present preoperatively, resection of the RLN is indicated.
    b. If the RLN is encased by tumor and the contralateral vocal fold is paretic or paralyzed, ipsilateral-involved RLN should be sacrificed.
    c. If the RLN is encased by tumor and the RLN is spared intraoperatively, then adjuvant therapy is indicated.
    d. If intraoperatively the tumor is found to be minimally adherent to the RLN (not encasing it), then the RLN should be preserved.

86. In MTC with RET mutation, the specific mutation type predicts which of the following?
    a. Age of onset
    b. Recurrence risk
    c. Association with other endocrine neoplasms
    d. Approach to surgical management
    e. All of the above

87. Which of the following is/are correct regarding MTC?
    i. Hereditary type is more common than sporadic.
    ii. Sporadic MTC may behave more aggressively than hereditary MTC.

iii. They uncommonly metastasize to cervical lymph nodes.
iv. Radioiodine, external beam radiation therapy, and conventional chemotherapy are not effective treatment options.
   a. i, ii, and iii
   b. ii and iv
   c. i and iii
   d. None is correct.
   e. All are correct.

88. MEN2A comprises all of the following *EXCEPT:*
   a. Pheochromocytoma
   b. Hyperparathyroidism
   c. Cutaneous lichen amyloidosis
   d. Marfanoid habitus
   e. Hirschsprung disease

89. Differential diagnosis of a fine needle biopsy specimen showing poorly differentiated large cell malignancy includes all of the following *EXCEPT:*
   a. Diffuse large cell lymphoma
   b. MTC
   c. Sarcoma
   d. Melanoma
   e. Anaplastic thyroid carcinoma (ATC)

90. In ATC, all of the following are associated with improved prognosis *EXCEPT:*
   a. Male gender
   b. Age <60 years
   c. Tumor size <7 cm
   d. Less extensive disease at presentation
   e. Coexistence of differentiated thyroid carcinoma

91. Which of the following are correct regarding ATC?
   i. If there is extrathyroidal invasion, an en bloc resection with the goal of achieving gross negative margins should be considered.
   ii. If complete resection can be performed with minimal morbidity, it should be performed because it may be associated with improved survival.
   iii. Incomplete tumor resection of tumor debulking should not be performed because it is unlikely to be beneficial for local control and/or survival.
   iv. With extrathyroidal extension into the larynx, total laryngectomy should be performed because this may improve survival.
   a. i, ii, and iii
   b. ii and iv
   c. i and iii
   d. All of the above are correct.

92. Symptoms and signs of hypercalcemia include all of the following *EXCEPT:*
   a. Bone fractures
   b. Renal calculi
   c. Fatigue
   d. Band keratopathy
   e. Diarrhea

93. In PHPT, surgery is advised for patients with which of the following?
   a. Nephrolithiasis
   b. Serum calcium >1.0 mg/dL above the reference limit
   c. T score <−2.5
   d. Creatinine clearance <60 cc/min
   e. All of the above

94. Complications of PHPT in pregnancy include all of the following *EXCEPT:*

   a. Low birth weight
   b. Hyperemesis gravidarum
   c. Spontaneous abortion
   d. Aortic stenosis
   e. Neonatal tetany

95. Normal serum calcium with elevated serum PTH can occur in which of the following?
   i. Secondary hyperparathyroidism (SHPT) resulting from hypercalciuria
   ii. SHPT resulting from renal insufficiency
   iii. PHPT with vitamin D deficiency
   iv. Parathyroid carcinoma
   a. i, ii, and iii
   b. ii and iv
   c. i and iii
   d. All of the above

96. On ultrasound, parathyroid adenomas are most commonly:
   a. Hyperechoic relative to thyroid follicular nodules
   b. Avascular
   c. Hypoechoic relative to thyroid follicular nodules
   d. Calcified
   e. Round in shape

97. Which of the following is/are correct regarding use of sestamibi for parathyroid localization?
   i. It is highly sensitive for the detection of double parathyroid adenomas.
   ii. Combining dual phase and subtraction single photon emission CT (SPECT) imaging can decrease false positive rates.
   iii. High mitochondrial content in parathyroid tumors can cause false-negative results.
   iv. False positives can occur with oxyphilic thyroid nodules.
   v. Four-dimensional CT is less sensitive for localization.
   a. i, ii, and iii
   b. ii and iv
   c. i and iii
   d. v
   e. All are correct.

98. Important questions to ask when evaluating a patient for hyperparathyroidism include all of the following *EXCEPT:*
   a. History of nephrolithiasis or osteoporosis
   b. Use of thiazide diuretics or lithium
   c. History of neck irradiation
   d. History of amyloidosis
   e. Family history of hypercalcemia

99. Which of the following is/are correct regarding parathyroid glands?
   i. The upper weight limit is 40 to 60 mg and the typical color is mahogany.
   ii. Supernumerary glands occur in 5% of cases.
   iii. Inferior and superior glands are usually supplied by the inferior thyroid artery (ITA).
   iv. They exhibit positional symmetry within the neck (upper glands > lower glands).
   v. Superior glands are dorsal and inferior glands are ventral to the RLN; this relationship is more constant than that between parathyroid glands and the ITA.
   a. i, ii, and iii
   b. ii and iv
   c. i and iii
   d. v
   e. All are correct.

100. Conditions that can be associated with SHPT include all
     of the following *EXCEPT*:
     a. Long-term lithium therapy
     b. Vitamin D deficiency
     c. Pseudohyperparathyroidism
     d. Impaired gastrointestinal absorption

CORE KNOWLEDGE

THYROID

Applied Surgical Embryology, Anatomy, and Physiology

- The medial thyroid anlage appears between weeks 2 and 3
  gestation from a ventral diverticulum of first and second
  pharyngeal pouch endoderm and descends into the neck
  from the foramen cecum at the base of tongue. TDCs may
  arise from persistence of this tract. Approximately 55% to
  76% of people have a pyramidal lobe extending superiorly
  from midline or either lobe. TDCs are lined by
  pseudostratified ciliated columnar epithelium, squamous
  epithelium, or both. The supporting cyst wall contains
  heterotopic thyroid tissue in approximately 20% of cases.
- The lateral thyroid anlage arises from a proliferation of
  pharyngeal endoderm, and the ventral portion of the
  fourth pharyngeal pouch becomes attached to the
  posterior thyroid surface during week 5 gestation. Neural
  crest cells are the source of the parafollicular C cells that
  secrete calcitonin. C cells derive from the ultimobranchial
  bodies that fuse with the middle to upper portion of
  the medial thyroid anlage. In patients with medullary
  carcinoma of the thyroid, total thyroidectomy should be
  performed to excise all C cells.
- The tubercle of Zuckerkandl projects posterolaterally from
  the thyroid lobe where the medial and lateral thyroid
  components fuse. Enlargement of the tubercle usually

occurs lateral to the RLN so that the nerve appears to
pass into a cleft medial to the enlarged tubercle. However,
the RLN can also run ventral to an enlarged tubercle
occasionally.
- The ITA is a branch of the thyrocervical trunk and lies
  anterior to the RLN in 70% of people. It is the main
  supply to the parathyroid glands. The superior thyroid
  artery, a branch of the external carotid, lies posterolateral
  to the external branch of the superior laryngeal nerve.
- The RLN carries motor, sensory, and autonomic fibers.
  It innervates all intrinsic muscles of the larynx with the
  exception of the cricothyroid muscle, which is innervated
  by the external branch of the superior laryngeal nerve.
  It also innervates the inferior constrictor muscle of the
  pharynx and cricopharyngeus muscle and carries sensory
  fibers from the larynx, upper esophagus, and trachea.
- After branching from the vagus nerve, the right RLN
  loops around the subclavian artery and returns back to
  the thyroid bed approximately 2 cm lateral to the trachea.
  The left RLN loops around the aortic arch, lateral to the
  obliterated ductus arteriosus, and returns to the neck to
  travel in the tracheoesophageal groove, following a more
  medial course than the right RLN.
- Figure 22-1 shows neural and vascular anatomy of the neck
  base.

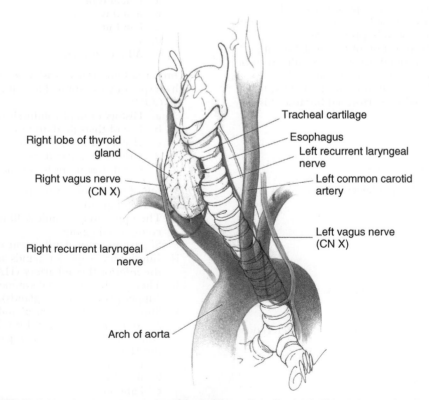

FIGURE 22-1 Neural and vascular anatomy of the neck base. (From Randolph GW, ed. *Surgery of the Thyroid and Parathyroid Glands.* 2nd ed. Philadelphia: Elsevier Saunders; 2013.)

- Three anatomic variants of a nonrecurrent laryngeal nerve (NRLN) have been identified:
  - Type 1: NRLN arises directly from cervical vagus and descends into the larynx at the level of the superior thyroid pole.
  - Type 2A: NRLN arises directly from cervical vagus, following a transverse path parallel to and over the trunk of the ITA, at the isthmus level.
  - Type 2B: NRLN makes a downward curve, following a transverse path parallel to and under the ITA trunk.
- Vagal nerve stimulation during surgery can help identify an NRLN where vagal stimulation high in neck → +laryngeal electromyogram activity and vagal stimulation low in neck → no laryngeal electromyogram activity.
- Thyroid hormones are iodinated derivatives of tyrosine and are produced by the thyroid gland in two forms: 3,5,3′-triiodothyronine (T3) and 3,5,3′,5′-tetraiodothyronine (thyroxine, T4).
- Within the gland, iodide is attached to thyroglobulin (Tg), a large glycoprotein that is stored as a colloid in the interior of each thyroid follicle. The process of hormone synthesis involves iodide oxidation → transfer of oxidized iodide to tyrosyl residues on Tg to produce monoiodotyrosine (MIT) and diiodotyrosine (DIT) → coupling of two iodotyrosine molecules to form T3 (MIT + DIT) or T2 (DIT + DIT). This process is catalyzed by thyroid peroxidase.
- To release hormone, thyrocyte cells take up Tg from the extracellular space via micropinocytosis or macropinocytosis and cleave it in lysosomes to release free T4 and T3 (plus MIT and DIT, which is deiodinated). Serum Tg rises with increased mass of normal or malignant thyroid tissues, increased thyrotropin (TSH) stimulation of thyroid tissue, and injury of thyroid tissue.
- Thyrotropin-releasing hormone (TRH) from the hypothalamus stimulates TSH release. Circulating levels of T3 and T4 negatively feed back on the anterior pituitary gland and hypothalamus to control TSH secretion and TRH gene expression, respectively.

Benign Thyroid Disease

- Subclinical and overt hypothyroidism occurs in 4.6% to 9.5% of the population, whereas subclinical and overt hyperthyroidism occurs in 1.3% to 2.2%.
- In the ambulatory patient, serum TSH is a recommended initial diagnostic test for evaluation of thyroid hypodysfunction or hyperdysfunction, with approximately 98% sensitivity and 92% specificity.
- Serum total T4 (TT4) or T3 (TT3) should never be used alone to indicate thyroid function, because alterations in amounts or avidity of thyroid hormone–binding proteins can affect measured TT4/TT3 levels without altering bioactive free levels or thyroidal status. When serum thyroid hormone–binding protein levels are normal, the free T4 index provides a reliable measure of the patient's thyroid status. However, in conditions where thyroid-binding protein levels markedly change (e.g., pregnancy, malnutrition), free T4 index is a poor estimate of the free T4 level. T3/T4 ratio may be useful to distinguish Graves disease (T3/T4 ratio > 20) from subacute thyroiditis (T3/T4 ratio < 12).
- Hyperthyroidism and hypothyroidism in adults are often secondary to autoimmune disease where IgG antibodies are formed against thyroid proteins (e.g., thyroglobulin, thyroid peroxidase, the TSH receptor). In the absence of thyroid dysfunction, measurement of thyroid antibodies is generally unnecessary. Although thyroid peroxidase antibody (TPOAb) is diagnostic of autoimmune disease, its presence does not guarantee development of autoimmune

hypothyroidism or hyperthyroidism for patients with normal TSH. Patients with elevated TPOAb and ultrasound changes of chronic thyroiditis have a threefold increased risk of developing overt hypothyroidism.
- The utility of Tg in evaluating thyroid function or thyroid disease is limited. It may be useful to distinguish between true endogenous hyperthyroidism (serum Tg elevated) and factitious thyrotoxicosis from exogenous thyroid hormone ingestion (serum Tg low). The Tg assay can be made more sensitive by stimulation with either recombinant human TSH (rhTSH) or endogenous hypothyroidism, both of which result in an approximate eightfold increase in Tg.
- Radionuclide thyroid imaging studies can be useful to determine the cause of hyperthyroidism but are not recommended for evaluation of hypothyroidism. I-123 is the preferred diagnostic isotope for noncancer imaging because it emits only gamma rays, compared with I-131, which also emits tissue-damaging beta particles. I-123 scans have 5% to 8% fewer false-negative results than technetium-99m pertechnetate (Tc-99m) scans; however, because Tc-99m scans are easier, faster, more widely available, and cheaper, they are used instead of I-123 scans at some institutions. Correlation between the two imaging modalities is high.

Hypothyroidism

- The most common adult causes of hypothyroidism, excluding iatrogenic causes, are Hashimoto thyroiditis and the hypothyroid phase of subacute thyroiditis (including postpartum thyroiditis).
- Hashimoto thyroiditis aggregates in families, possibly associated with human leukocyte antigen genes, and a defect in immunoregulation may be important in the pathogenesis.
- Serum TSH is almost always elevated in primary hypothyroidism and should be ordered as the initial diagnostic test. A rise in TSH occurs before a fall in T4 or T3. TSH should not be used to assess patients with known or suspected hypothalamic disease (i.e., secondary hypothyroidism). Diagnosis is confirmed by the presence of antithyroid antibodies.
- If TSH is between 0.3 and 4.5 mIU/L, the patient does not have hypothyroidism. TSH > 10 mIU/L → initiate treatment with L-thyroxine (unless recovering from acute illness or subacute thyroiditis when TSH may transiently rise to elevated levels before normalizing). TSH 4.5 to 10 mIU/L → repeat labs in 1 month including TSH, free T4, TPOAb level → if FT4I is low, commence L-T4 therapy. Measuring T3 is not indicated because it will be maintained within the normal range in mild to moderate hypothyroidism.
- The goal of treatment is to normalize the serum TSH level to 0.5 to 2.5 mIU/L.
- Approximately 15% of people >60 years of age will have TSH between 4.5 and 10 mIU/L; of these, 27% to 33% will have spontaneous normalization of TSH over 3 to 4 years.
- There are no case-controlled studies that show a significant physiologic benefit from adding T3 to L-T4 therapy.

Hyperthyroidism

- Graves disease is the most common cause of adult hyperthyroidism in North America. Other causes include toxic multinodular goiter, toxic adenoma, and the thyrotoxic phase of subacute thyroiditis, including postpartum thyroiditis.

- Serum TSH measurement is the most sensitive diagnostic test for hyperthyroidism and is always suppressed in primary hyperthyroidism, generally to levels <0.1 mIU/L. If TSH < 0.3, thyroid hormone levels should be measured, including total T3 and FT4I.
- The findings of diffuse goiter, exophthalmos, and biochemical tyrosinemia are diagnostic of Graves disease. However, if the etiology is unclear, a radionuclide thyroid uptake scan is diagnostically helpful. Radioactive iodine uptake will be greatly increased and diffuse in Graves, patchy in toxic multinodular goiter (increased within the hyperactive nodule and inhibited in surrounding tissues), suppressed in the thyrotoxic phase of subacute thyroiditis, normal with a "hot" nodule for toxic adenoma, and low with metastatic thyroid carcinoma.

Graves Disease and Toxic Nodular Goiter

- Graves syndrome comprises hyperthyroidism, goiter, ophthalmopathy, and, occasionally, a dermopathy (pretibial myxedema).
  - Hyperthyroidism is caused by autoantibodies to the TSH receptor that activate the receptor. There is an underlying genetic predisposition.
  - Histology shows follicular hyperplasia, patchy lymphocytic infiltration, and rare lymphoid germinal centers.
- Development of hyperthyroidism in toxic nodular goiter takes many years and predominantly occurs when single autonomous nodules are >2.5 cm in diameter.
- CT should be ordered in any patient with compressive or obstructive symptoms, with iodinated contrast as long as TSH is not suppressed.
- Treatment of hyperthyroidism includes antithyroid drugs (ATDs), radioactive iodine ablation, and thyroidectomy. ATDs methimazole and propylthiouracil block thyroid hormone synthesis, and beta-blockers are useful to ameliorate cardiovascular and neuromuscular symptoms.
  - In Graves disease, methimazole (or sometimes carbimazole in Europe and Asia) is a first-line pharmacologic option either for primary treatment or to prepare a patient for radioactive iodine (RAI) therapy or surgery. Propylthiouracil is indicated as a first-line medication in pregnancy and in patients with adverse reactions to methimazole. Treatment with ATDs for 12 to 18 months results in long-term remission in 40% to 60% of patients with Graves disease. If hyperthyroidism recurs, RAI or surgery should be considered.
  - RAI is the treatment of choice for toxic nodular goiter (TNG) if radioiodine uptake is adequate and the patient is a poor surgical candidate. However, the standard RAI dose may need to be increased due to TNGs having lower I-131 uptake. After RAI, most patients are euthyroid within 2 to 4 months with many eventually becoming hypothyroid. There is a 20% chance of recurrence with RAI for TNG. In Graves disease, RAI is the treatment of choice; in the United States it is generally administered as a single large dose.
  - Bilateral near total or total thyroidectomy is recommended for patients with large TNGs with obstructive upper aerodigestive symptoms, coincidental suspicious/cold/growing thyroid nodules, and contraindication or refusal of I-131 or ATDs. Subtotal thyroidectomy is associated with higher relapse rates in Graves disease and thus should not be performed. Preoperatively, patients should be treated with ATDs to restore euthyroidism with or without beta-blockers.
  - Iodine given in pharmacologic doses inhibits thyroid hormone release for days to weeks and can be useful in preparing patients for surgery and in the treatment of thyrotoxic crises. Normal dose of potassium iodide is 60 mg (one drop) three times daily.

Thyroglossal Duct Cysts

- Thyroglossal duct cysts are located between hyoid and thyroid cartilage > hyoid/suprahyoid > suprasternal > base of tongue.
- The Sistrunk procedure is the standard surgical treatment.
- Incidence of malignancy is 1%, primarily PTC; management is controversial → incidentally discovered thyroglossal duct cyst PTC may be managed by the Sistrunk procedure alone provided there is no evidence of suspicious thyroid pathology or cervical adenopathy. Alternatively, total thyroidectomy plus the Sistrunk procedure may be performed given the incidence of concomitant occult primary thyroid carcinoma is 11% to 56%. This also allows postoperative treatment with radioiodine due to a high risk of lymph node metastasis.
  - Prognosis is excellent: overall 10-year survival >95%.

Cervical and Substernal Goiter

- The incidence of cervical and substernal goiters increases with age.
- Anterior mediastinum is affected in approximately 85% of patients; posterior mediastinum in 15% (Figure 22-2).
- Posterior mediastinum extension → trachea displaced and great vessels splayed anteriorly → mass excavates region

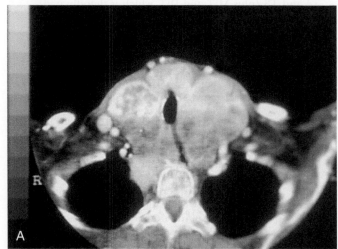

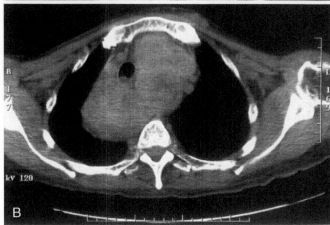

FIGURE 22-2 Computed tomography (CT) of the neck showing **(A)** anterior and **(B)** posterior substernal goiters. (From Randolph GW, ed. *Surgery of the Thyroid and Parathyroid Glands.* 2nd ed. Philadelphia: Elsevier Saunders; 2013.)

posterior to RLN, ITA, innominate and subclavian arteries, innominate vein, carotid sheath → care must be taken to avoid RLN injury.

- Mediastinal thyroid masses can exist without connection to the normal orthotopic cervical gland, and vascular supply may be through mediastinal arteries and veins.
- Symptoms include cough, dyspnea, foreign-body sensation, neck tightness, or wheezing; 25% may be asymptomatic.
  - Approximately one-third of goiter patients have upper airway obstruction.
- The presence of airway compression, malignancy, and hyperthyroidism are important to address during preoperative workup.
  - Plain chest radiography is of limited value.
  - CT or MRI should be performed in all patients.
  - Thyroid function must be tested; hyperthyroidism may occur in up to 30% of goiter patients.
- Of patients with cervical goiter, 3% (3% to 7% with substernal extension) have vocal fold paralysis, and all patients must have preoperative laryngeal examination. Symptomatic vocal assessment does not predict objective laryngeal examination findings.
- Treatment:
  - T4 suppressive therapy: variable efficacy in reducing goiter size; associated with high regrowth rates when treatment is discontinued; limited in the elderly population (higher risk of atrial fibrillation and accelerated bone loss)
  - Radioiodine: the larger the goiter, the less responsive to radioiodine. Can cause a transient increase in goiter size by 11% to 60% in up to 7% of patients treated. Thus, it should be considered only for smaller goiters without airway impact and for patients who are unable to have surgical excision.
  - Surgery: indications include upper aerodigestive tract symptoms without other cause, radiographic evidence of tracheal compression, masses >5 cm, goiter with subclinical hyperthyroidism, suspicion for carcinoma, and substernal extension. Awake, sitting up, flexible transnasal or transoral intubation are the safest methods of intubation where concerns exist regarding tracheal compression and laryngeal deviation. In most cases (excluding invasive malignant disease), tracheal compression will yield to a reasonably sized endotracheal tube. The extent of surgery is determined by the initial disease; for unilateral enlargement, total unilateral lobar resection is reasonable; however, there may be a recurrence rate of between 15% to 42%. Carotid sheath dissection is helpful during goiter removal and allows vagal nerve stimulation to monitor RLN function. RLN may be splayed over the surface of a goiter or entrapped on the surface through fascial band fixation.

THYROID NEOPLASMS

Thyroid Nodules

- Nodule prevalence has increased over the past two decades, which has been attributed to an aging population and increased detection through use of radiological imaging modalities.
- Approximately 8% to 15% of nodules >1 cm in size harbor malignancy.
- Expected rate of growth of solid nodules is 1 to 2 mm in each dimension per year.
- Ultrasound is the preferred method of radiologic visualization (Figure 22-3). Many distinctive, highly sensitive ultrasound characteristics of malignant thyroid

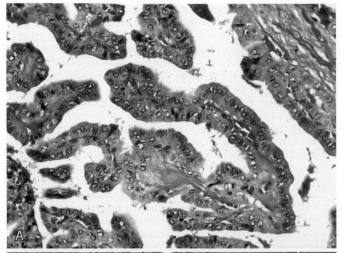

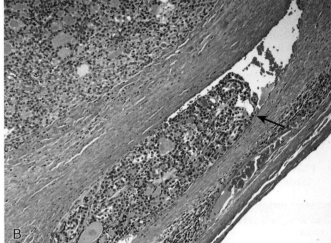

FIGURE 22-3 Histological findings in thyroid carcinoma. **A,** Papillary thyroid carcinoma (PTC) characterized by papillary architecture with fibrovascular cores and cells showing diagnostic nuclear features. **B,** Follicular neoplasm *(upper left)* showing the presence of vascular invasion, including tumor within an intracapsular endothelial-lined vascular space *(arrow).* The presence of invasive growth and absence of nuclear features diagnostic for PTC confers the diagnosis of follicular carcinoma. (Courtesy Bruce M. Wenig MD, Department of Pathology, Mount Sinai Health System.)

nodules have been identified (e.g., microcalcifications, indistinct nodule margins, hyperechogenicity, central nodule vascularity, irregular/spherical/tall shape, abnormal lymphadenopathy); however, specificity is lower and no single feature is diagnostic.
  - Specificity of microcalcifications for thyroid carcinoma is 71% to 94%, with sensitivity of 35% to 72%.
- Serum TSH measurement is indicated in the initial work-up of a patient with a thyroid nodule; if subnormal, I-123 or technetium Tc-99m pertechnetate scintigraphy can be performed.
- According to the 2015 American Thyroid Association (ATA) guidelines, fine needle aspiration (FNA) is indicated for nodules >1 cm in greatest dimension with high or intermediate suspicion sonographic findings, and nodules 1.5 cm in greatest dimension with low suspicion sonographic findings. FNA cytology (FNAC) may be considered for nodules >2 cm in greatest dimension with very low suspicion sonographic patterns (e.g., spongiform). High suspicion ultrasonic appearance (malignancy risk, 70%-90%) refers to solid hypoechoic nodules or partially cystic nodules with a solid hypoechoic

component with one or more of the following features: irregular margins (specifically defined as infiltrative, microlobulated, or spiculated), microcalcifications, taller than wide shape, disrupted rim calcifications with small extrusive hypoechoic soft tissue component, or evidence of extrathyroidal extension. Intermediate suspicion ultrasound appearance (malignancy risk 10-20%) refers to hypoechoic solid nodules with smooth regular margins, without microcalcifications, extrathyroidal extension, or taller than wide shape. Low suspicion nodules on ultrasound (malignancy risk, 5%-10%) are isoechoic or hyperechoic solid nodules, or partially cystic nodules with eccentric uniformly solid areas without microcalcifications, irregular margins, or extrathyroidal extension, or taller than wide shape. Very low suspicion (malignancy risk, <3%) nodules appear spongiform or partially cystic on ultrasound without any of the sonographic features described in the low, intermediate, or high suspicion patterns.

- The 2014 British Thyroid Association Guidelines state that ultrasound-guided FNAC should be performed if ultrasound appearances are equivocal, indeterminate, or suspicious of malignancy.
- Fine needle aspiration is not indicated for
  - "Hot nodules" on I-123 scintigraphy
  - Nodules <1 to 1.5 cm in size in ultrasonographic low risk nodules
  - Purely cystic nodules
  - "Pseudonodules" in patients with Graves or Hashimoto disease where clear nodule borders cannot be identified in all ultrasound planes
- FNAC results may be classified using the Bethesda or Thy classification systems:

Table 22-1 **Bethesda and Thy Classification Systems**

Grade	Interpretation	
	Bethesda	*Thy*
1	Nondiagnostic	Nondiagnostic
2	Benign (malignancy risk <5%)	Nonneoplastic
3	Atypia or follicular lesion of undetermined significance (malignancy risk, 5%-15%)	Neoplasm possible: 3a: atypical features present 3f: follicular neoplasm suspected
4	Neoplasm, either follicular or Hürthle cell (malignancy risk, 15%-25%)	Suspicious of malignancy
5	Suspicious for malignancy (malignancy risk, 60%-75%)	Diagnostic of malignancy
6	Malignant (malignancy risk, >95%)	

- Bethesda/Thy 1 nodules should undergo repeat FNAC under ultrasound guidance.
- Bethesda/Thy 2 nodules should have a serial ultrasound performed 6 to 18 months after initial ultrasound. Repeat FNAC is indicated for nodules that exhibit a >50% change in volume or >20% increase in at least two nodule dimensions in solid nodules or in the solid portion of mixed cystic–solid nodules. If a Bethesda 2 nodule has undergone repeat ultrasound-guided FNA with a second benign cytology result, ultrasound surveillance for this nodule for continued risk of malignancy is no longer indicated
- Many Thy 3a cases reflect suboptimal specimens and can be reallocated on repeat cytology. Therefore, ultrasound

assessment with repeat FNAC is usually indicated. The cytological interpretation of a 3a nodule should be clearly stated in the report and may include situations such as inability to exclude a follicular neoplasm or papillary carcinoma. For Thy 3f lesions, differential diagnoses include a hyperplastic nodule, follicular adenoma, or follicular carcinoma. These cannot be distinguished on cytology alone and a histology sample (e.g., diagnostic thyroid lobectomy) is required for diagnosis.

- For Bethesda 3 and 4 (Thy 3) "indeterminate" nodules, recent studies have confirmed the ability of genetic markers (including BRAF, Ras, RET/PTC) and protein markers (galectin-3) to improve preoperative diagnostic accuracy and potentially avoid the need for unnecessary operations.
  - 2015 ATA guidelines state that molecular testing may be used to supplement malignancy risk assessment data for Bethesda 3 and 4 nodules in lieu of proceeding directly with surgery, and that informed patient preference and feasibility should be considered in clinical decision making.
  - For suspicious (Bethesda 5) nodules, BRAF mutation testing may be considered as they are reported to confer a close to 100% probability of malignancy.
- Because of an increased risk for malignancy, current ATA guidelines state that total thyroidectomy may be preferred in patients with indeterminate nodules that are cytologically suspicious for malignancy, positive for known mutations specific for carcinoma, sonographically suspicious, or large (>4 cm), or in patients with familial thyroid carcinoma or a history of radiation exposure, if completion thyroidectomy would be recommended based on the indeterminate nodule being malignant following lobectomy. Additionally, patients with indeterminate nodules who have bilateral nodular disease, those with significant medical comorbidities, or those who prefer to undergo bilateral thyroidectomy to avoid the possibility of requiring a future surgery on the contralateral lobe may undergo total or near-total thyroidectomy, assuming completion thyroidectomy would be recommended if the indeterminate nodule proved malignant following lobectomy.
- 2-[19F]Fluoro-2-deoxy-D-glucose PET (^{18}FDG-PET) scans appear to have relatively high sensitivity for malignancy but low specificity and thus are not recommended for indeterminate nodules.

Differentiated Thyroid Carcinoma

- DTC encompasses papillary (PTC) and follicular (FTC) thyroid carcinomas.
- The incidence of PTC is increasing. Women : men = 3 : 1, peak incidence is at 40 to 50 years in women and 10 to 20 years higher in men.
- Childhood ionizing radiation exposure (including that used to treat benign conditions of the head and neck such as tonsillitis) is a risk factor for PTC. Approximately 5% of nonmedullary thyroid cancers are hereditary. Familial syndromes include familial nonmedullary thyroid Cancer, familial adenomatous polyposis, Gardner syndrome, Cowden disease, Werner syndrome, and Carney complex.
- Classic PTC has an indolent clinical course with low morbidity and mortality.
  - Histologic variants include follicular (behaves similarly to classical PTC), tall cell (increased mortality; radioiodine refractory), columnar cell (encapsulated form has very good prognosis; invasive form is very aggressive with high mortality), diffuse sclerosing (more frequent in children exposed to radiation at Chernobyl,

higher rates of lymph node metastases but possibly similar long-term prognosis to classic PTC), solid (more frequent in children exposed to radiation at Chernobyl, similar nuclear features to classic PTC, lymph node metastases common), and insular (large size at presentation, positive cervical nodes in >50%, 70% with distant metastases; 30 year cancer specific mortality rate = 25%).

- Larger primary tumor size is associated with poorer disease outcome (10-year tumor recurrence and cancer-specific mortality rates) and higher rates of locoregional and distant metastases.
- Up to 45% of patients with PTC in one lobe have contralateral lobe involvement; multifocality is common.

- Follicular thyroid lesions can be separated into three clinical entities: follicular adenomas, minimally invasive follicular carcinomas, and widely invasive follicular carcinomas. Differentiation between these requires tumor capsule evaluation, with capsule disruption being required for diagnosis of malignancy.
  - FTC more commonly undergoes hematogenous spread compared with lymphatic spread for PTC → higher distant metastasis rates and lower risk of cervical lymph node metastases compared with PTC.
- Thyroid cancer staging for differentiated thyroid cancer uses the tumor/node/metastasis (TNM) staging system and is dependent on the age of the patient, with those <45 years being limited to Stage 1 or 2 regardless of the presence of distant metastatic disease.
- Ultrasound can be used to detect macroscopic nodal metastases, particularly of the lateral neck; however, contrast-enhanced CT imaging has better sensitivity than ultrasound in localizing lymph node metastases. The combination of CT and ultrasound provides the most comprehensive preoperative assessment of nodal involvement. CT is also useful to assess for carcinoma invasion into surrounding tissues, trachea, and esophagus and thus to aid with surgical planning.
- Preoperative laryngeal examination should be performed for all patients with thyroid carcinoma or preoperative voice changes.
  - Subjective voice complaints and objective laryngeal examination findings have poor correlation → preoperative finding of vocal cord paralysis (VCP) correlates well with the presence of RLN invasion in cases of thyroid carcinoma
- The 2015 ATA guidelines recommend near-total or total thyroidectomy for patients with thyroid cancer >4 cm, gross extrathyroidal extension (clinical T4), or clinically apparent metastatic disease to nodes (clinical N1) or distant sites (clinical M1), with gross removal of all primary tumors, unless there are contraindications to this procedure.
  - For patients with thyroid cancer >1 cm and <4 cm without extrathyroidal extension and without clinical evidence of any lymph node metastases (cN0), the initial surgical procedure can be either a bilateral procedure (near-total or total thyroidectomy) or a unilateral procedure (lobectomy).
  - If surgery is chosen for patients with thyroid cancer <1 cm without extrathyroidal extension and cN0, the initial surgical procedure should be a thyroid lobectomy unless there are clear indications to remove the contralateral lobe. Thyroid lobectomy alone is sufficient treatment for small, unifocal, intrathyroidal carcinomas in the absence of prior head and neck irradiation, familial thyroid carcinoma, or clinically detectable cervical nodal metastases.

- Observation may be appropriate for patients at high surgical risk because of comorbid conditions, patients expected to have a relatively short remaining life span (e.g., with serious cardiopulmonary disease, other malignancies, very advanced age), or patients with concurrent medical or surgical issues that need to be addressed prior to treatment.
- The 2014 British Thyroid guidelines recommend total thyroidectomy for patients with tumors >4 cm in diameter, or tumors of any size in association with any of the following characteristics: multifocal disease, bilateral disease, extrathyroidal spread (pT3 and pT4a),familial disease, and those with clinically or radiologically involved nodes and/or distant metastases. The evidence for total thyroidectomy compared to hemithyroidectomy in patients with unifocal tumors >1 to ≤4 cm in diameter, age <45 years, with no extrathyroidal spread, no familial disease, no evidence of lymph node involvement, no angioinvasion and no distant metastases, is unclear. In such cases, personalized decision making is recommended.
- Completion thyroidectomy may be necessary when the diagnosis of malignancy is made following thyroid lobectomy for an indeterminate or nondiagnostic biopsy. Many studies of papillary cancer have observed a higher rate of cancer in the opposite lobe when multifocal (two or more foci), as opposed to unifocal, disease is present in the ipsilateral lobe, and thus completion thyroidectomy is recommended in the presence of multifocal disease.
- The benefit of central lymph node dissection for the management of PTC is controversial. Microscopic nodal metastases are common and may be present in up to 90% of patients with clinically negative preoperative neck radiographic assessments. The clinical significance of microscopically positive lymph nodes with regards to recurrence-free survival rates is controversial and unlikely to affect recurrence-free survival rates (RFS). ATA guidelines recommend:
  - Therapeutic central-compartment (level VI) neck dissection for patients with clinically involved central nodes as an accompaniment to total thyroidectomy.
  - Prophylactic central-compartment neck dissection (ipsilateral or bilateral) should be considered in patients with papillary thyroid carcinoma with clinically uninvolved central neck lymph nodes (cN0) who have advanced primary tumors (T3 or T4) or clinically involved lateral neck nodes (cN1b), or if the information will be used to plan further steps in therapy.
  - Thyroidectomy without prophylactic central neck dissection may be appropriate for small (T1 or T2), noninvasive, clinically node-negative PTC (cN0) and for most follicular carcinomas (Figure 22-4).
- Therapeutic lateral neck dissection of draining nodal bases is indicated in the case of macroscopically positive nodes due to associated decreased RFS rates
  - The benefit of radioiodine remnant ablation (RRA) with I131 after thyroidectomy for patients with low risk disease is controversial, with some studies citing improvement in recurrence and mortality rates and others finding no advantage. For high-risk patients, RRA reduces recurrence and cancer-specific mortality. The ATA recommends RAI ablation be considered after total thyroidectomy in ATA intermediate risk level differentiated thyroid cancer patients. RAI adjuvant therapy is routinely recommended after total thyroidectomy for ATA high risk differentiated thyroid cancer patients with known distant metastases, gross extrathyroidal extension of the tumor regardless of tumor size, or primary tumor size >4cm even in the absence of other high risk features.

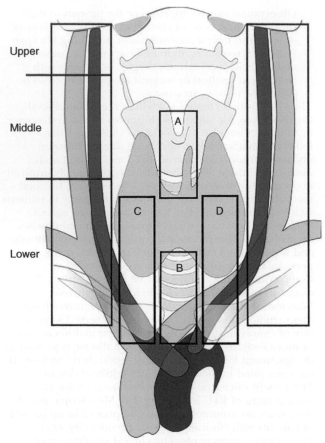

FIGURE 22-4 The four most important nodal-bearing regions within the central neck: prelaryngeal (Delphian) *(A)*, pretracheal *(C)*, and bilateral paratracheal *(B and D)*. (From Randolph GW, ed. *Surgery of the Thyroid and Parathyroid Glands*, 2nd ed. Philadelphia: Elsevier Saunders; 2013.)

- Successful remnant ablation refers to an absence of visible RAI uptake on a subsequent diagnostic RAI scan or an undetectable stimulated serum thyroglobulin.
  - The ATA recommends that the minimum activity (30-50 mCi) necessary to achieve successful remnant ablation be utilized, particularly for low-risk patients. A posttherapy RAI scan is recommended, usually 2 to 10 days following ablation.
- TSH suppression after thyroid surgery is recommended for high-risk patients, although the appropriate level and duration of TSH suppression are controversial. Patients with stages 3 and 4 disease may have improved overall survival after TSH suppression to <0.1 mIU/L, although no effect on disease-free survival is evident for any tumor stage.
- With respect to monitoring for disease recurrence using thyroglobulin, if basal Tg is <0.1 ng/mL, then 99.7% of rhTSH stimulated Tg will be <2 ng/m, suggesting absence of recurrent or persistent tumor. Thyroid carcinoma patients have a higher prevalence of antibodies to Tg (TgAbs) than euthyroid controls and TgAb positivity will make elevated Tg levels read as unmeasurable in commercially available assays. The TgAb level may be used as surrogate marker of tumor recurrence, and thyroid carcinoma patients with rising levels of TgAb need evaluation for disease recurrence.
- Ultrasound is the mainstay of radiological follow up for low-risk patients with undetectable Tg and negative antithyroglobulin antibodies. Diagnostic whole body scanning (DxWBS) 6 to 12 months after remnant ablation may be of value in the follow-up of patients with high or

intermediate risk of persistent disease. PETCT scanning may be useful to localize recurrent disease in Tg-positive, RAI scan–negative patients.

Medullary Thyroid Carcinoma

- Medullary thyroid carcinoma arises from parafollicular "C" cells of neuroendocrine origin and comprise 5% to 10% of all thyroid cancers. It occurs in hereditary (25%) and sporadic (75%) forms.
- Histology shows amyloid and spindle cells. Sporadic forms are bilateral or multifocal in one-third of cases; familial forms are bilateral or multifocal in 95% of cases.
- Germline mutations in the RET protooncogene are responsible for hereditary forms and have prognostic significance relative to the clinical behavior of MTC. Somatic mutations involving RET exist in 40% to 50% of sporadic MTC and 40% to 50% of sporadic PTCs.
- MEN2A → MTC/pheochromocytoma/ hyperparathyroidism/Hirschsprung disease/cutaneous lichen amyloidosis. MEN2B → MTC/pheochromocytoma (in >50% of patients)/presence of ocular, oral intestinal, and musculoskeletal ganglioneuromas, and unique musculoskeletal disorders. In MEN2B, MTC is present in almost every patient and is associated with poorer prognosis than other MTC forms.
- Tumors most commonly present as a palpable thyroid or neck mass. Early spread to central compartment and ipsilateral and contralateral jugular nodes (levels II to V) is common; nodal metastases occur in >70% of patients with palpable thyroid disease.
- The most sensitive predictors of survival in MTC are age at diagnosis and tumor stage. Age is not reflected in the TNM staging system, unlike well-differentiated thyroid cancer.
- Preoperative evaluation should include serum calcitonin and carcinoembryonic antigen measurement, serum calcium, RET protooncogene analyses, biochemical screening for pheochromocytoma (for any patient >10 years of age), and neck ultrasound. Imaging for distant metastatic disease (CT neck/chest/abdomen, PET-CT) should be considered in patients with cervical lymph node metastases or those with basal calcitonin >150 to 500 pg/mL.
  - Calcitonin is generally elevated (especially in sporadic MTC), and measurement of calcitonin helps screen patients at risk for MTC and in follow-up of patients after treatment. Carcinoembryonic antigen has lower diagnostic specificity for MTC than calcitonin.
- Surgery is the mainstay of treatment because MTC does not take up radioiodine and hormone suppression is ineffective.
  - Sporadic forms: total thyroidectomy plus central neck dissection. Ipsilateral lateral neck dissection can be considered based on degree of preoperative calcitonin elevation.
  - MEN syndromes: total thyroidectomy plus individualized lymph node dissection on the basis of pretherapeutic basal calcitonin serum levels
    - ≤200 pg/mL: no lymph node metastases present in contralateral neck, thus ipsilateral lateral and central neck dissection is adequate.
    - >200 pg/mL: bilateral lymph node metastases are increasingly present, plus mediastinal and distant metastases.
  - RET gene carriers without clinical disease should have prophylactic total thyroidectomy before basal calcitonin elevation.
  - Parathyroid glands may be autotransplanted locally into the sternomastoid muscle for sporadic, familial, or

MEN2B MTC or distantly into the nondominant forearm in cases of MEN2A.

- Biochemical cure refers to patients with normal calcitonin levels after MTC surgery. For recurrent disease, surgery is recommended in the absence of distant metastases. External beam radiation therapy to the neck has not shown any survival benefit. Tyrosine kinase inhibitors (e.g., sorafenib) that target RET hold promise for the palliation of locally advanced or metastatic disease.

Anaplastic Thyroid Carcinoma

- ATC comprises 17% of all thyroid cancers; median survival is 5 months and 1-year survival is 20%.
- All patients are TNM stage 4 (A, B, or C) at presentation.
- ATCs exhibit wide variations in appearance with several morphologic patterns recognized. All patterns are highly proliferative with numerous mitotic figures and atypical mitoses, usually with extensive necrosis. The three main patterns are spindle cell, pleomorphic giant cell, and squamoid.
- Ultrasound, cross-sectional imaging of neck and chest (CT or MRI) and PET-CT may be useful for preoperative evaluation. The larynx should be examined in all patients with suspected ATC because vocal fold paralysis is common.
- ATC resectability should be determined by routine preoperative imaging studies. If locoregional disease is present and grossly negative resection margins can be achieved, surgery should be considered: total thyroidectomy with therapeutic central and lateral neck dissection. In patients with systemic disease, resection of the primary tumor for palliation should be considered to avoid current or eventual airway or esophageal obstruction.
- If preoperative staging and primary tumor assessment deem that surgical resection is not possible, neoadjuvant external beam radiotherapy and/or chemotherapy should be considered to permit possible delayed primary surgical resection.
- Definitive postoperative radiation (with or without concurrent chemotherapy) should be offered to patients with good performance status and no metastatic disease if no microscopic or macroscopic residual tumor remains.
- For small intrathyroidal ATC found within a DTC, a total lobectomy or total/near-total thyroidectomy is appropriate. The need for adjuvant systemic therapy in these cases is controversial; close postoperative observation with frequent imaging studies in the first 12 months may be suitable.

PARATHYROID

Embryology and Anatomy

- Inferior parathyroid glands (PIII) derive from third pharyngeal pouches, and superior glands (PIV) derive from dorsal portions of the fourth pharyngeal pouches between weeks 5 and 12 of gestation.
- In approximately 80% of cases, PIV are located on the posterior aspect of the thyroid lobe in a 2-cm area centered located 1 cm above the ITA and RLN intersection (Figure 22-5). The gland is often freely movable on the thyroid surface but may adhere closely to the thyroid capsule; in 15% of cases, they may be located on the posterolateral surface of the superior thyroid pole. Rarely, they may be located above the upper thyroid pole or in retroesophageal or retropharyngeal locations.
- PIII are more variable in location due to their longer embryologic migration. In 50% of cases, they rest on a fat lobule at the level of the inferior thyroid pole on its

anterior, lateral, or posterior aspect. They can also be located in the cervical or mediastinal thymus, high up on the posterior thyroid lobe surface, superior to PIV in the neck (often along the carotid sheath at the level of the carotid bifurcation), adjacent to the aortic arch or pericardium, or can be intrathyroidal (0.5% to 4% of cases).

PRIMARY HYPERPARATHYROIDISM

- Characterized by hypercalcemia with inappropriately elevated PTH levels. Peak incidence 50 to 60 years. Women : men = 3 : 1.
- Hypercalcemia of malignancy is a differential diagnosis. This may be associated with elevated PTH and/or elevated levels of parathyroid hormone-related protein (PTHrP).
- Organ systems affected by elevated PTH include:
  - Skeleton: PTH is catabolic at cortical sites (e.g., distal one-third radius) and anabolic at cancellous sites (e.g., lumbar spine). In PHPT, dual energy radiograph absorptiometry reveals decreased bone density at distal one-third radius with close to age-appropriate bone density in lumbar spine. This is the opposite of typical postmenopausal estrogen-deficiency bone changes. Incidence of fractures of vertebrae and wrist but not hip is increased by PHPT. Parathyroidectomy leads to increases in bone density of vertebrae and femoral neck.
  - Nephrolithiasis is the most common manifestation of symptomatic disease, occurring in 15% to 20% of all PHPT patients with hypercalciuria in 40%. Surgery for PHPT reduces the incidence of recurrent nephrolithiasis.
  - Other: fatigue, depression, anxiety, weakness are possible associations.
- Risk factors for development of PHPT are history of neck irradiation and prolonged lithium usage.
- Pathology: single parathyroid adenoma in 80% to 90% of cases, double adenomas in 2% to 4%. All four glands are involved in 6% to 10% (four-gland parathyroid hyperplasia).
- Preoperative testing should include calcium, albumin, PTH, 25-hydroxyvitamin D, alkaline phosphatase, albumin, phosphate, magnesium, chloride, 24-hour urinary calcium/creatinine, and bone densitometry. In the case of family history of PHPT or Zollinger-Ellison syndrome, consider MEN1 genetic testing. In case of pheochromocytoma/MTC in the patient or family member, consider RET gene testing.
  - Urinary calcium : creatinine clearance ratio is important to rule out benign familial hypercalciuric hypercalcemia. In familial hypercalciuric hypercalcemia, total 24-hour urine calcium is <100 mg, and calcium/creatinine clearance ratio is low.
  - Serum chloride : phosphate ratio >33 may support a diagnosis of PHPT.
  - Measurement of ionized calcium is important if normocalcemic PHPT is a possible diagnosis. Normocalcemic PHPT diagnosis requires 25-hydroxyvitamin D within normal physiologic range (>30 ng/mL) and secondary causes of hyperparathyroidism to be ruled out.
- Surgical intervention is advised for patients with any overt manifestation of PHPT or, for asymptomatic patients with serum calcium >1.0 mg/dL above reference limit, creatinine clearance <60 cc/min, markedly reduced bone density at any site (T score <2.5 or fragility fracture), and age <50 years.

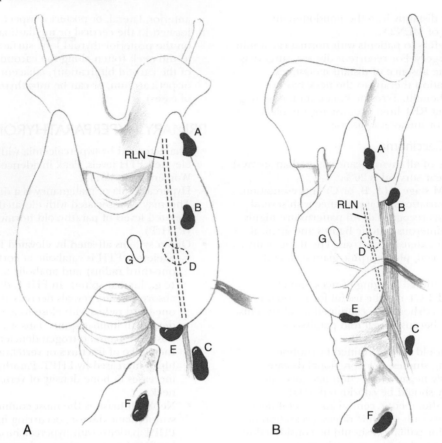

FIGURE 22-5 A, Anteroposterior view of the cervical region showing the relationship of the parathyroid glands to the recurrent laryngeal nerve. *A*, *B*, and *C* glands are superior glands; *E* and *F* glands are inferior glands. *D* glands are those closest to the recurrent laryngeal nerve (RLN) and cannot be easily deciphered as superior or inferior without intraoperative assessment of the pedicle in relation to the RLN. The *G* gland is intrathyroidal. **B,** Lateral view. (From Randolph GW, ed. *Surgery of the Thyroid and Parathyroid Glands.* 2nd ed. Philadelphia: Elsevier Saunders; 2013.)

- Preoperative localization can include:
  - Ultrasound: adenomas appear hypoechoic to thyroid follicular nodules (occasionally mixed hyperechoic and hypoechoic), oval, and occasionally cystic.
  - CT may be useful for lesions that are nonlocalizing on ultrasound and sestamibi and for glands in ectopic locations (e.g., anterior mediastinum/ tracheoesophageal groove). Four-dimensional CT uses the timing of contrast perfusion to identify the adenoma and gives both anatomic and physiologic information about the abnormal gland (parathyroid glands have rapid uptake and early contrast washout compared with thyroid).
  - MRI may be useful for ectopic glands or reoperative surgery. Adenoma will enhance with increased T2 signal intensity and isointense T1 signal.
  - Nuclear medicine studies:
    - No radiotracer is specific for the parathyroid glands. Double tracer subtraction imaging improves specificity by administering two tracers (one thyroid specific [I-123] and one that accumulates in both parathyroid and thyroid tissues [technetium pertechnetate]) and using a computer to subtract the thyroid-only image from the combined image. This technique is subject to motion artifact and thus can be used only with planar images.
    - Sestamibi accumulates in mitochondria. Parathyroid adenomas often have a high concentration of oxyphilic cells that contain a high mitochondrial content → increased sestamibi uptake compared with normal thyroid tissue (lower mitochondrial content), and thus sestamibi washes out of thyroid faster than from parathyroid. Images are taken at 10 minutes, then at 2 to 3 hours (dual-phase imaging). Sestamibi subtraction imaging is more sensitive than dual-phase imaging (89% versus 70%); however, dual-phase imaging is not affected by motion artifact. Sestamibi is sensitive for large single adenomas but less sensitive for hyperplasia (sensitivity 45%), double adenomas (30%), and small single adenomas.
    - SPECT reconstructs planar, two-dimensional images taken from multiple angles with gamma cameras to produce three-dimensional tomographic images. It is used with dual-phase imaging techniques. SPECT increases the sensitivity of dual-phase planar imaging; however, it is still less sensitive than subtraction images. SPECT images can be fused with CT images to provide better anatomical localization.
    - Combining ultrasound and sestamibi imaging provides complementary functional (sestamibi) and structural (ultrasound) assessment.
- Medical management: 50% of patients with PHPT do not meet surgical guidelines. If < 50 years of age, progression of disease may occur with overt clinical disease. Thus, close follow-up of such patients is advisable with annual blood tests and bone densitometry. Bisphosphonates can reduce urine and serum calcium levels and, when used in PHPT, increase bone density in lumbar spine and hips. For PHPT in postmenopausal women, estrogen replacement therapy can reduce total serum calcium by 0.5 to 1.0 mg/dL without any effect on PTH. Calcimimetic

medications (e.g., cinacalcet) reduce serum calcium concentrations to normal in PHPT, useful in intractable PHPT and inoperable parathyroid carcinoma.

- Surgical management: optional procedures for parathyroid surgery include bilateral four-gland exploration and minimally invasive parathyroidectomy (MIP). MIP uses preoperative sestamibi and/or ultrasound to localize the hyperfunctioning parathyroid gland, thus enabling targeted gland removal.
  - Intraoperative PTH (iPTH) provides an additional functional criterion for uniglandular versus multiglandular disease and can be used to verify that the correct gland has been excised in presumed uniglandular disease approached via MIP. A baseline PTH level should be sent prior to skin incision and a second baseline level taken just before the adenoma's vascular supply is ligated and the adenoma resected. PTH half-life is 3 to 7 minutes, and if the postexcision level at 10 to 15 minutes reduces by >50% from baseline values and into the normal range, the operation can be considered successful. If the intraoperative PTH drop at 10 minutes is not significant, the neck can be reexplored. If the 10-minute fall is significant but does not fully meet the >50% criteria, a 20-minute postexcision assay can be performed prior to proceeding with neck exploration. Jugular venous sampling for intraoperative PTH assay may be useful in patients with negative preoperative localization studies to lateralize the side of the neck harboring the most hypersecreting parathyroid gland. Operative failure is defined by hypercalcemia associated with elevated PTH levels occurring within 6 months of the operation. Recurrent hyperparathyroidism has hypercalcemia and elevated PTH levels >6 months after a period of eucalcemia.
  - For multiglandular disease, conservative resection of only grossly enlarged glands results in high cure rates; aggressive subtotal resections in these patients can lead to permanent hypoparathyroidism.

SECONDARY AND TERTIARY HYPERPARATHYROIDISM

- SHPT results from an abnormality in calcium homeostasis leading to a compensatory increase in parathyroid hormone secretion. It is commonly seen with progressive chronic kidney disease and long-term lithium therapy.
  - Pathogenetic factors leading to SHPT in chronic kidney disease include hypocalcemia, hyperphosphatemia, and active vitamin D deficiency.

- Histopathologic findings include asymmetrical glandular enlargement, nodularity, and increased oxyphilic cell concentrations.
- Rates of parathyroidectomy in SHPT are influenced by available medical therapies such as vitamin D receptor activators and calcimimetics; most patients can be managed with medical treatment alone.
- Surgery should be considered for persistent high serum intact PTH >500 pg/mL with hypercalcemia or hyperphosphatemia that is refractory to medical therapy. Surgery is also indicated for patients with severe osteitis fibrosa, progressive ectopic calcification, calciphylaxis, or disabling subjective symptoms (e.g., bone pain, arthralgia, depression, pruritus).
- Surgical methods can include total parathyroidectomy with autograft into the brachioradialis muscle, total parathyroidectomy without autograft, or subtotal parathyroidectomy, depending on the clinical scenario.
- Tertiary hyperparathyroidism (THPT) refers to clinically persistent SHPT after successful renal transplantation.
  - Parathyroidectomy is the most successful treatment for resolving advanced HPT cases in THPT. Indications include persistent hypercalcemia >6 months after renal transplant, low bone mineral density, nephrolithiasis, deterioration of kidney graft due to THPT, symptomatic HPT, or enlarged parathyroid gland detected on ultrasound.
  - Subtotal and total parathyroidectomy with autograft are accepted surgical treatment options.

PARATHYROID CARCINOMA

- Parathyroid carcinoma comprises <0.5% of cases of PHPT.
- The etiology is unknown. Metastases occur late (lung > lymph nodes > liver). There is no gender predominance. The average age of presentation is 49 years. Patients generally present with end-organ disease. There are no accepted staging criteria.
- Surgery is the only effective treatment option. Regional nodal metastases are uncommon. Distant metastases occur in 10% to 20% of patients during long-term follow-up. Frozen section is not useful for intraoperative diagnosis. Immunohistochemical testing is utilized to confirm the diagnosis.
- In inoperable disease, hypercalcemia is controlled with bisphosphonates and calcimimetic agents. Radiotherapy may be of use. Chemotherapy is not effective. Most common causes of death are complications related to intractable hypercalcemia.

ANSWERS

TRUE OR FALSE QUESTIONS

1. F	14. F	27. T	40. T
2. F	15. T	28. F	41. T
3. F	16. T	29. T	42. F
4. T	17. F	30. T	43. F
5. F	18. F	31. F	44. T
6. T	19. T	32. F	45. T
7. F	20. T	33. F	46. T
8. T	21. F	34. T	47. F
9. T	22. T	35. T	48. T
10. F	23. F	36. T	49. F
11. T	24. T	37. T	50. T
12. F	25. T	38. F	
13. T	26. F	39. F	

SINGLE BEST ANSWER QUESTIONS

51. d	64. e	77. a	90. a
52. d	65. d	78. b	91. a
53. b	66. a	79. c	92. e
54. c	67. d	80. d	93. e
55. a	68. c	81. b	94. b
56. c	69. a	82. d	95. a
57. e	70. b	83. e	96. c
58. a	71. e	84. c	97. b
59. d	72. d	85. b	98. d
60. b	73. d	86. e	99. e
61. c	74. b	87. b	100. c
62. e	75. c	88. d	
63. a	76. c	89. c	

SUGGESTED READINGS

1. Haugen B, Alexander E, Bible K, et al. American Thyroid Association management guidelines for patients with thyroid nodules and differentiated thyroid cancer. The American Thyroid Association (ATA) guidelines taskforce on thyroid nodules and differentiated thyroid cancer. *Thyroid.* 2015; DOI: 10.1089/thy.2015.0020.

2. Chandrasekhar SS, Randolph GW, Seidman MD, et al. Clinical practice guideline: improving voice outcomes after thyroid surgery. *Otolaryngol Head Neck Surg.* 2013;148 (suppl 6):S1-S37.

3. Randolph GW, Dralle H, Abdullah H, et al. Electrophysiologic recurrent laryngeal nerve monitoring during thyroid and parathyroid surgery: international standards guideline statement. *Laryngoscope.* 2011;121(suppl 1): S1-S16.

4. Thyroid Carcinoma. National Comprehensive Cancer Network Clinical Practice Guidelines in Oncology. Version 2, 2014. <http://www.nccn.org/professionals/physician _gls/pdf/thyroid.pdf>.

5. Shindo ML, Kandil E, McCaffrey JC, et al. Management of invasive well-differentiated thyroid cancer: an American Head and Neck Society consensus statement. AHNS consensus statement. *Head Neck.* 2014;36(10):1379-1390.

6. Carty SE, Cooper DS, Doherty GM, et al. Consensus statement on the terminology and classification of central neck dissection for thyroid cancer. *Thyroid.* 2009;19(11): 1153-1158.

7. Yeh MW, Bauer AJ, Bernet VA, et al. American Thyroid Association statement on preoperative imaging for thyroid cancer surgery. *Thyroid.* 2015;25(1):3-14.

8. Randolph GW, ed. *Surgery of the Thyroid and Parathyroid Glands.* 2nd ed. Philadelphia: Elsevier Saunders; 2013.

9. Attie JN, Khafif RA. Preservation of parathyroid glands during total thyroidectomy. *Am J Surg.* 1975;130(4): 399-404.

10. Halsted WS. The operative story of goiter. *Johns Hopkins Hosp Rep.* 1920;19:152-153.

11. Perros P, Colley S, Boelaert K, et al. British Thyroid Association. Guidelines for the management of thyroid cancer. *Clin Endocrinol.* 81(s1):1-122.

Anesthesia for Otolaryngology | 23

Howard Meng | Gerard Curley

TRUE OR FALSE QUESTIONS

PHARMACOLOGY OF ANESTHETIC AGENTS

T/F 1. Ketamine as an induction and analgesic agent can cause increased oral secretions.

T/F 2. Muscle relaxants will significantly reduce the firmness of laryngeal tissue that has undergone radiation.

T/F 3. Drugs that have higher lipid solubility (e.g., benzodiazepines, barbiturates) are dosed based on total body weight, whereas hydrophilic drugs, which have a tendency to remain in the intravascular space, are dosed based on ideal body weight.

T/F 4. Opioids may indirectly cause raised intracranial pressure.

T/F 5. Histamine release after morphine administration is an idiosyncratic rather than a dose-dependent reaction, which can lead to a decrease in blood pressure or bronchospasm.

T/F 6. Remifentanil has a context-sensitive half-time of 3 to 4 min, which increases with increasing infusion duration.

T/F 7. Protective airway reflexes are not as depressed with propofol as with thiopental, so patients are more likely to "buck" or cough during airway instrumentation in the absence of a muscle relaxant.

T/F 8. The use of meperidine (pethidine) in patients taking monoamine oxidase inhibitors may lead to the development of the potentially lethal serotonin syndrome.

T/F 9. Ketamine maintains upper airway tone and airway protective reflexes.

T/F 10. Ketamine decreases pulmonary vascular resistance and is the agent of choice in patients with pulmonary hypertension.

T/F 11. Application of local anesthetic appears to decrease postoperative pain in tonsillectomy and myringotomy tube placement.

T/F 12. Local anesthetic overdose with cocaine can lead to arteriolar dilation and hypotension.

T/F 13. The maximum recommended dose of epinephrine with local anesthetic agents or used alone in adult otolaryngologic surgeries is 200 mcg.

PHYSIOLOGY AND BASIC MONITORING

T/F 14. The nostrils account for as much as 50% of all airway resistance during quiet breathing.

T/F 15. Patients with obesity and an increased neck circumference are at increased risk for upper airway collapse during and after general anesthesia.

T/F 16. The tendency for airway collapse is mitigated by chemoreceptors activated by both hypercapnia and hypoxemia that preferentially stimulate the airway dilator muscles over the diaphragm, resulting in an increase in negative inspiratory pressure.

T/F 17. The larynx is innervated by the superior laryngeal and recurrent laryngeal nerves.

ANESTHETIC EQUIPMENT AND OXYGEN DELIVERY SYSTEMS

T/F 18. Jet ventilation pressure for adults should be 20 lb/in² or less.

T/F 19. General anesthesia can be maintained by jet ventilation alone, without supplementation via IV anesthetics.

T/F 20. Barotrauma associated with jet ventilation can result in subcutaneous emphysema, pneumothorax, and pneumomediastinum.

T/F 21. Suboptimal frequency of jet pulses in ventilation correlates with mucosal edema, congestion, and epithelia cell flattening, all of which contribute to necrotizing tracheobronchitis.

T/F 22. Polyvinyl chloride endotracheal tubes (ETTs) are flammable and can ignite and vaporize, producing hydrochloric acid, when in contact with a laser beam.

T/F 23. In airway surgery, jet ventilation is an accepted and feasible method even in those with severe small airway disease.

PREOPERATIVE ASSESSMENT AND POSTOPERATIVE CARE

T/F 24. Adults experience less postoperative pain from tonsillectomy than children.

T/F 25. Preoperative apnea-hypopnea index is a reliable indicator of difficult intubation in uvulopalatopharyngoplasty patients.

T/F 26. IV acetaminophen is as effective as intramuscular meperidine in the treatment of posttonsillectomy pain.

T/F 27. The addition of 0.5 to 1 mcg/kg of dexmedetomidine infused during tonsillectomy/adenoidectomy may help to attenuate emergence delirium in toddlers at the conclusion of the anesthetic.

T/F 28. There is a difference in the incidence of airway complications on emergence between patients who are extubated awake and those who are deeply anesthetized.

T/F 29. Patient pain profiles after adenoidectomy and tonsillectomy are very similar.

T/F 30. Infiltration of peritonsillar space with local anesthetic and epinephrine has been shown to be effective in reducing intraoperative blood loss, but not in decreasing postoperative pain.

T/F 31. Induction and maintenance of middle ear surgery with propofol has been shown to decrease risk of postoperative nausea and vomiting (PONV).

T/F 32. Postoperative emesis and oral intake on postoperative day 1 are improved post tonsillectomy with the use of a single intraoperative dose of steroids.

T/F 33. Postoperative pain is improved by a single intraoperative dose of steroids.

T/F 34. The positive predictive value of coagulation testing is high for identifying patients undergoing tonsillectomy who will have intraoperative or postoperative bleeding.

T/F 35. Patients receiving total intravenous anesthesia (TIVA, propofol and remifentanil) for middle ear surgeries have better pain profiles than anesthesia provided by volatile anesthetics and fentanyl.

T/F 36. Among atropine, scopolamine, and glycopyrrolate, the anticholinergic drug with the least effect on heart rate is scopolamine.

INTRAOPERATIVE CARE DURING EAR, NOSE, AND THROAT (OTOLARYNGOLOGY) SURGERY

T/F 37. In Zenker diverticulum surgery, a rapid sequence induction is usually performed, and cricoid pressure is applied only when the neck of the diverticulum is below the cricoid cartilage.

T/F 38. Inhalation induction can be prolonged secondary to foreign obstruction of the airway. Nitrous oxide should be avoided to prevent air trapping distal to the obstruction.

T/F 39. Volatile-based anesthesia involving isoflurane and fentanyl provides better surgical visualization and less blood loss than total IV anesthesia at equal reduction in blood pressure.

T/F 40. Ludwig angina often causes dental abscesses that extend into the submandibular, submental, and sublingual areas. Involvement of the submandibular spaces results in the greatest risk of compromising the airway.

T/F 41. The ETT cuff should be pressurized to at least 25 mmHg to prevent seepage of blood and tissue into the airway when operating in the oropharynx.

T/F 42. When controlled hypotension is desired, administration of vasodilation drugs is associated with better operating conditions than beta-adrenergic blockade.

T/F 43. Manipulation of the carotid sheath can cause asystole.

T/F 44. Phenylephrine can be used safely in flap reconstruction to facilitate perfusion of the flap.

T/F 45. Manipulation of the right-sided carotid sheath and stellate ganglion during neck dissection is associated with greater hemodynamic instability than in the left side.

T/F 46. Heliox administration is superior to oxygen in stridorous patients because it has lower density and viscosity compared with oxygen.

T/F 47. In patients requiring ETT placement with history of neck radiation therapy, the gold standard method of intubation is video laryngoscopy.

T/F 48. The types of ETTs used for fiberoptic intubation are limited compared with ETTs used for GlideScope (video laryngoscopy) intubation.

T/F 49. When providing opioid-based muscle relaxation, at least 50% of muscle response should be preserved, as determined by a twitch monitor.

T/F 50. Bilateral radical neck dissection for head and neck cancer may result in postoperative hypertension and loss of hypoxic drive.

SINGLE BEST ANSWER QUESTIONS

51. All of the following are determinants of eye injury with laser use *EXCEPT:*
    a. Pupil size
    b. Degree of pupil pigmentation
    c. Wavelength of laser
    d. Diameter of eye

52. In middle ear surgery, especially tympanoplasties, which anesthetic gas should be avoided to decrease the risk of graft disruption?
    a. Sevoflurane
    b. Nitrous oxide
    c. Isoflurane
    d. Desflurane

53. Which of the following statements is correct regarding LeFort fractures and nasotracheal intubation?
    a. Nasotracheal intubation is contraindicated in LeFort I fractures.
    b. Nasotracheal intubation is contraindicated in LeFort II fractures.
    c. Nasotracheal intubation is contraindicated in LeFort III fractures.
    d. Nasotracheal intubation is not contraindicated in any of the types of LeFort fractures.

54. Patients with obstructive sleep apnea will have worsened apneic episodes peaking postoperatively during what time?
    a. Within the first 4 hours
    b. Within the first 24 hours
    c. Within the first 48 hours
    d. Within the first 72 hours

55. In instances such as vocal cord surgery where profound muscle relaxation is required for a relatively brief procedure, which of the following drugs will best facilitate this?
    a. Fentanyl
    b. Remifentanil
    c. Pancuronium
    d. Rocuronium

56. Which of the following is *NOT* a common complication of high-frequency jet ventilation?
    a. Hypertension
    b. Bronchospasm
    c. Hypercarbia
    d. Pneumothorax

57. Cuffed ETTs are sometimes used in children for tonsillectomy and adenoidectomy to prevent blood from leaking into the trachea. Which of the following complications does high cuff pressure often predispose the patient to?
    a. Postextubation croup
    b. Tracheomalacia
    c. Laryngospasm
    d. Mucosal bleeding

58. All of the following are advantages of laryngeal mask airway over endotracheal intubation for tonsillectomy and adenoidectomy *EXCEPT*:
    a. Decrease in incidence of postoperative stridor
    b. Decrease in postoperative laryngospasm
    c. Increase in immediate postoperative oxygen saturation
    d. Decreased surgical site bleeding

59. Laryngospasm can sometimes occur on awakening due to light levels of anesthesia. Which of the following statements is *INCORRECT*?
    a. An ETT puts a healthy patient at greater risk of laryngospasm than a laryngeal mask airway.
    b. Active asthma puts the patient at 10 times increased risk for laryngospasm than a normal patient.
    c. Of the ENT surgeries, adenotonsillectomy carries the greatest risk for laryngospasm.
    d. Risk of laryngospasm inversely correlates with age.

60. Which of the following is a benefit of using a video laryngoscope over fiberoptic scope for intubation?
    a. Faster time to ETT placement
    b. Can provide confirmation of ETT placement
    c. Allows for use in patients with limited mouth opening
    d. Can be accomplished with the patient awake and asleep

61. For airway laser surgery, which of the following combination of gases is/are most appropriate?
    i. Air and 21% oxygen
    ii. 30% Oxygen and nitrous oxide
    iii. 30% Oxygen and helium
    iv. 50% Oxygen and sevoflurane
    v. 50% Oxygen and nitrous oxide
    a. i
    b. ii
    c. iii
    d. iv
    e. v
    f. i and ii
    g. i and iii

62. Topical cocaine for vasoconstriction should not exceed what dose?
    a. 1 mg/kg
    b. 3 mg/kg
    c. 4 mg/kg
    d. 6 mg/kg
    e. 10 mg/kg

63. The use of oxymetazoline as a topical vasoconstrictor should be avoided with concurrent use of which class of medication?

a. Calcium channel blockers
b. Beta-blockers
c. Monoamine oxidase inhibitors
d. Thyroid hormone replacements

64. Posttonsillectomy hemorrhage usually occurs within which period of time?
    a. 4 hours
    b. 6 hours
    c. 12 hours
    d. 24 hours
    e. 48 hours

65. Which of the following drugs should *NOT* be used intraoperatively when a nerve integrity monitor is to be used?
    a. Succinylcholine
    b. Rocuronium
    c. Propofol
    d. Remifentanil

66. Which of the following ETT tube materials is most likely to be flammable on contact with laser?
    a. Rubber
    b. Stainless steel
    c. Polyvinyl chloride
    d. Silicone

67. Which of the following steps is *NOT* consistent with the American Society of Anesthesiologists guidelines for managing airway fires?
    a. Remove the ETT.
    b. Stop flow of anesthetic gas.
    c. Maintain FiO_2 of at least 30%.
    d. Remove all flammable and burning materials from the airway.
    e. Pour saline or water into patient's airway.

68. Which of the following anesthetic gases is known to increase the risk of PONV?
    a. Sevoflurane
    b. Desflurane
    c. Isoflurane
    d. Nitrous oxide
    e. Halothane

69. Which of the following is *NOT* a disadvantage of jet ventilation?
    a. Need for total IV anesthesia
    b. Increased risk of barotrauma
    c. Inability to accurately measure $ETCO_2$
    d. Inability to easily measure tidal volume
    e. Inability to accurately assess for level of oxygenation

70. Following tracheostomy for facial trauma, an increase in peak inspiratory pressure does *NOT* indicate which of the following?
    a. Malpositioned ETT
    b. Bronchospasm
    c. Debris or secretions in the trachea
    d. Pneumothorax
    e. Edematous upper airway

71. Bilateral neck dissection can result in which of the following combinations postoperatively?
    a. Hypertension and loss of hypoxic drive
    b. Hypertension and loss of hypercapnic drive
    c. Hypotension and loss of hypoxic drive
    d. Hypotension and loss of hypercapnic drive
    e. Hypotension with no change in respiration

72. Controlled hypotension is generally advocated in many ENT surgeries and can be accomplished with slight head-up tilt. Which of the following complications requires the closest intraoperative monitoring?
    a. Decreased cerebral perfusion
    b. Formation of venous air embolism
    c. Increased lung atelectasis
    d. Increased dependent edema
    e. Compression of cervical nerves

73. In a patient with head-up tilt to improve controlled hypotension, at which level should the arterial pressure monitoring transducer be fixed?
    a. Level of the heart
    b. Level of the brain
    c. Level of the surgical field
    d. Level of the arterial cannulation

74. A patient post functional endoscopic sinus surgery becomes hypotensive secondary to bleeding and requires reintubation. Which of the following drugs is/are most appropriate for induction?
    i. Etomidate
    ii. Ketamine
    iii. Propofol
    iv. Sevoflurane gas induction
    a. i
    b. ii
    c. i and ii
    d. ii and iii
    e. iv
    f. iii and iv

75. Which of the following is the best predictor of a difficult intubation in morbid obesity?
    a. Mallampati score
    b. Neck circumference
    c. Limited neck movement
    d. Thyromental distance
    e. Body weight

76. Which of the following statements regarding infection control is *INCORRECT*?
    a. Devices to be used in the upper airway that may cause bleeding must remain sterile until used.
    b. Provided there is an adequate filter between the patient and the breathing circuit, the circuit can be reused for subsequent patients on an operating list.
    c. When performing central neural blockade, the anesthetist must adopt a full aseptic technique.
    d. When performing central venous cannulation, the anesthetist must adopt a full aseptic technique.
    e. When performing vascular cannulation, the anesthetist must wash hands and should wear gloves.

77. Increased alveolar-arterial oxygen gradient can be caused by which of the following?
    a. Endotracheal intubation
    b. Decreased cardiac output
    c. Second gas effect
    d. Atelectasis

78. Lignocaine spray to the vocal cords reduces laryngospasm by:
    a. Blocking parasympathetic afferent receptors
    b. Paralyzing the smooth muscle
    c. Blocking the sympathetic response
    d. Blocking the parasympathetic and sympathetic responses

79. Which of the following statements is correct regarding the management of a 65-year-old man who requires neck dissection for a tumor previously treated with large doses of bleomycin?
    a. A chest radiograph is essential to exclude pulmonary fibrosis.
    b. Oxygen therapy should be given by face mask soon after narcotic premedication.
    c. Impairment of renal function is common.
    d. Surgery should be delayed for 48 hours after lymphangiography.

80. Application of cricoid pressure with a force of 40 newtons will resist reflux with an intraesophageal pressure of:
    a. 30 mm Hg
    b. 40 mm Hg
    c. 50 mm Hg
    d. 60 mm Hg
    e. 70 mm Hg

81. Which of the following statements is correct regarding personnel working in an operating room environment?
    a. Levels of volatile anesthetic agents of less than 5 parts per million are considered safe.
    b. Chronic exposure to trace levels of anesthetic agents causes significant cognitive impairment.
    c. The risk of abnormal pregnancy is higher than that of smokers.
    d. The risk of cancer is increased in males.
    e. None of the above

82. All of the following are predictors of difficult intubation *EXCEPT*:
    a. Interincisor distance <3 cm
    b. Prominent C1 spinous process
    c. Prominent maxillary canines
    d. Mallampati classification Class IV
    e. Thyromental distance <6 cm

83. A 60-year-old man with a 45 pack year history of smoking and heavy drinking presents with stridor. He has had a hoarse voice for about 4 months. He has been waking at night for a week with difficulty breathing, relieved by sitting up. He is sitting upright in bed with moderate inspiratory stridor. His SaO_2 on air is 95%. Which of the following should be the next step in his management?
    a. Awake fiberoptic intubation
    b. Computed tomography scan of the neck
    c. Examination under anesthesia following gaseous induction
    d. Nasendoscopy under topical anesthesia
    e. Tracheostomy under local anesthetic

84. In performing an awake fiberoptic intubation it is most important that care is taken to avoid which of the following?
    a. Causing any bleeding that will obstruct view
    b. Oversedation, because this leads to posterior pharyngeal wall collapse
    c. Trauma to nasal turbinates
    d. Contact with vocal cords, because this will induce coughing
    e. Oral route, because the patient may bite the fiberoptic scope

85. What is the most distant anatomy seen on Cormack-Lehane grade III laryngoscopy?
    a. Soft palate
    b. Hard palate
    c. Epiglottis

d. Arytenoid cartilage
e. Subglottis

86. In apneic oxygenation sometimes used for rigid bronchoscopy, how much does $PaCO_2$ increase in the first minute?
    a. 6 mm Hg
    b. 4 mm Hg
    c. 2 mm Hg
    d. There is no measurable increase in $PaCO_2$.

87. Which of the following lasers require(s) use of clear protective eyewear?
    i. Potassium titanyl phosphate (KTP)
    ii. Argon
    iii. CO_2
    iv. Neodynium:yitrium aluminium garnet (Nd:YAG)
    a. i
    b. ii
    c. iii
    d. iv
    e. i and ii
    f. i and iii
    g. iii and iv

88. All of the following are effective for reducing probability of emesis in patients following tonsillectomy *EXCEPT*:
    a. Decompressing stomach with orogastric tube
    b. Treatment with ondansetron
    c. Use of total IV anesthesia
    d. Administration of meperidine postoperatively

89. Advancing the ETT over the fiberoptic bronchoscope sometimes fails due to ETT impingement on which of the following anatomical structures?
    a. Vocal cords
    b. Arytenoid cartilages
    c. Epiglottis
    d. Tongue

90. General anesthesia with muscle relaxant use and microlaryngeal tube is the most common practice for panendoscopy. Which of the following is *NOT* an advantage to using this method?
    a. It provides a secure airway.
    b. It allows capnographic measurements.
    c. Airway pressures are reduced.
    d. There is no pollution of the operating room by anesthetic gases.

91. Jet ventilation entrains a mixture of oxygen and room air into the airway. The entrainment process occurs according to which of the following properties of physics?
    a. Poiseuille's law
    b. Boyle's law
    c. Venturi effect
    d. Charles's law
    e. Gay-Lussac's law

92. Which of the following nerve(s) can be regionally blocked to reduce intraoperative irritation during endoscopic procedures?
    i. Glossopharyngeal nerve
    ii. Superior laryngeal nerve
    iii. Supraclavicular nerve
    iv. Recurrent laryngeal nerve
    a. i
    b. ii
    c. iii
    d. iv
    e. i and ii
    f. i and iv

93. Which of the following is mostly commonly injected into the ETT cuff in order to identify a cuff leak from laser use?
    a. Lidocaine
    b. Methylene blue
    c. Propofol
    d. Diluted epinephrine 1:100,000
    e. Sodium bicarbonate

94. On full mouth opening, the soft palate and the base of the uvula are visible. To which modified Mallampati class does the view correspond?
    a. Class I
    b. Class II
    c. Class III
    d. Class IV

95. Which of the following is *NOT* a risk factor for PONV?
    a. Young age
    b. Smoker
    c. Female sex
    d. Intraoperative use of opioids

96. In patients diagnosed with malignant hyperthermia intraoperatively, which of the following medications is best used for treatment?
    a. Dantrolene
    b. Nifedipine
    c. Verapamil
    d. Propranolol
    e. Rocuronium

97. In patients with cardiac instability secondary to local anesthetic toxicity, which of the following is the *LEAST* appropriate action?
    a. Administer IV intralipid.
    b. Prepare resuscitation cart for possible cardiac arrest.
    c. Give reduced dose of epinephrine.
    d. Stop local anesthetic infusion or further administration of local anesthetics.
    e. Administer vasopressin.

98. In performing local anesthesia, which of the following maximum doses of local anesthetics is *NOT* correct?
    a. Lidocaine 5 mg/kg
    b. Lidocaine with epinephrine 7 mg/kg
    c. Bupivacaine 3 mg/kg
    d. Prilocaine 2 mg/kg

99. In a patient taking paroxetine, administration of which of the following antiemetics could precipitate serotonin syndrome?
    i. Dimenhydrinate
    ii. Ondansetron
    iii. Metoclopramide
    iv. Droperidol
    a. i
    b. ii and iii
    c. ii and iv
    d. ii, iii, and iv
    e. All of the above

100. In a patient with QTc of 520 ms, which of the following medications is most appropriate for intraoperative use to prevent PONV?
    a. Dexamethasone
    b. Dimenhydrinate
    c. Ondansetron
    d. Metoclopramide
    e. Droperidol

CORE KNOWLEDGE

PREOPERATIVE ASSESSMENT FOR OTOLARYNGOLOGY

- A focused medical history is the cornerstone of preoperative evaluation and should establish the patient's general state of health; present illness; exercise tolerance; current medications; drug allergies; surgical and anesthetic history; history of tobacco, alcohol, or other drug use; and a physical examination, including an airway assessment.
- Perioperative cardiac complications are among the most common and concerning potential risks of surgery and anesthesia. The standard of care for preoperative cardiac evaluation is established by the 2014 update of the American College of Cardiology/American Heart Association guidelines on Perioperative Evaluation and Management of Patients Undergoing Noncardiac Surgery. The guidelines take into consideration three variables: the patient's history, exercise capacity, and relative risk of the planned surgery.
- For moderate and high-risk surgeries, the patient's functional capacity should be assessed, and if adequate (i.e., ability to perform four metabolic equivalents or greater, equivalent to climbing two flights of stairs without symptoms), no further workup or treatment should be necessary.
- If functional capacity is limited or cannot be assessed, and if two or more clinical risk factors are present (Lee Index, or Revised Cardiac Risk Index), further testing should be considered, with either a stress echocardiogram or nuclear stress test, potentially followed by cardiac catheterization if a significant abnormality is found.
- Patients who are already taking beta-blockers should continue them perioperatively to avoid rebound hypertension and tachycardia that will lead to increased myocardial oxygen demand and potentially myocardial ischemia, myocardial infarction, or sudden cardiac death. It is reasonable to initiate beta blockade in patients with three or more nonoperative Revised Cardiac Risk Index factors for typical otolaryngologic surgery with a target heart rate less than 60 beats per minute, but caution should be exerted to avoid hypotension secondary to overzealous beta-blocker administration.
- Although there is no consensus to withdraw angiotensin-converting enzyme inhibitors and angiotensin receptor blockers routinely in the perioperative period, several authors recommend that they should not be taken on the day of surgery if a prolonged high blood loss procedure is planned (e.g., extensive cancer case with microvascular free flap), and they should be avoided the night before surgery too.
- Effective perioperative interventions to reduce risk for obstructive sleep apnea patients include (1) meticulous preoxygenation given that these patients may be more difficult to ventilate and intubate; (2) judicious use of intraoperative and postoperative opioids and other sedatives; (3) extubation only when the patient is wide awake, easily follows commands, and appears to have airway reflexes completely intact; (4) close monitoring of oxygen saturation in the postanesthesia care unit; (5) postoperative admission to a step-down unit where oxygen saturation can be monitored; (6) continuation of preoperative continuous positive airway pressure or bilevel positive airway pressure use; and (7) admitting most patients for overnight observation.
- Perioperative management of patients who require temporary discontinuation of anticoagulants must weigh the risk of a thrombotic event during interruption of the medication against the risk of bleeding related to the procedure. The American College of Chest Physicians has published consensus guidelines, most recently updated in 2012, for the perioperative management of patients receiving antithrombotic therapy. According to these guidelines, all high-risk patients (atrial fibrillation, mechanical heart valve, or thromboembolic disease) should receive bridging anticoagulation therapy with subcutaneous therapeutic-dose low-molecular-weight heparin or IV unfractionated heparin.
- Patients on antiplatelet therapy because of coronary stents have a high risk of stent thrombosis in the perioperative period if therapy is interrupted. Following placement of a bare metal stent, nonurgent procedures should be delayed for at least 4 to 6 weeks; following placement of a drug-eluting stent, nonurgent procedures should be delayed for at least 1 year. For patients with a recent drug-eluting stent placement in whom surgery cannot be delayed, aspirin and clopidogrel treatment should be continued without interruption if the stent was placed within the previous 6 months. If stenting occurred greater than 6 months prior, consideration can be given to continuing aspirin without interruption, continuing clopidogrel until 5 days before surgery, and resuming therapy as soon as possible after surgery.
- Many patients presenting with cancers of the head and neck have prolonged tobacco and alcohol use as risk factors. Overall, the available evidence overwhelmingly supports that cessation of smoking in the perioperative period is advantageous, and though the optimal preoperative duration of abstinence is not clear, it appears that the greater the duration, the better, with at least 2 weeks or, preferably, 4 weeks for best results.
- Malignancies in the head and neck area may have been previously treated with radiation. Radiation-induced scarring of the head and neck area can present with significant fibrosis, leading to reduced mobility of tissues and joints. Obliteration of the lymph nodes can lead to significant postoperative edema. In otolaryngology patients particular attention is paid to any upper airway deformities that may make mask ventilation and/or intubation with direct laryngoscopy difficult. These include oropharyngeal masses, neck masses, thyromegaly, and postradiation changes in soft tissue of the head and neck. Often the otolaryngologist has performed indirect laryngoscopy during the preoperative assessment, and discussion of the findings can aid in planning for airway management.
- Voice changes or abnormal breath sounds, such as stridor, need to be evaluated thoroughly for the location and degree of obstruction. The surgical and anesthesia teams may review preoperative imaging (Figure 23-1) together to best identify ways of securing the airway.
- Preoperative testing should be directed by the history and physical examination, and the need for any tests should be considered in light of the planned surgery, including expected hemodynamic instability and blood loss. In general, tests should be ordered only if the results have the potential to change management. Many centers use age as a criterion for routine electrocardiography testing. There is no routine indication for preoperative chest radiograph, but a chest radiograph should be obtained to assess abnormalities that are present in the patient's history or on physical examination.

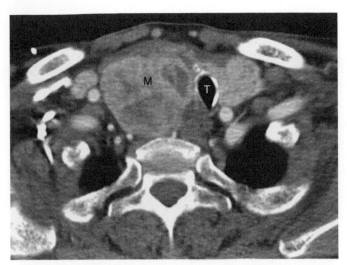

FIGURE 23-1 Axial computed tomography images demonstrating marked enlargement of the right thyroid lobe (*M*), with leftward deviation and mild narrowing of the trachea (*T*).

DIFFICULT AIRWAY

- Otolaryngologists will routinely care for patients with complex upper airway anatomy and pathology, including acute infection, angioedema, trauma, malignancy, and prior surgery and radiation therapy of the head and neck. These cases demand meticulous preoperative history and physical examination targeted to determine those patients at risk for difficult intubation, difficult ventilation, and risk of aspiration. Communication between the otolaryngologist and anesthesiologist to devise and safely employ effective airway management strategies is paramount.

- Particular factors pertinent to airway management include a history of head and neck malignancy, surgery, or trauma; requiring prolonged time on a ventilator; history of tracheostomy; reported "difficult" intubations during previous surgeries; problems with cervical spine mobility or mouth opening; the presence of loose or missing teeth; and a history of personal or familial congenital or genetic syndromes.

- A targeted physical examination should be performed with a focus on physical attributes associated with difficult intubation and mask ventilation, including overall body habitus; neck proportion and extensibility; oral excursion and the presence of potential oral cavity and/or oropharyngeal obstruction; any prominent, loose, or missing dentition; thyromental distance; and jaw projection.

- Several classification schemes have been devised to assist in grading the degree of airway "difficulty," including the widely used Mallampati score. Other predictors commonly used include small mouth opening (<3 cm), short thyromental distance (<6 cm), inability to protrude the mandible, limited neck movement, and large neck circumference (>40 cm). It should be noted that no grading system or physical attribute is 100% predictive of a difficult intubation, and they are best applied together and in proper clinical context. The presence of a beard, obesity, lack of teeth, and a history of snoring are strong indicators of difficult bag mask ventilation.

- Endotracheal intubation is most commonly performed by conventional laryngoscopy with either the Macintosh-style or Miller-style blades. The Macintosh-style blade is curved and designed for insertion into the vallecula anterior to the epiglottis in order to retract upward, thereby revealing the larynx. In contrast, the straight Miller-style blade is placed posterior to the epiglottis to compress the tongue base and supraglottis anteriorly. This is particularly useful in patients with excessive soft tissue in this region or a floppy, elongated epiglottis, as commonly found in pediatric patients.

- Oral and nasal airways are adjunctive devices commonly used in airway management. Inserted blindly following the induction of general anesthesia, these devices can mechanically augment airflow and thereby facilitate mask ventilation or spontaneous breathing. A major advent in modern anesthesiology has been the incorporation of the supraglottic airway, most commonly the laryngeal mask airway for routine care. Although the supraglottic airway creates a reliable and effective airway, it does not protect against aspiration and may prove unreliable in patients with decreased lung or chest wall compliance (e.g., asthma, chronic obstructive pulmonary disease, obesity).

- The most common device used by anesthesiologists to intubate the patient with a difficult airway is a flexible bronchoscope. This instrument has the advantage of being able to be advanced and manipulated in a 360-degree manner, thus facilitating use in both transnasal and transoral routes, depending on clinical and anatomical characteristics. Video laryngoscopy is the most recent technology used for airway management, and a variety of devices offer improved success in difficult and routine intubations.

- There are an array of bougies, stilettes, and introducers that can be used with traditional or video laryngoscopy for difficult or emergent intubations. They may be placed when there is limited laryngeal visualization and depend on tactile feedback to confirm proper placement within the trachea.

- In cooperative patients who are likely to be difficult to mask ventilate after the induction of general anesthesia, it is advisable to proceed with an "awake" method of securing the airway. There are many methods to prepare the patient for an awake intubation, but in general, they include a combination of airway local anesthesia topicalization, often using nebulized lidocaine, local anesthetic nerve blocks, and judicial doses of IV sedatives and analgesics, while assuring the patient remains awake, responsive, and spontaneously breathing. Common local blocks include bilateral superior laryngeal nerve blocks along with the transtracheal administration of local anesthesia that targets the recurrent laryngeal nerve. This is often combined with a flexible fiberoptic technique, especially for cases involving known and significant upper airway obstruction.

- Management of the difficult airway does not end with placement of an ETT; the anesthesiologist and otolaryngologist must share in the decision-making process and strategy for the management of tracheal extubation. In general, the lack of a cuff leak may suggest a higher likelihood of postextubation stridor or the need for reintubation or tracheotomy, although this remains controversial. When airway edema or other pathology is suspected, there are several techniques for evaluating the anatomy prior to tracheal extubation, including use of the fiberoptic bronchoscope or video laryngoscope (Figures 23-2 and 23-3). Use of an airway exchange catheter to maintain access to the airway has been described and offers some advantages.

- In cases when noninvasive strategies fail or the patient is clinically unstable, invasive means of ventilation and airway access are required. These include transtracheal needle ventilation, in which a large bore (14-gauge)

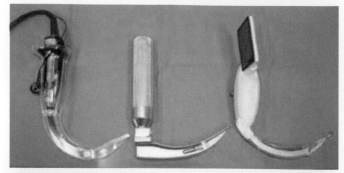

FIGURE 23-2 Example of GlideScope with its angulated blade to 60 degrees.

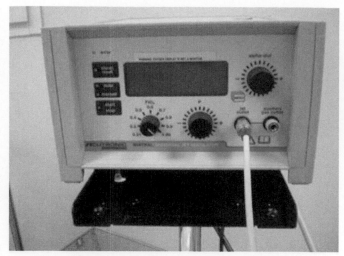

FIGURE 23-4 Example of automatic jet ventilator.

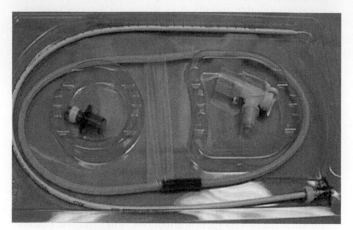

FIGURE 23-3 Example of video laryngoscope.

angiocatheter is inserted directly into the tracheal lumen. There are a number of commercially available cricothyrotomy kits that are inserted based on the Seldinger technique. Although the point of entry is midline and may be performed through the anterior tracheal wall, the cricothyroid membrane is preferred in emergent situations due to the presence of the complete ring of cricoid cartilage, which can prevent unintended puncture through the posterior tracheal wall and resultant esophageal injury or mediastinal insufflation.

SHARED AIRWAY DURING LARYNGOLOGY AND PHONOSURGERY

- Microlaryngeal surgery means that both the otolaryngologist and anesthesiologist must share the airway. While the anesthesiologist must be secure in providing adequate oxygenation, ventilation, analgesia, amnesia, and a relaxed environment free from motion, the otolaryngologist must work in a constricted space where millimeters of extra room can mean the difference between surgical success and failure.
- For the most part, these procedures will require general anesthesia with good access to the airway and aerodigestive structures provided by a small ETT and adequate muscle relaxation or a plane of anesthesia deep enough to allow for good surgical access. As most of these procedures are of short duration, judicious use of paralytics and short-acting anesthetic agents are of great value. For very short procedures the use of neuromuscular blockade is often omitted and larger doses of remifentanil and propofol are employed to achieve excellent laryngoscopic conditions.
- Small-diameter tracheal tubes are required to allow for optimal surgical visualization and manipulation. Internal

diameter tracheal tubes of 5.5 mm generally satisfy this requirement and allow for adequate gas exchange. Controversy exists over the use of such small tracheal tubes in large adults. Adequate minute ventilation delivered through small tracheal tubes is accompanied by high readings on inspiratory pressure monitors. This is generally of little clinical importance because the small tube acts as a resistor across which there is a substantial pressure drop. Actual intratracheal pressures approximate those seen with larger tracheal tubes. Consequently, the risk of barotrauma is no greater using small tubes than large ones despite high measured peak inspiratory pressures on the anesthesia machine. Nevertheless, increasing time spent in inspiration (i.e., adjusting the I:E ratio from 1:2 to 1:1) will decrease pressures required to achieve adequate tidal volumes.

- Ventilatory modes for modern laryngology practice are divided into two categories: closed systems and open systems. Closed systems, which are familiar to all anesthesiologists, protect best against aspiration, allow for positive pressure ventilation, and minimize operating room pollution from anesthetic gases. Closed systems do, however, limit surgical visibility, interfere with surgical manipulations, risk tracheal tube–related laryngeal damage, and predispose to fire during laser applications. Open systems maximize laryngeal visualization, reduce risk of tracheal tube trauma, and provide the best laser safety. Open techniques of ventilation can include spontaneous ventilation, apneic oxygenation, and jet ventilation. Open systems fail to protect lower airways against aspiration. The selection of the use of an open system is also determined by the lesion's location, size, mobility, and vascularity.
- Jet ventilation usually involves administration of 100% oxygen under approximately 20 lbs/in² (psi) pressure, via a catheter or blunt needle. Anesthesia maintained with remifentanil 0.05 to 0.5 mcg/kg/min and propofol 50 to 150 mcg/kg/min is used widely. Supraglottic (proximal) jet ventilation entails attaching the jetting needle to a suspension laryngoscope. Potential problems associated with supraglottic jet ventilation include malalignment of jet stream; gastric insufflation; possible blowing of blood, smoke, and infectious debris into the airway; vocal cord movement; and barotrauma. Subglottic jet ventilation involves placing a 2 to 3 mm diameter jetting catheter into the trachea. Oxygen is delivered directly to the trachea. Advantages of subglottic jet ventilation include vocal cord immobility and ample time to establish rigid (suspension)

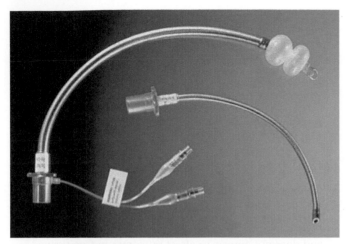

FIGURE 23-5 Example of laser endotracheal tube.

laryngoscopy. Disadvantages of subglottic jet ventilation include slight obstruction to surgical field and barotrauma.

- High-frequency jet ventilators (Figure 23-4) are set to deliver approximately 110 breaths/minute for this purpose. High-frequency jet ventilation provides for continuous gas flow out of the airway, which tends to carry away small amounts of blood and debris as well as reducing peak and mean airway pressures, which could minimize ventilator-related hypotension. Ventilator rate, percentage inspiratory time, and driving pressure affect $PaCO_2$. Continuous positive airway pressure and FIO_2 contribute to oxygenation.
- Although oxygenation during jet ventilation is adequately measured by pulse oximetry, ventilation cannot be quantitatively assessed by noninvasive means. $PaCO_2$ evaluation requires arterial blood gas analysis. If jet ventilation is to be used for extensive periods of time, then arterial catheters are indicated.
- It is best to maintain high-frequency jet ventilation catheters as far from the carina as possible to prevent jets from stimulating the carina. Immediate consequences of carinal stimulation can be hypertension, tachycardia, and/or bronchospasm. Long-term consequences include postoperative coughing and/or bleeding.
- Laser airway surgery is associated with a 0.5 to 1.5% incidence of fire. Laser fires can occur with the CO_2 laser and the Nd:YAG lasers. These fires typically start at the tracheal tube, tracheal tube cuff, or cottonoids in the airway. Fires can result from direct impact, reflected light, heated dry cloth, or hot dry tissues. If the ETT is pierced by the laser or flame, two important problems can arise. First, polyvinyl chloride is degraded into toxic constituents. Second, inspired gases with high oxygen concentrations are easily ignited. Flames are directed down the airway into trachea and lungs. Puncture of the tracheal tube cuff can allow inspired gases to surround laser fields and predispose to fire in the newly created local, oxygen-enriched atmosphere.
- Laser-resistant tracheal tubes (Figure 23-5) reduce the chances of converting the tracheal tube into a hospitable environment for a fire. Many laser tubes are equipped with two inflatable cuffs (inflated with water/saline). If the upper cuff is punctured by the laser and deflated, the lower cuff should continue to seal the trachea, allowing for positive pressure ventilation and preventing inspired gases from reaching the laser field.
- The lowest FIO_2 (<0.3) that provides adequate oxygenation is employed as the inspiratory gas mixture for all surgeries

involving lasers. Nitrous oxide is not used. Helium has been used to dilute oxygen. Helium does not support combustion, flows through small tracheal tubes better than other gases, and minimally delays ignition if the tracheal tube is punctured.
- On making the diagnosis of airway fire, the burning element (usually the tracheal tube or cottonoid) should be removed once the oxygen source is eliminated. The most recent 2013 American Society of Anesthesiologists guidelines suggest removal of the ETT, cessation of flow of all airway gases, and removal of all flammable and burning materials from the airway. Saline or water should be poured into the patient's airway. Consider rigid bronchoscopy after extinguishing fire for assessment of airway damage or if concerned about residual debris. Oxygenation can be resumed by face mask and the patient should be reintubated as soon as possible.
- Laser surgery exposes everyone in the operating room to burns from errant beams, and this includes the patient. The body part most susceptible to injury is the eye. Determinants of eye injury include pupil size, degree of pigmentation, size of retinal image, pulse duration, pulse repetition rate, and wavelength. CO_2 laser causes limited tissue penetration, capable of damaging only the cornea. Nd:YAG laser has deeper penetration and may cause retinal injury and scarring. The patient's eyes should be covered with wet gauze to prevent damage.

OTOLOGIC SURGERY

- The use of nitrous oxide has previously been contraindicated in middle ear surgery due to its potential to diffuse from blood into middle ear space, increasing compartmental pressure and dislodging grafts. Middle ear pressure rises with nitrous oxide administration, and because it is reabsorbed negative pressure may develop in the middle ear cavity. Tympanic membrane rupture, nausea, vomiting, or serous otitis may result from use of nitrous oxide. Nitrous oxide is not the only anesthetic agent that can have an effect on middle ear pressure; desflurane and sevoflurane may increase middle ear pressure.
- For mild hypotension, the combination of anesthetic gas and remifentanil infusion can help to optimize surgical field view and reduce blood loss. Slight head-up position is also helpful.
- Even where the facial nerve electromyography monitor is not being used, it is vastly preferable in ear surgery that the patient not be paralyzed, so that even unanticipated facial nerve issues can be recognized promptly.
- For controlled emergence, remifentanil infusions are generally used throughout the case and patients are extubated while on a low infusion. Application of lidocaine through the ETT with the cuff deflated in a deeply anesthetized patient can achieve similar results.

NASAL AND SINUS SURGERY

- An important objective for the anesthesiologist is to minimize nasal mucosal bleeding during nasal and sinus surgery; this can be achieved through a variety of anesthetic management options. The reduction of bleeding will facilitate surgical visualization and reduce the formation of nasal and subcutaneous septal hematomas. In general, the anesthetic goal should be to achieve a reduction in cardiac output while preserving systemic vascular resistance. Reducing the blood pressure via vasodilation with isoflurane, sevoflurane, desflurane, sodium nitroprusside, nitroglycerine, or hydralazine does not improve surgical conditions and may in fact create a worsened state. This is in comparison with the reduction of blood pressure by cardiac output depression with beta-blockade therapy or with the use of high-dose remifentanil and its resulting bradycardia from a sympathectomy and high parasympathetic tone.

- Nasal surgery can be accomplished via inhalational anesthesia or TIVA. TIVA has been shown to reduce blood loss and improve visualization of the surgical field. TIVA also has the added benefit of reducing coughing on emergence and decreasing the risk of PONV.
- Patients with significant cardiopulmonary disease may not tolerate a reduction in cardiac output. These patients should be identified early, and the risks and benefits of the proposed anesthetic and procedure should be discussed in the presence of the patient, anesthesiologist, and surgeon.

THYROID, PARATHYROID, AND PAROTID SURGERY

- Patients presenting for thyroid surgery may have large goiters. These can lead to tracheal deviation, tracheal compression, and stridor. Radiologic assessments (ultrasound, computed tomography) are useful in determining the extent of airway disturbance by the mass of the goiter and determining the need for an awake fiberoptic intubation. In long-standing goiter, extubation following surgery can be complicated by tracheomalacia and airway obstruction.
- Before surgery is to be performed, a euthyroid state should be achieved. It is therefore incumbent on the anesthesiologist to review thyroid function tests in the preoperative period.
- Prior to thyroid, parathyroid, and parotid surgery, it must be clearly established whether monitoring of the recurrent laryngeal nerve and/or the facial nerve is required. If nerve monitoring is to be carried out, paralysis should be avoided.
- Bilateral superficial cervical plexus blockade has been shown to significantly reduce postthyroidectomy pain as compared with placebo.
- Airway compromise after thyroid and parathyroid surgery can result from a variety of causes, including airway invasion, vocal cord paralysis, and tracheomalacia. In addition, postoperative bleeding can occur suddenly and without warning and can lead to a dramatic and life-threatening loss of airway from direct tracheal compression from the hematoma along with venous and

lymphatic compression, resulting in impressive airway edema. Due to the proximity of the recurrent laryngeal nerve during dissection, vocal cord paralysis is also a potential complication.

- Hypocalcemia can occur in the immediate postoperative period after thyroid and parathyroid surgery. Signs and symptoms of hypocalcemia include muscle spasm, tetany, bronchospasm, and laryngospasm. Treatment is airway control as necessary and calcium chloride administration (1 g IV over 10 to 15 minutes).

HEAD AND NECK CANCER SURGERY

- Patients with a fixed larynx from radiation therapy are known to be difficult to ventilate and intubate and have a high GlideScope failure rate.
- Intermittent intraoperative vasopressor use is acceptable and does not appear to affect outcomes in free tissue transfer procedures. The timing of administration should not coincide with microvascular anastomosis, if possible. Vasopressor infusions should be avoided, if possible. Large volume resuscitations are generally unnecessary and should be avoided; they can lead to increased edema and complications. There is no current evidence to support the routine use of volume expanders in major head and neck surgery. Moderate hemodilution with transfusion to maintain hematocrit of 25 to 30 is generally preferred.

POSTOPERATIVE PAIN MANAGEMENT

- Preemptive analgesia with acetaminophen, cyclooxygenase-2 selective inhibitors (celecoxib, meloxicam), gabapentinoids, or clonidine 1 to 2 hours prior to surgery can reduce postoperative pain.
- The use of local anesthetic, via application of swabs in the tonsillar bed post excision, provides a reduction in posttonsillectomy pain.
- Dexamethasone IV prior to incision and ketorolac and acetaminophen perioperatively reduce postoperative pain.
- Inpatients with moderate to severe levels of pain should receive IV patient-controlled analgesia (not nursing-administered boluses).
- Consider intraoperative IV lidocaine infusion, ketamine infusion, and/or methadone for opioid-tolerant patients, those with significant preoperative pain, and extensive surgeries. Consider postoperative low-dose ketamine in patients with poorly controlled pain (especially patients with chronic pain on opioid therapy).

ANSWERS

TRUE OR FALSE QUESTIONS

1. T	14. T	27. T	40. F
2. F	15. T	28. F	41. F
3. T	16. F	29. F	42. F
4. T	17. T	30. T	43. T
5. F	18. T	31. T	44. F
6. F	19. F	32. T	45. T
7. F	20. T	33. F	46. F
8. T	21. T	34. F	47. F
9. F	22. T	35. F	48. T
10. F	23. F	36. T	49. F
11. T	24. F	37. T	50. T
12. F	25. T	38. T	
13. T	26. T	39. F	

SINGLE BEST ANSWER QUESTIONS

51. d	64. b	77. d	90. c
52. b	65. b	78. a	91. c
53. c	66. c	79. a	92. e
54. d	67. c	80. b	93. b
55. b	68. d	81. e	94. c
56. d	69. e	82. b	95. b
57. a	70. e	83. d	96. a
58. d	71. a	84. b	97. e
59. a	72. b	85. d	98. d
60. a	73. b	86. a	99. d
61. g	74. c	87. g	100. a
62. b	75. b	88. d	
63. c	76. a	89. b	

SUGGESTED READINGS

1. Apfelbaum J, Hagberg C, Caplan R, et al. Practice guidelines for management of the difficult airway: an updated report by the American Society of Anesthesiologists task force on management of the difficult airway. *Anesthesiology.* 2013;118(2):251-270.

2. English J, Norris A, Bedforth N. Anesthesia for airway surgery. *Contin Educ Anaesth Crit Care Pain.* 2006;6(1): 28-31.

3. Apfelbaum J, Caplan R, Barker S, et al. Practice advisor for the prevention and management of operating room fires: an updated report the american society of anesthesiologists task force on operating room fires. *Anesthesiology.* 2013; 118(2):271-290.

4. Won Y, Yoo J, Chae Y, et al. The incidence of postoperative nausea and vomiting after thyroidectomy using three anaesthetic techniques. *J Int Med Res.* 2011;39(5):1834-1842.

5. Evans E, Biro P, Bedforth N. Jet ventilation. *Contin Educ Anaesth Crit Care Pain.* 2007;7(1):2-5.

6. Chaaban M, Baroody F, Gottlieb O, et al. Blood loss during endoscopic sinus surgery with propofol or sevoflurane: a randomized clinical trial. *JAMA Otolaryngol Head Neck Surg.* 2013;139(5):510-514.

7. Sommer M, Geurts J, Stessel B, et al. Prevalence and predictors of postoperative pain after ear, nose, and throat surgery. *Arch Otolaryngol Head Neck Surg.* 2009;135(2): 124-130.

8. Doyle DJ. Anesthesia for ear, nose, and throat surgery. In: Miller R, ed. *Miller's Anesthesia.* 8th ed. Philadelphia: Elsevier Saunders; 2014:2523-2549.

9. Jefferson N, Riffat F, McGuinness J, et al. The laryngeal mask airway and otorhinolaryngology head and neck surgery. *Laryngoscope.* 2011;121(8):1620-1626.

10. Kellman R, Losquadro W. Comprehensive airway management of patients with maxillofacial trauma. *Craniomaxillofac Trauma Reconstr.* 2008;1(1):39-47.

24 | Maxillofacial Trauma

Robert M. Kellman | Matthew D. Johnson

TRUE OR FALSE QUESTIONS

T/F 1. Repair techniques have progressed from wiring across fractures to rigid fixation with plates and screws.

T/F 2. The advancement of imaging has hindered the progression of the treatment of facial fractures, confusing the determination of fractures as studies progressed from plain radiograph to computed tomography (CT) and onward to high resolution and 3D reconstructions and intraoperative imaging.

T/F 3. The paired frontal sinuses, housed within the frontal bones centrally, are present in approximately 85% of the population.

T/F 4. The following nerves traverse the frontal bone: branches of the olfactory nerves, supratrochlear nerves, and supraorbital nerves.

T/F 5. The malar eminence and zygomatic arch are key components of facial projection and contour.

T/F 6. Enophthalmos can result from minor changes in zygomatic position as a result of malposition of the lateral rim of the orbit.

T/F 7. Restoration of primary occlusion is dependent primarily on proper repair of mandibular fractures; correct repositioning of the maxilla following trauma is less important.

T/F 8. The nasal bones are the most frequently fractured bones of the human body.

T/F 9. The orbital shape has inferolateral concavity and medial convexity.

T/F 10. A blowout fracture implies that the orbital rims have been fractured, altering the orbital volume.

T/F 11. The maxillofacial skeleton has specific areas that serve as crumple zones, preventing injury to some vital structures; energy is dissipated prior to reaching the brain, but the eyes are often at risk.

T/F 12. The mandible is a U-shaped bone with two hinge points; in significant trauma, it is designed to absorb impact forces rather than transmit these to the middle fossa and cranial floor.

T/F 13. With loss of dentition, mandibular bone atrophies in a uniform pattern, evenly throughout the mandible.

T/F 14. There is no indication for early intervention in orbital injury; progressive vision loss and increasing intraorbital pressure should be evaluated by an ophthalmologist.

T/F 15. Quality of facial examination diminishes with time from injury due to swelling, hematoma, tubes, packing, and cervical collar or other treatment devices.

T/F 16. Soft tissue swelling can obscure examination of the zygoma and nasal bones, making assessment of malposition difficult.

T/F 17. The horizontal palpebral width should be the same on each side and is roughly equal to the intercanthal distance.

T/F 18. Mixed Le Fort fractures, such as II and III, are more difficult to treat than a Le Fort III fracture combined with a zygomaticomaxillary complex fracture.

T/F 19. With CT imaging, the plane of section relates to best visualization of fractures as follows: vertical structures are better seen on coronal scans, and horizontal structures are better seen on axial scans.

T/F 20. Fracture through the pterygoid plates is highly suggestive of the presence of a Le Fort type fracture.

T/F 21. Type I and type II medial canthal tendon injuries can be repaired by securing fragments containing the ligament into position, whereas type III injuries require resuspension.

T/F 22. Most maxillofacial injuries are considered contaminated; therefore, antibiotic treatment is initiated at the time of presentation and continued for a minimum of 24 hours after surgery.

T/F 23. In consideration of the management of facial fractures, it is best to take a piecemeal approach.

T/F 24. Wide elevation is considered to have an impact on soft tissue redraping following facial fracture repair; therefore, it is important to consider suspension of the soft tissues during closure.

T/F 25. Approaches and incision choices should be based on access needed to properly repair the injury, the ability to camouflage scars, and the surgeon's experience.

T/F 26. After completion of a repair through lower lid incisions, a Frost stitch can be placed in the lower lid and taped to the forehead to prevent lid malposition; this is removed when sutures are taken out 1 week later.

T/F 27. Primary bone healing occurs after rigid fixation when there is no motion across a fracture line; secondary bone healing occurs following callus formation and bone ingrowth.

T/F 28. Biomechanics of the facial skeleton is designed with the facial form to support its function, with alternating pillars/buttresses and areas of weakness.

T/F 29. The middle third of the face is composed of four vertical buttresses and three horizontal buttresses; these act as load paths of forces of mastication to this region.

T/F 30. Zygomatic fractures are most frequently hinged at the zygomaticomaxillary interface.

T/F 31. The primary determinants of facial projection are the maxilla and nasal bones.

T/F 32. Mandibular compression and tension zones have been found to vary depending on the location of the food bolus placement, changing from inferior to superior.

T/F 33. Mandibulomaxillary fixation (MMF) is used for repair of mandibular fractures; following fracture reduction and rigid fixation, the wires are clipped and the arch bars removed, allowing the patient to function.

T/F 34. In comminuted posterior wall fractures of the frontal sinus, the anterior fossa should be repaired and reconstructed when possible, followed by sinus obliteration.

T/F 35. All skull base defects with cerebrospinal fluid (CSF) leak and rhinorrhea are ideally repaired at the time of facial fracture repair.

T/F 36. The risk of meningitis from CSF leak increases the longer the leak persists.

T/F 37. Le Fort I fracture repair necessitates reestablishing the two medial and two lateral buttresses for stable repair.

T/F 38. Bone deficits in the region of the buttresses requires replacement only if more than one buttress or pillar is deficient.

T/F 39. The amount of fixation of zygomatic fractures is dependent on the amount of instability and can range from percutaneous reduction to multipoint fixation.

T/F 40. In repair of orbital floor fractures, slight overcorrection of enophthalmos and hypoglobus is important to account for intraoperative swelling.

T/F 41. Arch bar placement can be performed with successive wires alternating across the fracture; a tension band will result across the fracture and along the superior surface of the mandible.

T/F 42. Load sharing places the functional forces onto the plates, whereas load bearing places the majority of the forces onto the mandibular bone.

T/F 43. The priority in mandibular fracture treatment is alignment of the fracture fragments.

T/F 44. Symphyseal fractures require load-bearing repairs; therefore, lag screw and miniplating techniques are not appropriate.

T/F 45. Fracture of the mandibular body can be fixed in a load-sharing fashion with a single miniplate, provided the patient does not chew on the side of the fracture during healing.

T/F 46. Mandibular fractures in the line of dentition that are nondisplaced may be treated with 4 to 6 weeks of MMF.

T/F 47. When teeth are in the line of a fracture, they should always be pulled due to risk of infection and subsequent osteomyelitis, followed by nonunion.

T/F 48. Panfacial fracture repair should employ the principles of maxillofacial trauma and proceed beginning with establishing occlusion, from known to unknown and from lateral to central.

T/F 49. Inadequate reconstruction of the orbital floor can result in hypoglobus and proptosis.

T/F 50. When a mandibular fracture has healed as a fibrous union, stabilizing with prolonged MMF may still allow bone to heal across the fracture.

SINGLE BEST ANSWER QUESTIONS

51. Which of the following is used in the treatment of facial fractures?
    a. Stainless steel wires
    b. Stainless steel plates and screws
    c. Titanium plates and screws
    d. Miniplates
    e. All of the above

52. All of the following are biocompatible *EXCEPT*:
    a. Porous polyethylene
    b. Hydroxyapatite cement
    c. Silastic
    d. Titanium plates and wires
    e. Stainless steel plates and wires
    f. All of the above are biocompatible.

53. The face is divided arbitrarily into thirds; each third contains:
    a. Upper third (frontal bones), middle third (maxilla, zygoma, orbits, nose, nasoorbital ethmoids [NOEs]), lower third (mandible)
    b. Upper third (frontal bones, NOEs, orbit), middle third (maxilla, zygomas), lower third (mandible)
    c. Upper third (frontal bones, NOEs), middle third (orbits, zygoma, vertical ramus of mandible), lower third (maxilla, body of mandible)
    d. Upper third (frontal bones, orbit), middle third (NOEs, zygoma, maxilla, vertical ramus mandible), lower third (horizontal body of mandible)

54. The zygoma participates in formation of all of the following structures *EXCEPT*:
    a. Lateral orbital rim
    b. Inferior orbital rim
    c. Maxillary sinus
    d. Origin of masseter muscle

55. Maxilla-related structures include which of the following?
    i. Nasal process
    ii. Nasolacrimal duct
    iii. Pyriform rim
    iv. Lacrimal crest
    v. Infraorbital nerve
    a. i, iii, and v
    b. i and iii
    c. i, ii, iii, and v
    d. All of the above

56. Which of the following is/are the most significant risk factor(s) for development of infection after midface fractures?
    a. Any fracture through the maxillary sinus
    b. Preexisting obstruction of the sinus outflow tract

    c. Concomitant fracture of the nasal bones
    d. Impingement of the infraorbital nerve

57. The medial canthal ligament:
    a. Has two components (superior and inferior) and attaches to the lacrimal crest
    b. Has two components (superior and inferior) and attaches to the lamina papyracea
    c. Has three components (anterior, posterior, and superior) and attaches to the lacrimal crest
    d. Has three components (anterior, posterior, and superior) and attaches to the lamina papyracea

58. Pressure injury at the orbital apex results in superior orbital fissure syndrome, affecting which of the following?
    a. CN III, IV, V2, VI
    b. CN II, III, X
    c. CN III, IV, VI
    d. CN II, III, V3

59. Which of the following statements is/are correct regarding the nose and central face?
    a. They provide airway, sense of smell, and contribute to overall cosmesis.
    b. They provide structure for the nasoethmoid complex (NEC).
    c. The surrounding thin bone allows for telescoping posteriorly with fracture.
    d. All of the above

60. From most frequent to the least, what is the order regarding the frequency of mandibular fractures by location?
    i. Condyle and subcondylar fractures
    ii. Ramus fractures
    iii. Angle fractures
    iv. Body fractures
    v. Symphysis and parasymphysis
    a. ii, v, iii, iv, i
    b. i, ii, iii, iv, v
    c. i, v, iii, iv, ii
    d. i, iii, iv, v, ii

61. Occlusion can be assessed by Angle classification; which of the following is the correct description of class I occlusion?
    a. Mesiobuccal cusp of the maxillary first molar is anterior to the buccal groove of the first mandibular molar.
    b. Mesiobuccal cusp of the maxillary first molar is posterior to the buccal groove of the mandibular first molar.
    c. Mesiobuccal cusp of the maxillary first molar is sitting in the mesiobuccal groove of the first mandibular molar.
    d. Mesiobuccal cusp of the maxillary molar falls lingual to the mandibular molar mesiobuccal groove.

62. Which of the following is the first step in assessing a patient with facial trauma?
    a. Observe for gross deformations.
    b. Evaluate airway, breathing, and circulation.
    c. Review the CT scan.
    d. Secure the cervical spine.

63. In a patient with orbital trauma, papillary examination shows decreased ipsilateral and contralateral response to stimulus of the right pupil and normal ipsilateral and contralateral response to stimulus on the left. There does not appear to be gaze restriction. Which of the following would be the next best step in management?
    a. Emergency surgical decompression
    b. Ophthalmologic consultation
    c. Neurosurgical consultation
    d. Magnetic resonance imaging (MRI) of the orbits

64. Increased intraocular pressure of 4 mmHg or more most likely suggests which of the following?
    a. Entrapment
    b. Impingement by bone fragments
    c. Orbital hematoma
    d. Normal orbital status

65. Enophthalmos can be recognized by which of the following?
    a. Posterior globe position
    b. Deepening of the upper lid crease
    c. Hertel exophthalmometer
    d. Any of the above

66. Intranasal examination shows swelling of the septum bilaterally; this is suggestive of which of the following?
    a. Septal abscess
    b. Septal hematoma
    c. Subluxed septal cartilages
    d. Soft tissue swelling

67. Injury of the NEC resulting in canthal avulsion or displacement of the bony fragment most often results in the tendon moving to which of the following positions?
    a. Inferior and posterior
    b. Lateral, inferior, and posterior
    c. Lateral, inferior, and anterior
    d. Lateral and anterior

68. Presence of mandibular fracture is suggested on examination by which of the following findings?
    a. Mental nerve paresthesia, drooling, and oral drainage
    b. Sensitive areas, mucosal tears, chin deviation, and anterior open bite
    c. Mandibular swelling, Angle class I occlusion, and mild tenderness
    d. Lip asymmetry and tongue protrusion

69. High-resolution CT is not helpful in determining the significance of which of the following features regarding frontal sinus fractures?
    a. Anterior table depression
    b. Posterior table fracture and displacement
    c. Displaced posterior table and soft tissue density in the sinus
    d. Outflow tract patency

70. CT imaging of the orbit allows which of the following?
    a. Anticipation of enophthalmos
    b. Estimation of extent of repair needed
    c. Assessment of the status of the orbital apex
    d. All of the above

71. Which of the following is the most important initial step in the management of facial trauma?
    a. Physical examination
    b. Evaluation of airway, breathing, and circulation
    c. Surveying for source and control of hemorrhage
    d. CT imaging to delineate details of fractures

72. The timing of fracture repair should be delayed according to which of the following?
    a. Presence of soft tissue swelling
    b. Surgeon preference
    c. Presence of neurologic instability
    d. Until after 48 hours of antibiotics

73. In the coronal approach, which of the following is the most important structure to avoid?
    a. Supraorbital nerve
    b. Supratrochlear nerve
    c. Pericranium
    d. Temporal (frontalis) nerve

74. Which of the following is the best initial choice regarding an isolated zygomatic arch fracture?
    a. Transoral reduction
    b. Gillies incision with reduction
    c. Coronal incision with reduction and plating
    d. Preauricular incision with reduction and plating

75. Extraoral incision is associated with all of the following *EXCEPT*:
    a. Risk of visible scar
    b. Risk of facial nerve injury
    c. Limited exposure
    d. Direct visualization

76. Which of the following is the order of events in biologic bone healing?
    i. Hematoma
    ii. Fibroblast migration/differentiation to chondroblasts
    iii. Deposition of callus to stabilization
    iv. Osteoid ingrowth
    v. Vessel ingrowth
    vi. Differentiation into osteoblasts
    a. i, ii, vi, v, iv, iii
    b. iii, i, iv, ii, vi, v
    c. i, v, ii, iii, vi, iv
    d. i, iii, ii, v, vi, iv

77. Wolf's law states which of the following?
    a. Bone can be directed to grow across a fracture using compression.
    b. Bone will remodel according to the forces acting on it.
    c. Bone healing requires stability.
    d. Facial bones cannot heal without intervention.

78. Repair of the displaced anterior wall fracture of the frontal sinus:
    a. Needs to be held in position without resistance to force
    b. Is positioned within a vertical pillar and requires strength in its fixation
    c. Must always be rigidly fixed into position
    d. Should be combined with endoscopic sinus surgery to open the frontal outflow tract

79. The zygoma is exposed to masticatory forces acting on the following regions *EXCEPT*:
    a. Zygomaticomaxillary medial buttress
    b. Zygomaticomaxillary lateral buttress
    c. Lateral orbital rim
    d. Zygomatic arch

80. All of the following are challenges to mandibular fracture repair *EXCEPT*:
    a. Tooth roots
    b. Inferior alveolar nerve
    c. Tension and compression zones
    d. Bony irregularities

81. Which of the following is the most significant determinant of facial height?
    a. Maxillary position
    b. Vertical buttresses
    c. Mandibular ramus
    d. Skull base position

82. When treating frontal sinus fractures, which of the following is/are the main principle(s) involved?
    a. Identification of the least invasive method for treatment
    b. Observation, obliteration, and cranialization
    c. Determination of the need for exploration and obliteration
    d. Cosmesis and maintenance of anterior cranial fossa

83. Of the following frontal sinus fractures, which of the following should warrant frontal sinus obliteration?
    a. Minimally displaced anterior wall, patent outflow tract, and nondisplaced posterior table
    b. Depressed anterior wall, fractured outflow tract, intact posterior wall, and air-fluid levels in frontal sinus
    c. Displaced anterior wall, patent outflow tract, displaced posterior wall, and aerated frontal sinus
    d. Nondisplaced anterior wall, fractured and collapsed outflow tract, displaced posterior wall, and soft tissue density throughout frontal sinus

84. With fractures of the skull base, which of the following locations is most likely to have an associated CSF leak?
    a. Posterior table frontal sinus
    b. Sphenoid sinus
    c. Orbital roof
    d. Lateral cribriform

85. When the palate is fractured, which of the following is of significant concern for proper repair?
    a. Loss of bone fragments
    b. Lingual or buccal version of teeth and rotated segment
    c. Severe laceration with avulsion of mucosa over intact bone
    d. Mobile alveolar segment

86. Le Fort II fractures should be stabilized with 1.5- to 2.0-mm plates with two screws on either side of the fracture in which of the following locations?
    a. Along the infraorbital rim and nasal root
    b. Along the infraorbital rim and pyriform aperture
    c. Along the zygomaticomaxillary region, pyriform aperture, and nasal root
    d. Along the zygomaticomaxillary region and infraorbital rim

87. Maxillary and midface fractures can become impacted in certain injuries where MMF appears in good occlusion. Avoidance of fixation with incomplete reduction is best improved by using which of the following?
    a. Adams suspension wiring
    b. Rowe disimpaction forceps
    c. Halo with external fixation
    d. Multiple approaches

88. A patient presents after being assaulted. He is a 19-year-old male and was struck in the cheek and eye with a bat. CT imaging shows fracture of the anterior and medial maxillary wall, nondisplaced orbital floor fracture, and a depressed and rotated zygoma fracture that is rotated and depressed. To prevent postoperative issues with the orbit, repair should include which of the following?
    a. Endoscopic examination of the orbital floor via the maxillary sinus
    b. Plating along the infraorbital rim
    c. Repair of the orbital floor
    d. Avoidance of lower lid incisions and close postoperative follow-up

89. During transconjunctival or subciliary approach to orbital floor injuries, which of the following is the best method to prevent lower lid malposition postoperatively?
    a. Placement of a Frost stitch
    b. Avoidance of lateral canthotomy
    c. Maintenance of the integrity of the orbital septum
    d. Addition of midface suspension maneuvers

90. A 67-year-old woman was involved in a motor vehicle accident. She was the driver and the airbag did not deploy. She struck her nasal root against the steering wheel, resulting in a comminuted NEC fracture. On examination, she has telecanthus and laxity of the medial canthal ligament, right more than left. Appropriate repair includes which of the following?
    a. Direct resuspension medially and superiorly
    b. Rigid fixation of NEC bone fragments
    c. Percutaneous resuspension of the medial canthal ligaments
    d. Transnasal resuspension medially with slight overcorrection

91. In treating mandibular fractures, when prior attempts have been unsuccessful at achieving proper reduction and rigid fixation, which of the following is the best choice for fallback technique?
    a. External fixation
    b. Lag screw technique
    c. Mandibular reconstruction plate
    d. Compression plating

92. Which of the following is an acceptable repair when fixing fracture of the mandibular angle?
    a. Load-bearing placement of a reconstruction plate
    b. Load-sharing miniplate over the oblique line
    c. Load-sharing repair with two miniplates at the angle
    d. All of the above
    e. None of the above

93. A 52-year-old male with chin deviation to the right, premature contact on the right, and anterior open bite is found to have mandible fracture. His dentition is intact. Which of the following is optimal management?
    a. Physical therapy
    b. MMF

c. Preauricular approach to open reduction and internal fixation (ORIF)
d. Transoral endoscopic-assisted ORIF

94. After a fall, an 86-year-old male is found to have mandibular fractures at the angle and parasymphyseal region. His edentulous mandible is noted to be atrophic. Which of the following is the best strategy for management?
    a. Load-bearing ORIF with bicortical plating
    b. Load-sharing ORIF with monocortical miniplates
    c. Removal of the bone fragment, because it is likely devitalized, and bone graft reconstruction
    d. Positioning of dentures and MMF with screw fixation

95. Which of the following statements is correct when approaching panfacial fractures?
    a. It is helpful to repair each fracture individually.
    b. Repair must proceed from the bottom up superiorly, with occlusion as the foundation.
    c. Beginning with occlusion and then proceeding from stable to unstable allows for systematic repair.
    d. Proceeding from the top down, create a stable central component and stabilize onto this foundation.

96. Which of the following is the most common osseous complication?
    a. Pseudoarthrosis
    b. Malunion
    c. Nonunion
    d. Osteomyelitis

97. Which of the following is the most common orbital complication?
    a. Hypoglobus
    b. Enophthalmos
    c. Ectropion
    d. Entropion

98. Repair of mandible fractures from which of the following areas has the highest rate of complications?
    a. Symphysis
    b. Angle
    c. Body
    d. Ramus

CORE KNOWLEDGE

ANATOMY

- Upper third
  - The frontal bone forms the forehead contour (Figure 24-1).
    - Creates the junction between the cranium and the face
  - Contains paired frontal sinuses (85% of population)
    - Anterior wall and posterior wall
      - Anterior wall fractures can affect facial cosmesis and sinus outflow tract function.
      - Posterior wall fractures, considered true skull fractures, warrant neurosurgical evaluation.
    - Most common deformation from trauma is central forehead depression.

- Supraorbital rims and orbital roofs
  - Fractures impact orbital/ocular functions.
  - Glabella, region centrally between the supraorbital rims
    - Dense bone that protects sinus outflow tracts and cribriform plate, through which olfactory nerves pass
  - Sensory nerves: supraorbital and supratrochlear pass through notches or foramina of the superior orbital rim (Figure 24-2).
- Middle third
  - Maxilla, zygomas, orbits
    - Zygoma, malar eminence determines facial projection and contour.

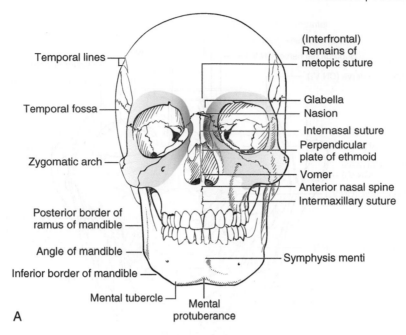

A

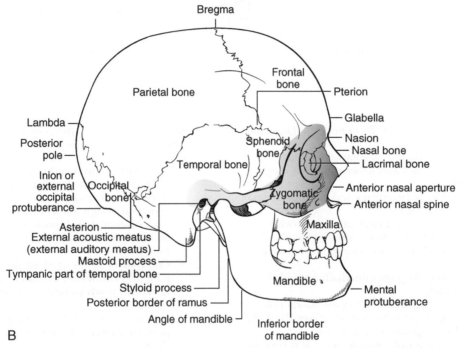

B

FIGURE 24-1 Frontal **(A)** and lateral **(B)** views of craniofacial skeleton.

- Projection posterolaterally as the zygomatic arch abutting the temporal bone; the masseter originates from this region.
- Superior and medial projections of the zygoma contribute to the lateral and inferior orbital rim, respectively, and associated portions of the orbital wall.
- Lateral buttress of midface is the inferomedial extension of the zygoma as it broadly contacts maxilla.
- Lateral orbital rim placement is near the equator of the globe; all other aspects of the orbital rim extend beyond the globe.
  - Fracture and incomplete repair of this region of the zygoma can result in globe malposition and enophthalmos.

- Maxilla
  - Located between zygoma laterally and nasal bones medially
  - Forms portion of inferior orbital rim and pyriform aperture
  - Maxillary dentition is important for mastication.
  - Houses the nasolacrimal duct and maxillary sinus
  - Anterior lacrimal crest is superior and medial projection of maxilla, attachment of medial canthus is located here.
  - Infraorbital nerve: terminal branch of V2, sensation to cheek, lateral nose, upper lip, and maxillary teeth
  - Nasal process interfaces with nasal bones.
    - Nasal bones are the most frequently fractured bones.

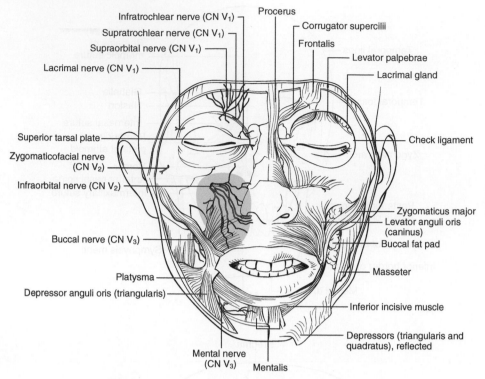

FIGURE 24-2 Frontal view of facial soft tissues, muscles, and nerves.

- Orbits
  - Structural contributions form multiple facial and skull bones.
    - Frontal, zygomatic, maxillary, lacrimal, palatine, greater and lesser sphenoid wing, and ethmoid
    - Lacrimal fossa (maxillary and lacrimal bones) houses lacrimal sac.
    - Maxillary bone and lacrimal crest provide attachment for medial canthal ligament (all three components: anterior, posterior, and superior).
    - Optic canal sits posteromedially behind the medial wall.
    - Optic foramen directed toward lateral rim
    - Orbital apex contains cranial nerves III, IV, V, and VI via superior orbital fissure.
    - Orbit shape is not a simple cone; it is concave inferolaterally and convex medially with significant convexity posteriorly.
    - Thin bones of the orbit protect the globe during injury by transmission of forces to the walls and blowout fractures.
- Central face
  - Trauma to the nasal root
    - Transmission posteriorly creates a telescoping injury.
    - NOE fracture or NEC
  - Nose and NEC (anterior and medial orbits)
    - Includes lacrimal crest and nasal process of maxilla
    - Nasal bones support the upper lateral cartilage and internal nasal valve.
    - Injury may result in nasal airway obstruction, dysosmia, or anosmia; this impacts taste, resulting in dysgeusia.

- Lower third
  - Mandible, including the posterior vertical ramus, temporomandibular joints, contains the mandibular dentition.
    - Mandible is a mobile hinge jointed at the skull base bilaterally; true arthrodial joint is able to slide/translate and swing/rotate.
    - U-shaped design allows for absorption of impact forces rather than transmission to the skull base.
    - Mandible most often fractures in more than one location.
    - Condylar head is seated within temporomandibular joint and connected to mandible by relatively weak neck; this tends to be a site of fracture, subcondylar region
    - Fractures of the vertical ramus are rare due to protective effect of the surrounding muscular sling.
      - Masseter along inferolateral surface
      - Pterygoids attach to the medial surface.
      - Temporalis attaches to the coronoid process.
    - Angle of mandible is located at the posterior aspect of the dentition.
      - Relatively common site for fractures
      - Extension through tooth-bearing mandible into thinner ramus bone
      - Fractures of this region are difficult to stabilize and have the highest rate of complications.
    - The tooth-bearing region has the thickest bone. It is divided into body and symphysis/parasymphysis region.
    - Inferior alveolar nerve, branch of V3, enters mandible at lingual and travels through the bone, supplying tooth roots; it becomes terminal branch as mental nerve exiting mental foramen beneath first bicuspid bilaterally.

- Loss of dentition results in atrophy of the alveolus and loss of bone from a top-down direction.
- Dental anatomy
  - There are 32 adult teeth; numbering begins with right maxillary third molar counting around the arch toward the left, then down to left mandibular third molar around the mandibular arch to the right mandibular third molar.
  - Overbite is vertical overlap of the maxillary incisors.
  - Overjet is the horizontal extension of the maxillary incisors beyond the mandibular incisors.
  - Dental direction
    - Mesial, toward the incisors
    - Distal, toward the posterior mandible or maxilla
    - Buccal, toward the cheek
    - Lingual, toward the tongue
  - Angle classification of occlusion
    - Class I: mesiobuccal cusp of the maxillary first molar sitting within the mesiobuccal groove of the mandibular first molar
    - Class II: maxillary molar is more anterior, chin is generally retruded
    - Class III: maxillary molar is more posterior, chin is relatively prognathic
  - Maxillary arch should be wider than the mandibular arch.
    - Crossbite is present if the maxillary buccal cusps fall lingual to the mandibular buccal cusps.

EVALUATION AND DIAGNOSIS

- Physical examination
  - Must address airway, breathing, circulation and any other potentially life-threatening injuries.
    - Laryngeal or tracheal trauma and airway compromise
    - Airway obstruction secondary to swelling or by blood
      - May require intubation, tracheotomy, fiberoptic assistance, retrograde intubation, temporizing with laryngeal mask airway, cricothyrotomy
      - Consider cervical spine status.
    - Bleeding
      - Nose and sinus bleeding can be managed by packing tamponade.
      - Carotid artery skull base bleeding requires angiography and balloon occlusion above and below.
  - Visual status
    - Progressive loss may indicate intraorbital pressure or optic nerve injury.
    - Early intervention is necessary for a chance to salvage vision.
  - Resultant quality of physical examination depends on time since injury, because swelling, hematoma, tubes, and treatment devices will hinder examination.
  - General facial appearance
    - Observe for presence of penetrating injury, laceration, possible foreign bodies.
    - Laceration should be evaluated by sterile wound examination when reasonable.
  - Facial nerve function
  - CSF otorrhea or rhinorrhea
  - Upper third
    - Evaluate sensation of V_1 branches: supraorbital, supratrochlear.
    - Observe and palpate for depression or step offs of forehead.

- Middle third
  - Orbit
    - As above, vision should be assessed as soon as possible.
    - Consider immediate ophthalmologic and/or neurosurgical evaluation.
    - Papillary response: assess afferent system (optic nerve) and efferent system (CN III oculomotor nerve and/or ciliary ganglion).
    - Forced duction testing, performed by anesthetizing the conjunctiva and using forceps to manipulate the globe in all directions
    - Applanation tonometer detects increase in pressure with directional gaze in the examination for entrapment shows >4 mmHg when looking in a direction
    - Globe position
      - Enophthalmos versus proptosis in anteroposterior plane
      - Hypoglobus versus superior displacement in vertical plane
      - Hertel exophthalmometer measures globe position but is dependent on intact lateral orbital rims.
      - Naugle device measures globe position relative to the external auditory canal.
      - Clinical signs of enophthalmos include posterior position of the globe, deepening of upper lid crease, and elongation of the upper lid.
    - Chemosis and subconjunctival hemorrhage and periorbital ecchymosis
      - Signs of orbital injury
    - Ophthalmologic evaluation should be obtained prior to repair of orbital injuries to clear the eye of severe conditions that may be subtle and pose a contraindication for surgery (e.g., retinal tear).
  - Zygoma
    - Malposition may be visible and palpable.
    - Deformation may be masked by soft tissue swelling.
    - Cutaneous cheek and lateral nasal paresthesia may be only indication of zygoma fracture.
  - Nose
    - Nasal fracture and deformation may be visible and palpable.
    - Also may be masked by swelling
    - Septum must be examined for hematoma and drained to avoid necrosis of cartilage.
    - There may be damage to upper lateral cartilage and loss of nasal valve function.
  - NOE/NEC
    - Careful evaluation of medial canthal relationship
    - Ligament can be attached to mobile bone fragment, partially avulsed on small bone fragment, or even totally avulsed.
    - Tends to displace laterally, anteriorly, and inferiorly
      - Displacement occurs gradually and can be missed acutely.
    - Measure horizontal palpebral widths and intercanthal distance.
      - Intercanthal distance should be approximately equal to each horizontal palpebral width (both of which should be equal).
    - An alternative measure is half the interpupillary distance.

- Examination findings include loss of nasal dorsal height and development of epicanthal folds.
- Direct traction (bowstringing) of the medial canthi tests the integrity of the attachment.
- Maxilla
  - Mobility is generally assessed at the dentition.
  - Alteration from premorbid occlusion suggests fracture of tooth-bearing bone.
  - Examination begins with dentition.
    - Observing for loose teeth
    - Mobility of alveolar segments
    - Mobility of entire midfacial segment suggests fracture.
  - Grasping maxilla and rocking gently back and forth
    - Motion suggests fracture.
    - Lack of motion does not assure intact bones; fracture may be impacted.
    - Anterior open bite is suspicious for fracture, especially if mandible is known to be intact.
  - Observe palate for mucosal tears or other evidence of fracture.
- Lower third
  - Observe mandible for sensitive areas, mucosal tears along gingival, mobile fragments, irregularities along the arch of dentition.
  - Subcondylar
    - Deviation to the ipsilateral side
    - Anterior open bite
    - Foreshortening of ipsilateral vertical ramus
    - Premature contact of molars
    - Bilateral subcondylar may only show anterior open bite and bilateral premature molar contact.
  - Assess sensation of mental nerve and document status.
  - Assess teeth for intrusions, subluxations, and avulsions.
    - Obtain dental consultation when appropriate.
- Radiographic evaluation
  - CT scan
    - Replaced other forms of imaging for craniomaxillofacial injuries
    - Necessary to assess nature and extent of injuries (involving the orbit)
    - Provides understanding of three-dimensionality of zygoma fractures
    - Isolated Le Fort fractures are rare; imaging helps delineate all levels involved.
    - The plane of CT determines how well select fractures are visualized.
      - Axial
        - Most frontal fractures, NOE fractures, zygomatic arch fractures, vertical orbital walls
        - Better for vertical structures
      - Coronal
        - Orbital roofs and floors, pterygoid plates
        - Better for horizontal structures
    - Three-dimensional reconstruction should be made with resolution >1.5 mm to avoid misrepresentations resulting from the computer algorithms.
      - Simple (isolated) nasal fractures likely do not need imaging.
    - If imaging is warranted, plain radiograph is sufficient.
  - Caldwell 6 foot view
    - Remains useful for creation of a template to be used intraoperatively for osteoplastic frontal sinus bone flap

- Upper third
  - Assessment of anterior and posterior walls
  - When posterior wall fracture is present, imaging cannot determine significance of soft tissue density within the sinus.
    - Direct visualization is recommended to assess for CSF leak or herniated brain tissue.
  - Fracture extending to floor of anterior fossa is best evaluated with high-resolution CT scan.
- Middle third
  - Coronal CT is best for orbital blowout fractures.
  - Axial scan to evaluate medial wall extension
  - Parasagittal reconstruction along plane of optic nerve (travels posteromedial to anterolateral) for orbital assessment
  - Imaging allows for assessment of orbital wall displacement and anticipation of volume change and outcome if unrepaired.
  - Visual loss and orbital apex neuropathies necessitate immediate CT imaging to evaluate for reversible injury.
  - Zygomatic arch fractures can be evaluated on plain radiograph with bucket handle views.
    - Normal arch is more flattened anteriorly; it is not a true convex arch.
  - Most zygoma fractures are best analyzed by CT scan related to the three-dimensional alterations in position.
  - Maxillary fractures are often seen on axial scans.
    - Horizontal components on coronal scans
    - Fractures through the pterygoid plates help identify and define presence of Le Fort fractures.
- Lower third
  - Many surgeons prefer panoramic tomography or plain radiographs to evaluate the mandible.
  - With high-resolution helical CT, sensitivity of CT scans has reached 100%; with Panorex it is 86%.
  - Three-dimensional reconstruction can assist with an appreciation of movement of fragments in complex fracture patterns.
  - Postoperative scanning is performed, particularly after endoscopic repair, to verify fracture fixation into reduction.
- Classification schema
  - Upper face
    - Frontal sinus fractures
      - Linear horizontal
      - Linear vertical
      - Comminuted anterior and posterior walls with/without NEC or supraorbital rim fractures
    - The above and multiple other classification systems exist; most have not shown to be clinically useful for planning and treatment approach.
    - Predicting CSF rhinorrhea
      - The more centrally located the skull base fracture, and the more severe the fracture, the greater the likelihood of CSF leakage.
  - Middle third
    - Craniofacial complex fractures (Figures 24-3 and 24-4)
      - Le Fort I: horizontal maxillary fracture, located above the maxillary dentition, separation of the upper jaw, through the posterior maxillary sinus wall, pterygoid plates, pyriform rims, and septum
      - Le Fort II: pyramidal fracture, starts at the zygomaticomaxillary buttress laterally and travels superomedially through the inferior orbital rim and orbital floor, involves medial orbit, crossed midline at the nasal root, traveling inferolaterally

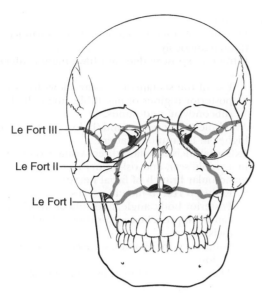

FIGURE 24-3 Le Fort fracture classification.

on the contralateral side; there is also fracture of the nasal septum, posterior maxillary sinus walls, and pterygoid plates
- Le Fort III: complete craniofacial separation, fracture at level of skull base, through zygomas, temporal and frontal bones, crosses lateral and medial orbits, traverses midline at nasofrontal junction; it also fractures through the septum, posterior maxillary sinus walls, and pterygoid plates
- Has been useful in communicating fracture patterns, often described by worst Le Fort present with specific details of fracture features
- NOE/NEC fractures
  - Type I: large central fragment containing the medial canthal ligament
    - Repaired by rigidly fixing the central fragment
  - Type II: there is significant comminution but the fragment containing the medial canthal ligament is still repairable.
    - Transnasal fixation of the fragment of tendon is necessary.
  - Type III: tendon is either detached or attached to an unusable fragment.
    - Tendon must be freed and directly repaired with transnasal fixation.
- Lower third
  - Mandibular fractures are classified by anatomic region and severity (Figure 24-5).
    - Severity: simple, comminuted, avulsive (bone loss)
    - Mandible features: dentulous, edentulous, atrophic edentulous
    - Anatomic region: subcondylar, condylar, angle, ramus, body, symphysis, parasymphysis
    - The designations "favorable" and "unfavorable" are no longer considered helpful.

MANAGEMENT

- Antibiotic therapy is initiated at the time of presentation, because most maxillofacial injuries are considered contaminated by communication with the nose, sinuses, and/or oral cavity.
  - Penicillins, cephalosporins, or clindamycin are sufficient for typical organisms.

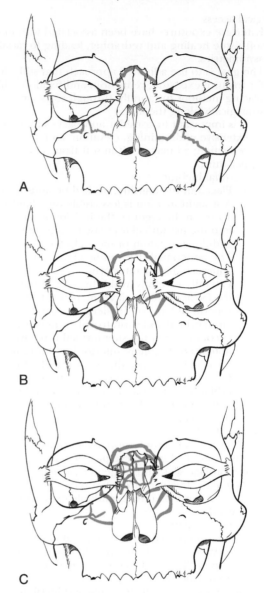

FIGURE 24-4 Nasoorbital ethmoid fracture classification.

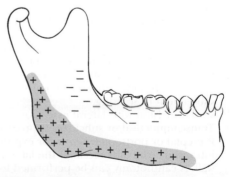

FIGURE 24-5 Simplified tension and compression areas of the mandible.

- Administered until 24 hours after surgery at a minimum
- Timing of repair
  - Antibiotics have reduced need for urgent repair.
  - Consider not waiting for swelling to reduce because CT imaging can assess fractures and operative intervention will reinsult the soft tissue envelope.

- Surgical access
  - Extensive exposures have been associated with difficult soft tissue healing and redraping, leading to facial asymmetries.
  - The goal is to use a limited approach that still allows for fracture exposure, reduction, and fixation, while placing incisions intraorally, through scars, or strategically along the face.
    - It is important to consider approaches that require extensive undermining, elevation, and/or significant retraction; all may result in soft tissue change.
  - Upper third
    - Coronal incision
      - Placed in the hairline, peaked or sinusoidal line
      - A straight incision is less visible on a bald scalp.
      - To reach the zygoma, the incision must extend into the preauricular crease to allow for additional rotation of the scalp flap.
      - The pericranial flap can be elevated via this approach, based anteriorly.
      - Laterally, carefully avoid the temporal branch of the facial nerve by elevating beneath the superficial layer of the deep temporal fascia.
      - Supraorbital and supratrochlear nerves are encountered at the supraorbital rim, either in notches or foramen; inferior lip of foramen is fractured to release the neurovascular bundle.
      - Elevation can reach the zygomatic arch, lateral orbital wall, the nasofrontal suture and nasal bones, medial orbital walls, and frontal process of the maxilla.
  - Middle third
    - There are numerous approach options; selection is based on need to achieve proper repair, location to camouflage scar, and surgeon experience.
    - Zygomatic fractures are often repaired at more than one site; therefore, multiple exposures are needed.
    - Gillies incision
      - Incision placed within temporal hairline, elevation beneath temporalis fascia, superficial to muscle. The instrument is passed underneath the zygomatic arch for reduction.
    - Gingivobuccal sulcus transmucosal incision
      - Access to anterior maxillary wall, piriform apertures, frontal process, zygomaticomaxillary junction
      - Approach to the zygomatic arch from below, intraorally
      - Avoid elevating bone fragments with the soft tissue. Avoid injury to infraorbital nerves.
      - Exposure can be extended by midfacial degloving approach; however, this risks nasal stenosis subsequent to scarring.
    - Lower lid incision with lateral extension
      - Transconjunctival or subciliary approaches
      - Preseptal or postseptal; allows for exposure of infraorbital rim and access to the lateral orbital wall. A canthotomy can be performed to widen exposure.
      - Orbital septal injury and scarring can lead to lower lid malpositions.
    - Transcaruncular or retrocaruncular incision
      - Access to medial orbital wall
      - Alternatively can be performed transcutaneously, similar to a Lynch incision.
    - Frost stitch may be used for 24 to 48 hours after approaches that traverse the lower lid, to reduce risk of malposition.

- Lower third
  - Exposure of fracture region either transmucosally or transcutaneously
  - Intraoral exposure does not have higher infection rate.
    - Use of transcutaneous trocar allows for access to posterior regions of mandible: angle, body, subcondylar, and ramus.
  - Avoid mental nerve around/below premolar region, higher in edentulous patient.
  - Extraoral incisions have direct visual exposure, result in a visible scar, and risk injury to marginal mandibular branch of facial nerve.
    - Reduced risk to mental nerves
    - Posterior body, angle, and subcondylar regions can be approached with submandibular incision.
    - Submental incision allows access to symphyseal region.
    - They can be combined by utilizing a Z incision.

BONE HEALING

- Begins immediately with development of a fracture hematoma
- Ingrowth of vessels brings fibroblasts and other progenitor cells.
- Then differentiation to chondroblasts, which lay down fibrocartilage and chondroid matrix
  - Leading to early stabilization and substrate for development of osteoid
- Next, differentiation into osteoblasts results in osteoid deposition and early callus formation.
  - Callus is deposited until the fracture is stable, stopping motion; with increased motion, there is increased callus formation.
- Once the fracture is stable, osteons with vessels grow across the fracture.
  - Bridging of the bone gap can occur only in the absence of motion.
- After bridging by bone, this is remodeled to match its function.
  - Wolff's law: bone remodels according to the forces acting on it.
    - Fails to account for aesthetics and dental function
    - Fractures healing on their own tend toward significant cosmetic deformity and compromised masticatory function.
- Principles relating to bone metabolism in facial skeletal repair
  - Realign bones to re-create aesthetic form and occlusal function.
  - Maximize the amount of stability created at the time of repair, with rigid fixation.
    - Minimize the development of callus and infection and allow for immediate function.
- Indirect or secondary bone healing: differentiation cascade with callus formation as described previously
- Direct or primary bone healing: occurs following rigid fixation when there is no movement along the fracture line.
- Unstable fractures heal without bone; instead, fibrous tissue spans the fracture, resulting in a nonunion, fibrous nonunion, or pseudoarthrosis.
  - This can occur if callus is unable to stabilize a fracture.

Biomechanics of the Facial Skeleton

- Facial form is designed to support its function, in that the facial skeleton will collapse in weaker areas to prevent

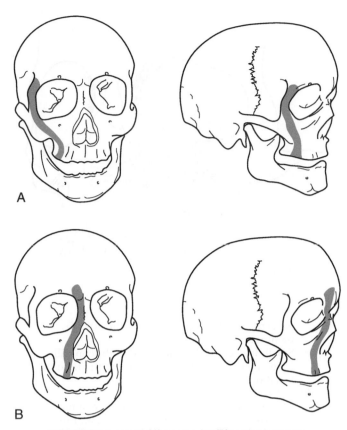

FIGURE 24-6 Lateral **(A)** and medial **(B)** vertical buttresses.

injury to vital structures, whereas there is strength in areas relevant to function (pillars and buttresses).

- The mandible articulates at the skull base and rotates during mastication, compressing the food bolus between the teeth by the force generated. Its fulcrum effect results in tension and compression zones in various areas of the mandible.
- Upper third
  - Anterior wall of frontal sinus is thin and provides cover for the sinus and aesthetic contour to the forehead. No significant forces act in this region.
  - Supraorbital rims, lateral frontal bone, and frontal bone superior to the sinus are dense, providing protection to the orbital and intracranial contents. There are still no significant forces acting in this region.
- Middle third
  - Pillars or buttresses (Figure 24-6) withstand the forces of mastication on the maxilla.
    - Vertical buttresses: lateral buttress passes from molar region superiorly along the zygomaticomaxillary suture through the malar eminence and up the lateral orbital rim; medial buttress passes from the canine region superior along the solid bone that borders the piriform aperture continuing upward along the solid frontal process of the maxilla into the frontal bone; posterior buttress is the pterygoid plates that transmit force to the skull base.
    - The goal of repair is to reconstruct these load-bearing regions that bear the impact of masticatory forces.
    - Horizontal buttresses: these serve as connections across the midface reinforcing the vertical buttresses. The palate forms an incomplete buttress,

malar eminence across the infraorbital rim to the contralateral malar eminence yet incomplete across the pyriform aperture, and the most superior is across the frontoorbital bar or bandeau.
  - These horizontal buttresses primarily reestablish facial architecture.
  - From anterior to posterior, the zygomatic arch buttresses between the temporal root and the malar eminence. It is the origin for the masseter muscle; this bone must be strong enough to withstand the muscular forces, yet able to crumple when needed.
- The zygoma has the solid malar eminence; however, the connections to other bones are not; this gives a crumple effect when significant force is applied. The arch and inferior orbital rim are thin; conversely the lateral rim is solid and the zygoma may remain hinged at this attachment. The final attachment is broadly to the maxilla (which is contiguous with the infraorbital rim). Zygoma repairs must be accomplished in three dimensions with multiple fixation points.
- Orbital biomechanics consist of reconstituting the orbital volume and shape to achieve proper positioning of the globe.
- When the central facial area is disrupted, the medial eyelids are pulled toward the intact lateral canthus, shortening the horizontal length of the eyelid. Reconstruction needs to withstand the constant lateral tension on the eyelid. Proper repositioning of nasal bones is pertinent for cosmesis and nasal function, given the relationship to the upper lateral cartilage and internal nasal valve.
- Lower third
  - There are multiple muscular attachments to the mandible that exert forces during contraction, even outside mastication. The mandible also supports the tongue and hyoid, participating in swallowing and airway function. The most significant forces acting on the mandible are produced during mastication.
  - Mandibular biomechanics can be simplified into tension forces superiorly and compression zones inferiorly. This causes distraction of the fracture superiorly and compression inferiorly. However, in reality, the mandible does not follow the simple beam model. Variability in the bone alters stability. There is greater torque and rotation potential in the symphysis region.
    - By controlling the distraction in the tension zone, the functional forces of mastication will maintain compression in the inferior region.
  - The presence of tooth roots and the inferior alveolar nerve limits placement of rigid fixation.
    - Champy: control of tension zone with monocortical mini plates positioned between tooth roots and inferior alveolar nerve
    - Spiessl: well-placed arch bar across the dentition to control the tension zone and a large bicortical compression plate. Must control the tension zone first to prevent distraction of the alveolar portion of the fracture.
  - The rotation in the symphysis region requires two plates to accomplish stable fixation.
  - The compression and tension zones vary in angle, depending on where mastication occurs. It has been observed in the angle region that forces are altered between compression and tension with the change in food bolus location. This has been confirmed for other areas of the mandible as well.
  - The angle remains difficult to repair; generally it is agreed that mandibular reconstruction plates offer the

most dependable repairs and highest overall success rate.
  • An alternative is two 2-mm miniplates.
• Vertical ramus is important as the only determinant of vertical facial height. In panfacial fractures, this is useful as a foundation to establish the correct height.

FRACTURE REPAIR

• Applying the principles of evaluation and understanding the biomechanical properties of the facial skeleton allow for proper analysis of the injury and appropriate repair.
• Most repairs currently are performed with titanium plates and screws. Other materials include stainless steel wires, absorbable plates and screws, polylactic acid, polyglycolic acid, and other polymers.
• Occlusion
  • Restoration of premorbid occlusal status is primary to visual alignment of bone fragments. Arch bars remain the standard for establishing and maintaining occlusion. Ivy loops stabilize only a few teeth rather than the entire arch without tension banding. Screws for MMF can be placed rapidly but carry the risk of tooth root injury.
  • MMF can be placed, then released after fracture plating. Arches should remain in place for the option of using guiding elastics during healing. MMF may be used in management of unfixed fractures, such as the subcondylar fracture.
• Upper third
  • Frontal sinus fractures
    • Key issues: is exploration necessary? Is obliteration necessary?
    • Anterior wall fractures are primarily cosmetic; they are repaired if significantly depressed. The smallest plate or absorbable plate is used because there are essentially no forces in this region. Select fractures can be repaired endoscopically.
    • Posterior wall fractures are managed to protect the anterior cranial fossa. Nondisplaced fracture without significant injury to duct or anterior wall can be observed. Instead, if the posterior wall is displaced, visualization of the sinus is warranted to assess for herniation of brain.
    • Sinus outflow tract must function, or the sinus must be obliterated. If the duct is involved and the posterior wall is intact, obliteration is acceptable. It is reasonable to allow the sinus to function and follow closely. Evidence of obstruction can be addressed endoscopically or obliteration can be performed. This approach requires follow-up.
    • Obliteration can be performed by removing mucosa, grinding down bone edges to remove mucosal nests, occluding the nasofrontal duct, rotating a pericranial flap, and filling the sinus with autologous fat graft or other materials. The sinus can be left empty to allow for osteoneogenesis. Indications for frontal obliteration include severe fractures affecting the outflow tract and failure of the outflow tract to function.
    • Cranialization is reserved for cases of severe posterior table comminution. Anterior fossa should be reconstructed and preserved whenever possible.
  • CSF rhinorrhea
    • May originate from frontal sinus, cribriform plate, fovea ethmoidalis, or sphenoid sinus. Transient leakage may have halted if herniated brain has plugged the defect. The longer the duration of CSF

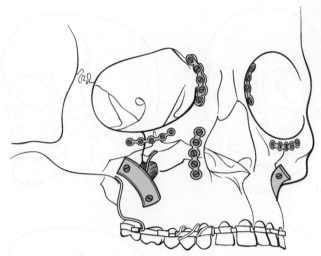

FIGURE 24-7 Diagram of rigid fixation of Le Fort I and II fractures.

leakage persistence, the greater the risk of meningitis.
  • Small defects can be addressed endoscopically.
  • Large defects should be repaired at the time of facial fracture repair.
• Skull base
  • CSF rhinorrhea and brain injury are common.
  • Neurosurgery evaluation is necessary, and repairs are performed in conjunction with neurosurgery.
• Middle third
  • Fractures involving the tooth-bearing maxilla are first placed into occlusion.
  • Le Fort I injuries require reestablishment of the medial and lateral buttresses with rigid fixation in line with masticatory forces (Figure 24-7).
  • Palatal fractures need to be evaluated for rotation; ensure that in-plane alignment is performed. Palatal splints are helpful to stabilize the dentition. Fixation is done with plates or along the premaxilla.
  • Le Fort II fractures should be stabilized along the infraorbital rims and the nasal root region bilaterally (see Figure 24-7). It important to verify that midface impaction is not present because MMF could place the patient in occlusion with the condyle outside the glenoid fossa.
  • Bony deficits in the region of buttresses should be replaced and/or grafted.
  • Zygoma repair depends on the severity of injury, ranging from reduction into position when hinged upon the frontozygomatic region to wide exposure and reconstruction of comminuted fractures. It is important to have good alignment, proper height, and correct rotation at the frontozygomatic region because this impacts the position of the malar eminence, the lateral orbital rim, and the orbit volume.
  • The zygomatic arch can be reduced by a closed approach intraorally in minor cases and through a Gillies incision in select cases. Severe cases that require fixation may require a bicoronal approach for exposure.
  • The goal of orbit repair is the restoration of the premorbid shape, taking into account the natural fluctuations of the orbital floor and walls. Repairs can be accomplished with autologous materials (septal bone, calvarial bone), porous polyethylene,

and titanium (but there is theoretical concern about tissue ingrowth into the plate).

- NOE, NEC fractures: type I repaired by stabilizing the bone segment where the medial canthal ligament attaches restoring the position (Figures 24-8 and 24-9). Type II and III injuries are typically addressed by exposing the ligaments and performing suture resuspension of the ligament to the posterior lacrimal crest across to the contralateral side, while protecting the globe, and fixed to the contralateral frontal bone (by plate, screw, or hole drilled in bone). Precise positioning of the medial canthus is important; symmetric positioning in bilateral injury is equally important.
- Lower third
  - Dentate mandible: first establish proper occlusal relationship between the maxillary and mandibular dentition, placing into MMF.
  - Principles of fracture repair
    - Load sharing: depends on integrity of underlying bone; plating is positioned such that the functional forces are directed to the bone while maintaining reduction and stability (miniplate, compression plate, lag screw).
    - Load bearing: must be used if bone is unable to share the load (thin, weak, comminuted, bone

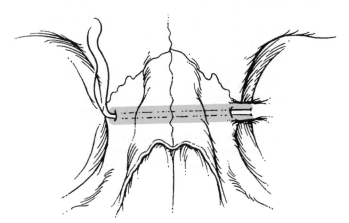

FIGURE 24-8 Suture passage through nasal root resuspending left medial canthus.

loss, atrophic). The repair then needs to be strong enough to tolerate the load across the fractured site while in function (long and strong plate, 2.4-mm titanium reconstruction plate). Requires three to four bicortical screws on each side of the fracture. A locking plate can be used to establish stability when the plate contour does not match the bone precisely.
- External fixation uses externally placed pins to hold bone in place across a fracture. Stability increases with the number of fixation points. This method is useful in the severely comminuted mandible.
- The lag screw technique can be used to compress two cortices together when they are overlapping, such as in an oblique fracture; it is also applicable to symphyseal fractures. Two screws are used and are oriented from opposite sides of the fracture.
- Symphysis
  - Load sharing: lag screws, two miniplates with minimum of two screws on each side
  - Load bearing: an arch bar (or miniplate) superiorly with a bicortical compression plate inferiorly
- Body
  - Load sharing: single miniplate is adequate if no chewing is done on the side of the fracture during healing.
  - Load bearing: a tension band (arch bar or miniplate) can be combined with a bicortical compression plate along the inferior border.
- Angle
  - Load sharing: miniplate technique (the best miniplate technique remains controversial)
    - 2 mm miniplate placed over the oblique line; patient instructed to chew on other side for 6 weeks.
    - Two miniplates, four-hole, 2 mm
  - Load bearing: reconstruction plate
- Ramus
  - Rigid fixation or functionally stable fixation, often two 2 mm miniplates
    - Closed reduction often insufficient to stabilize posterior mandible against forces of muscular sling, may cause rotation of ramus

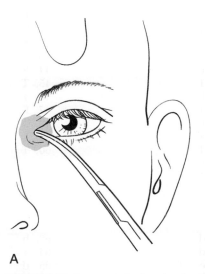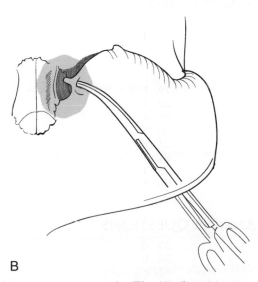

A   B

FIGURE 24-9 Placement of a clamp into the caruncle **(A)** and rotation of coronal flap **(B)** to identify medial canthus.

- Closed reduction with MMF lasts 6 to 8 weeks
- Subcondylar
  - Closed reduction with MMF, 10 to 14 days, followed by physiotherapy; training elastics can be instituted if malocclusion returns.
  - Open reduction carries a risk of injury to the facial nerve.
    - Indications
      - Condylar displacement into middle fossa
      - Inability to obtain reduction
      - Lateral extracapsular displacement of the condyle
      - Invasion by a foreign body
    - Relative indications
      - Bilateral condylar fractures in edentulous mandible without splint available
      - Condylar fracture when splinting is not recommended
      - Bilateral condylar fractures along with comminuted midface fractures
      - Bilateral condylar fractures associated with gnathologic problems
  - Endoscopic-assisted repair of subcondylar fractures reduces risk complications and has a high success rate; however, the procedure is technically challenging.
- Closed reduction with 4 to 6 weeks of MMF may be applied to fractures within the dentition and that are nondisplaced.
- Teeth: fractures through or around teeth have a higher incidence of infection; however, extracting the tooth does not decrease the infection rate. Only when the tooth is infected or abscessed does it require removal. Extracting the mandibular third molar may destabilize the angle and its repair.
  - Edentulous mandible
    - Repair is made difficult by the atrophy of the bone and the absences of teeth.

- Dentures can be used as splint to reposition segments properly.
- Mandibular atrophy has had unacceptably high complication rates, in part due to perceptions that a single small plate will suffice for a small mandible.
- Atrophic mandible is a contraindication to load-sharing repair.
- Panfacial fractures
  - If possible, establish the occlusal relationship first.
  - Reconstruction proceeds from the periphery toward the center, working from known to unknown, from stable to unstable.
  - More solid cranial areas are typically repaired first. The facial height is established by reconstruction of the mandible.

COMPLICATIONS

- The most common complication is failure to obtain ideal reduction, which can result in malocclusion, altered facial contour, and asymmetry. Malunion occurs once the bones have healed in the wrong position.
- The most common orbital complication is enophthalmos. Hypophthalmos or hypoglobus may be seen as well; both can be addressed with addition of graft material to the orbit.
- Nonunion most often results from motion at the fracture site. This predisposes the patient to infection and osteomyelitis, which in turn results in bone loss and fibrous union. It is important to treat with antibiotics and remove devitalized bone. Nonunion may heal across fibrosis with MMF or other rigid fixation.
- Soft tissue complications include scarring, midfacial ptosis, facial asymmetry, lid malpositions (ectropion, entropion), and nerve injury (supraorbital, supratrochlear, infraorbital, mental nerve, and facial nerve during transcutaneous approaches).
- Secondary revision or delayed fracture repair requires tedious assessment, evaluation, imaging, and planning, applying principles in craniofacial and orthognathic surgery.

ANSWERS

TRUE OR FALSE QUESTIONS

1. T	14. F	27. T	40. F
2. F	15. T	28. T	41. T
3. T	16. T	29. T	42. F
4. F	17. T	30. F	43. F
5. T	18. F	31. F	44. F
6. T	19. F	32. T	45. T
7. F	20. T	33. F	46. T
8. T	21. F	34. T	47. F
9. T	22. T	35. F	48. T
10. F	23. F	36. T	49. F
11. F	24. T	37. T	50. T
12. T	25. T	38. F	
13. F	26. F	39. T	

SINGLE BEST ANSWER QUESTIONS

51. e	55. d	59. d	63. b
52. f	56. b	60. d	64. a
53. a	57. c	61. c	65. d
54. c	58. a	62. b	66. b

67. c	75. c	83. d	91. c
68. b	76. c	84. d	92. d
69. c	77. b	85. b	93. b
70. d	78. a	86. a	94. a
71. b	79. c	87. b	95. c
72. c	80. d	88. a	96. b
73. d	81. c	89. c	97. b
74. a	82. c	90. d	98. b

SUGGESTED READINGS

1. Chen CT, Chen YR, Tung TC, et al. Endoscopically assisted reconstruction of orbital medial wall fractures. *Plast Reconstr Surg.* 1999;103(2):714-720.
2. Fox AJ, Kellman RM. Mandibular angle fractures: two-miniplate fixation and complications. *Arch Facial Plast Surg.* 2003;5:464-469.
3. Gonty AA, Marciani RD, Adornato DC. Management of frontal sinus fractures: a review of 33 cases. *J Oral Maxillofac Surg.* 1999;57:372-379.
4. Kellman RM. Endoscopically assisted repair of subcondylar fractures of the mandible: an evolving technique. *Arch Facial Plast Surg.* 2003;5:244-250.
5. Kellman RM. Safe and dependable harvesting of large outer-table calvarial bone grafts. *Arch Otolaryngol Head Neck Surg.* 1994;120(8):856-860.
6. Kellman RM. Use of the subcranial approach in maxillofacial trauma. *Facial Plast Surg Clin North Am.* 1998;6(4):501-510.
7. Le Fort R. Etude experimentale sur les fractures de la machoire supérieure. *Rev Chir Paris.* 1901;23:208, 360, 479.
8. Lee C, Mankani MH, Kellman RM, et al. Minimally invasive approaches to mandibular fractures. *Facial Plast Surg Clin North Am.* 2001;9:475-487.
9. Wilson IF, Lokeh A, Benjamin CI, et al. Contribution of conventional axial computed tomography (nonhelical), in conjunction with panoramic tomography (zonography), in evaluating mandibular fractures. *Ann Plast Surg.* 2000;45:415-421.
10. Wilson IF, Lokeh A, Benjamin CI, et al. Prospective comparison of panoramic tomography (zonography) and helical computed tomography in the diagnosis and operative management of mandibular fractures. *Plast Reconstr Surg.* 2001;107:1369-1375.